Clinical
Exercise

a case-based approach

Clinical Exercise

a case-based approach

Melainie Cameron
School of Exercise Science
Centre of Physical Activity Across the Lifespan (CoPAAL)
Australian Catholic University

Steve Selig
School of Exercise and Nutrition Sciences
Deakin University

Dennis Hemphill
School of Sport and Exercise Science
Institute of Sport, Exercise and Active Living
Victoria University

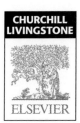

CHURCHILL LIVINGSTONE

ELSEVIER

Sydney   Edinburgh   London   New York   Philadelphia   St Louis   Toronto

Churchill Livingstone
is an imprint of Elsevier

Elsevier Australia. ACN 001 002 357
(a division of Reed International Books Australia Pty Ltd)
Tower 1, 475 Victoria Avenue, Chatswood, NSW 2067

National Library of Australia Cataloguing-in-Publication Data

---

Cameron, Melainie.

Clinical exercise : a case-based approach / Melainie
Cameron, Steve Selig, Dennis Hemphill.

9780729539418 (pbk.)
Includes index.

exercise therapy.
Clinical exercise physiology.
Physical fitness--Testing--Case studies.
Rehabilitation.

Selig, Steve.
Hemphill, Dennis Allan

613.71

Publisher: Melinda McEvoy
Developmental Editor: Rebecca Cornell
Publishing Services Manager: Helena Klijn
Project Coordinator: Natalie Hamad
Edited, proofread and indexed by Forsyth Publishing Services
Cover and internal design by Stan Lamond
Typeset by TNQ Books and Journals Pvt. Ltd.
Printed by 1010 Printing International Ltd.

Contents

Introduction

USING A CASE-BASED APPROACH

This book is divided into two sections. Section 1 is a brief review of the scientific evidence supporting the use of exercise as therapeutic intervention. The first chapter reviews our understanding of evidence-based practice, and introduces the concept of practitioners applying ethical and scientific reasoning in their clinical decision making. Practitioners cannot afford to rely on scientific data alone when making decisions that affect clients' lives. We argue that evidence-based practice is a good deal more than reliance on numbers, and we weave examples of the complexity of evidence-based practice throughout the theory chapters of Section 1.

To avoid repetition, chapters in Section 1 are cross-referenced, and some supporting information from other authors is provided in appendices. This section can be read as a whole, or in discrete chapters.

Section 2 is a collection of clinical tales. Most of these tales are presented as structured case studies, written using the familiar form of clinical note taking (SOAP: subjective, objective, assessment, plan), but a handful of the tales diverge from this format, including personal narratives and stories of times we (authors, clinicians) have got things wrong.

Case studies in Section 2 are structured for clinical teaching, and for continuing professional development of practitioners, but may also serve as bedtime reading. Be warned: many case studies do not draw neat conclusions; neither are all the answers included in Section 2. These case studies are intended to prompt discussion and fuel debate. We hope readers argue about them with their colleagues just as one might disagree with friends over a popular novel or a new film.

All the case studies are intended to represent the real, complex, human world of clinical exercise practice. We have not sanitised cases by removing confounding factors, ethical dilemmas, or unexpected outcomes. Rather, we draw attention to these peculiarities of clinical practice and ask readers to apply the *ethical reasoning skills* discussed in Chapter 1 to their reading of the remainder of the book.

Authors contributing to this book include exercise physiologists (or biokineticists as they are known in Southern Africa), exercise scientists, sport scientists, physiotherapists, physical educators, psychologists, an osteopath, a chiropractor, an occupational therapist, an ambulance paramedic, a sport and exercise ethicist, and a specialist medical practitioner (endocrinologist). Readers are likely to be drawn from similarly diverse backgrounds. Recognising that no one profession can claim ownership of clinical exercise, we have adopted the generic term 'clinical exercise practitioner' throughout the book. Also, we have used other generic labels such as therapist and clinician. Readers are invited to apply the content of this book as they see fit to their own work in clinical exercise.

ON TELLING STORIES ...

Story is engaging pedagogy. In stories we see ourselves, explore our worlds, and learn to tell our own tales. Case studies and other stories included in this book fall into one of three types: factual accounts, aggregates, and personal tales.

Factual accounts

Factual accounts are case reports of real clients, in real clinical encounters. The authors of these case studies are the clinicians who have consulted with these clients and have access to clinical data for inclusion in the case studies. Before preparing the case reports, either in writing or on film, clinicians have sought clients' express permission to tell their stories in this book. Where clients wished, names and identifying details have been altered to protect clients' privacy but, in all important ways, these case reports are real.

Aggregates

Experienced clinicians will, over years of clinical practice, have seen many clients with common complaints. Over time, recalling a single client may become difficult, but identifying and describing a 'type' becomes easy. Some of the clinician authors in this section of the book have chosen to write fictitious accounts, each telling a story not of a single person, but of an aggregate client created from the recollections of many consultations with real clients. Any data included in these case studies are fictitious, but plausible, given the clinical presentations described. Similarly, although the stories are not real, they could be.

To offer maximum privacy to the clients who have allowed their stories to be told in this book, we have not distinguished between aggregate case studies and factual account case studies.

Personal tales

Some authors have chosen to tell personal tales of their work as clinicians or of their experiences as clients. Their deep honesty is touching and adds personal character to this book. Authors were under no pressure to give personal accounts — they have shared generously and freely. For example, the authors of Chapter 10 have presented personal accounts of their own self-care (or lack thereof) as professionals. This chapter has the voice of letters rather than clinical case studies; although the authors are practitioners, they have written personally about themselves rather than clinically about their clients.

CAVEAT

The classification of disease is open to debate. In each chapter we consider several conditions that might have just as easily been included in other chapters. For example, osteoporosis and arthritis are considered in musculoskeletal conditions rather than in chapters on metabolic or chronic and complex conditions, respectively. We have made some arbitrary decisions about where conditions will appear and cross-referenced chapters to avoid repetition.

Melainie Cameron

Foreword

It is a great pleasure and an honour for me to commend this timely book: *Clinical exercise, a case-based approach*. There is no doubt that this eminently readable book will make an important contribution to sharpening the edges of good practice among health practitioners and allied health professionals who apply exercise as the basis of their treatment plans.

Studying the human in motion and the influence of motion on the human is a fascinating, complex and rapidly expanding field. Many different professionals have an interest in the mechanisms of human volitional movement and apply tailored domains of this field of study to classify and characterise the work and expectations of its professionals. Physical educators, exercise physiologists, physical therapists, biokineticists, physiotherapists, psychologists and clinicians, especially those working in orthopaedics, physical medicine and rehabilitation, are examples. Each extracts and applies a particular slant of this field of knowledge, yet, all of these specialists will find this book entirely relevant as it considers and reveals the essence and intricacies of human movement in the context of health enhancement.

Most remarkable about the human moving is how easily our neuromuscular system just does it, unless of course the system is compromised, has failed in some way, or is in pain. Prescribing movement as a therapeutic modality not only makes sense, but is gaining ground thanks to the importance and priority attached by agencies, professionals and advocates in our respective social systems. Emerging is a new, exciting, undisputed view that accords the recognition that exercise is medicine.

Although convincing scientific evidence substantiates the relationship between activity and health, the challenge for the practitioner lies in the detail of the intervention. Sharing and learning through a case-based approach sensitises clinicians to engage critically, compassionately and carefully in the lived experience of the storyteller. From the words used, the context described, and the observations made, a personalised health trajectory, using exercise at the centre of the therapy, can be constructed. This approach will assist practitioners to explore causation, examine similarities, recognise trends, record episodes and reflect on decisions in their quest to guide their practice. Exercise practitioners, who apply principles to recommend dose-specific activity prescriptions, are sought-after professionals who are increasingly positioning themselves as indispensable in clinical practice.

The time for this approach is both opportune and pressing. While we fail to weave sufficient, regular physical activity into the fabric of our daily lives, we will increasingly need the direction of clinicians to prescribe, guide, monitor and evaluate the best exercise dose for health protection. There is no doubt that activity prescriptions are fundamental in rehabilitation and vital for enhancing and advancing precious life.

The detail of how much, what specifically, and when remain important issues. This book considers and recommends the dose, modality, progression and execution-specific selection of exercise in therapeutic applications. The rich, honest and deeply human tales in this book, set alongside readily digestible theory skilfully extracted via lessons learned from clients, patients and seasoned professionals in practice, enables the reader to quickly gain wisdom from the stories told. This approach will persuade reflective practitioners to apply therapeutic solutions for their clients with clarity, confidence and kindness.

This is a vital read for students in the field of human movements studies, exercise science and sports medicine. Contributing authors and the editors are congratulated on this excellent text and Melainie Cameron is applauded for her leadership and direction given to its production.

Dr Claire M Nicholson
Exercise Scientist
Immediate past head of Human Movement Science,
University of the Witwatersrand,
Johannesburg, South Africa

Contributors

Mark B Andersen
BA, MS, PhD
Professor, School of Sport and Exercise Science,
Institute of Sport, Exercise and Active Living, Victoria University

Suzanne Broadbent
BEducation, BExScience (Hon), PhD
Senior Lecturer, School of Sport and Exercise Science,
Institute of Sport, Exercise and Active Living, Victoria University

Melainie Cameron
BAppSc (Ost), MHSc, PhD
Associate Professor, School of Exercise Science, Centre of Physical Activity Across the Lifespan
(CoPAAL), Australian Catholic University

Natalie Chahine
BAppSc (Biomed Sc), Grad Dip (Exercise Rehab), MAppSc (Exercise Rehab)
Exercise Physiologist, Community Health Team Leader, Western Region Health Centre

Garry Francis-Pester
BPhysiotherapy, MAPA, BEd, Grad Dip Ergonomics
Managing Director, Physiotherapy & Human Movement Clinic Pty Ltd

Cadeyrn J Gaskin
BBS (Hons), MBS, PhD
Research Fellow, Deakin University

Marek Gorski
MEd (PE) (Poland), Grad Dip (Exercise Rehab)
Exercise Physiologist, Acute Rehabilitation Unit, Kingston Centre, Southern Health

Dennis Hemphill
BA (Hons), MA, PhD
Associate Professor, Head of School, School of Sport and Exercise Science,
Institute of Sport, Exercise and Active Living, Victoria University

Loretta Konjarski
BEd (PE), MEducation
Lecturer, School of Sport and Exercise Science,
Institute of Sport, Exercise and Active Living, Victoria University

Itamar Levinger
BEd, MSc, PhD
Research Fellow, School of Sport and Exercise Science,
Institute of Sport, Exercise and Active Living, Victoria University

Christian Lorenzen

BAppSci (HumMov) (Hons), PhD
Lecturer, School of Exercise Science, Centre of Physical Activity Across the Lifespan
(CoPAAL), Australian Catholic University

Gina Mendoza

BAppSc (Hons), Grad Dip (Exercise Rehab)
Lecturer, School of Sport and Exercise Science
Institute of Sport, Exercise and Active Living, Victoria University

Meg Morris

BAppSc, Grad Dip (Geron), MAppSc, FACP, PhD
Professor, Head of School, Melbourne School of Health Sciences,
The University of Melbourne

Sarah-Johanna Moss

MSc (Biochemistry), PhD (Biokinetics), MBA
School of Biokinetics, Recreation, and Sport Sciences, North-West University
(Potchefstroom)

Geraldine Naughton

BAppSci (Distinctions), BEd (Primary), MAppSci (Exercise Physiology), PhD
Professor, Research Fellow, Centre of Physical Activity Across the Lifespan (CoPAAL),
Australian Catholic University; Murdoch Children's Research Institute,
Royal Children's Hospital, Melbourne

Belinda Parmenter

BHlthSc (ExSc)
Associate Lecturer, Exercise, Health and Performance Research Group, University of Sydney

Alan Pearce

BSc (Spt Sci) Hons, PhD
Senior Lecturer, School of Sport and Exercise Science, Institute of Sport,
Exercise and Active Living, Victoria University

Henry Pollard

BSc, Grad Dip Chiro, Grad Dip AppSc, MSportSc, PhD
Adjunct Associate Professor, School of Medicine, University Notre Dame (Sydney)

Jacqueline Raymond

BAppSci (HMovt), PGD (Sci), PhD
Lecturer, University of Sydney

Robert Robergs

FASEP, EPC, PhD
Lecturer, Exercise Physiologist and Biochemist, Division of Physical Performance
and Development, Center For Exercise and Applied Human Physiology,
University of New Mexico

Mark Sayers

BAppSc, MAppSc, PhD
Senior Lecturer in Sports Biomechanics, School of Health & Sport Sciences,
University of the Sunshine Coast

Steve Selig
BSc, PhD
School of Exercise and Nutrition Sciences, Deakin University

Nigel Stepto
BSc, BSc (Hons) BSc (Med) (Hons), MSc, PhD
Lecturer, School of Sport and Exercise Science, Institute of Sport, Exercise and Active Living, Victoria University

Helena Teede
MBBS, FRACP, PhD
Professor, Director of Research, The Jean Hailes Foundation, Southern Health, School of Public Health & Preventative Medicine, Monash University

Dan van der Westhuizen
BPE (Hons), MHMSc, PhD, PGDipSportsMed, PGDipTeaching
Lecturer, School of Sport and Exercise Science
Institute of Sport, Exercise and Active Living, Victoria University

Helen Webb
BEd, MHlthSci (Hons), Teach Cert
Senior Lecturer, School of Nursing and Midwifery, Australian Catholic University

Cilas Wilders
BJur, PhD
Professor in Biokinetics, School of Biokinetics, Recreation, and Sport Sciences, North-West University (Potchefstroom)

Ida Yiu
Cert. OSH, BSc (OT), MSc (Ergonomics)
Rehabilitation Manager, Jardine Lloyd Thompson Ltd

Reviewers

Kade Davison
BAppSc (Hmn Mvt), BHSc (Hons), PhD
Lecturer, School of Health & Human Sciences, Southern Cross University

Ian Gillam
BSc (Hons), MSc, PhD, Dip PE
Exercise Physiologist and Sports Nutritionist,
Wellness Clinic, National Institute of Integrative Medicine, Hawthorn East

Herbert Groeller
BEd (PHE), MSc(Hons), PhD
Senior Lecturer, School of Health Sciences, University of Wollongong

Frank Marino
BPE, MEd, PhD, SpecCertClinRese(Neuro)
Head of School, School of Human Movement Studies, Charles Sturt University

Tim D Noakes
DSc(Med) in Exercise Science, MD, MBChB
Professor, Director, UCT/MRC Research Unit for Exercise Science and Sports Medicine (ESSM),
Department of Human Biology, Faculty of Health Science, University of Cape Town

Rebecca Sealey
B.SpExSc (Hons) ESSAM AEP
Lecturer (Clinical Exercise Physiology), Institute of Sport and Exercise Science,
School of Public Health, Tropical Medicine and Rehabilitation Sciences, James Cook University

E Gail Trapp
DipTeach, AssDip AppSc, BSpSc, MSpSc (Hons), PhD, AEP
Lecturer, Exercise Physiology Program, School of Medical Sciences, University of NSW

Acknowledgments

This book was a team effort, and our thanks go out to all who participated. Plans for this book were conceived when we worked as colleagues at Victoria University (VU). Much of our writing was undertaken there, and we recruited several VU colleagues as chapter authors. Part way through the development of this book, Dennis took a more senior position within VU, and I moved to the Australian Catholic University. Almost a year later, Steve moved to a new appointment at Deakin University.

As editors, Steve, Dennis, and I shared the load. I managed the writing side of the project, buoying chapter and case study authors along, understanding their trials and delays in writing, keeping them focussed on this project, and binding their offerings together in (largely) consistent styles. Steve took care of the filming of case studies, and recruiting clinicians, clients and students to create the visual stories that add much to this book. Dennis applied his mind as an ethicist and philosopher to each of the case studies, to ensure that they were rich, complex narratives filled with lessons of life and humanity as well as clinical education. Like most of the authors, each of us held full-time academic positions while completing this project. We worked together, as do horses harnessed to pull a cart. Thank you gents — I couldn't have done it alone.

Each of the chapter and case study authors deserves thanks. Their writing was of high quality right from the start; even the earliest drafts were gems worth keeping. They tolerated well my requests for revisions, and their (mostly) timely responses kept the project moving along.

The editorial and production team at Elsevier were helpful, generous, and respectful every step of the way, even when we changed plans, appointed new authors, and sent the wrong information. Their kindness and patience were blessings throughout the project.

Our colleagues in the School of Sport and Exercise Science at Victoria University, the School of Exercise Science at the Australian Catholic University, and the School of Exercise and Nutrition Sciences at Deakin University also deserve our gratitude. These fine people put up with us talking about 'the book' ad nauseum and accepted our excuses for bowing out of other jobs. Thank you for giving us time and space; we're coming back to work now.

Melainie Cameron
(on behalf of the editorial team: Melainie Cameron, Steve Selig and Dennis Hemphill)

Abbreviations

6MWT	6-minute walk test
ABI	acquired brain injury
ACE	angiotensin-converting enzyme
ACE-inhibitors	angiotensin converting enzyme inhibitors
ACLS	advanced cardiac/cardiopulmonary life support
ACR	American College of Rheumatology
aF	atrial fibrillation
AGS	American Geriatrics Society
ALS	amyotrophic lateral sclerosis
ANS	autonomic nervous system
APB	abductor pollicis brevis
ARBs	angiotensin II receptor blockers
AS	aortic stenosis
ASMP	arthritis self-management program
BCLS	basic cardiac/cardiopulmonary life support
BMD	bone mineral density
BMI	body mass index
CAD	coronary artery disease
CDCP	Centers for Disease Control and Prevention
CF	cystic fibrosis
CFTC	cystic fibrosis transmembrane conductance
CHF	chronic heart failure
CNS	central nervous system
COPDs	chronic obstructive pulmonary diseases
CP	cerebral palsy
CPT	conventional chest physiotherapy
CVA	cerebrovascular accident (stroke)
DAS	Disease Activity Score
DBP	diastolic blood pressure
DMARDs	disease modifying anti-rheumatic drugs
DXA	dual-energy X-ray absorptiometry
EDD	end-diastolic diameter
EF	ejection fraction
EIB	exercise induced bronchoconstriction
EMG	electromyogram
ESD	end-systolic diameter
FAI	free androgen index
FES	functional electrical stimulation
FEV_1	forced expiratory volume in one second
FFA	free fatty acid
fMRI	functional magnetic resonance imaging
FPG	fasting plasma glucose
FRC	functional residual capacity

FS	fractional shortening
FVC	forced vital capacity
GI	glycaemic index
HADS	Hospital Anxiety and Depression Scale
HAES	health at every size
HAQ	Health Assessment Questionnaire
HbA1c	glycosylated haemoglobin
$HbO_2sat\%$	percentage of oxygen saturation in blood (oxyhaemoglobin)
HDL	high density lipoprotein
HMG-CoA	3-hydroxy-3-methylglutaryl coenzyme A
HOCM	hypertrophic obstructive cardiomyopathy
HT	hypertension
IGT	impaired glucose tolerance
IHD	ischaemic heart disease
ILD	interstitial lung diseases
IMT	inspirational muscle training
LBM	lean body mass
LDL	low density lipoprotein
LTD	long-term depression
LTI	long-term inhibition
LTP	long-term potentiation
MACTAR	McMaster Toronto Arthritis Patient Preference Disability Questionnaire
MEG	magnetoencephalography
MEP	motor evoked potential
MetS	metabolic syndrome
MMRC scale	Modified Medical Research Council scale
MND	motor neuron disease
MRI	magnetic resonance imaging
MS	multiple sclerosis
MST	modified shuttle test
NO	nitric oxide
NSSQA program	National Sports Science Quality Assurance program
OA	osteoarthritis
OGTT	oral glucose tolerance test
PAD	peripheral arterial disease
PCOS	polycystic ovary syndrome
PD	Parkinson's disease
PEF	peak expiratory flow
PEP	positive expiratory pressure
PET	positron emission tomography
POTS	postural tachycardia syndrome
pQCT	peripheral quantitative computed tomography
PTCA	percutaneous coronary angioplasty
PVC	premature ventricular contraction
QCT	quantitative computed tomography
QoL	quality of life
QUS	quantitative ultrasound
RA	rheumatoid arthritis
RAS	renin-angiotensin-aldosterone
RCT	randomised controlled trial

RPE	rating of perceived exertion
RT	resistance training
SAH	subarachnoid haemorrhage
SBP	systolic blood pressure
SHBG	steroid/sex hormone binding globulin
SOAP	subjective, objective, assessment, plan
SV	stroke volume
T2DM	type 2 diabetes mellitus
TBI	traumatic brain injury
TLC	total lung capacity
TMS	transcranial magnetic stimulation
UPDRS	Unified Parkinson's Disease Rating Scale
VC	vital capacity

Review of the scientific evidence

Chapter 1

Doing evidence-based practice

Melainie Cameron and Dennis Hemphill

TO BE AN EXPERT, OR NOT TO BE — THAT IS THE QUESTION

In planning and preparing this book we have been prompted to consider expertness, and ask some difficult questions about its utility. To begin with, we (the editors) sought a 'big name' in the field to write this opening chapter on evidence-based practice. David Sackett replied to our invitation with the most interesting refusal we have ever received. He explained that he no longer wrote anything about evidence-based medicine because, simply being identified as an expert in the field, his opinion might be overvalued, thereby undermining a principle of evidence-based practice that clinical decisions are based on sound research and data (ie: evidence) rather than on opinions (of experts or otherwise). A decade ago David had argued, somewhat controversially, for the compulsory retirement of experts (Sackett 2000), but for our work at least he recommended a couple of other leaders who continue to write extensively on this topic.

In preparing our book proposal, Elsevier required that we demonstrate our capacity to undertake this project. Two of the four (unidentified) proposal reviewers made comments that the editors were not recognised leaders in the field of exercise science. Consequently, this would make it difficult to recruit other authors who are themselves leaders in the field.

We do not consider ourselves 'big-name' experts in the field, and we concede that the reputation of the editors and authors will not be a major selling point of the book. The editors do, however, bring to the project a variety of professional experiences that inform this work. Each of us is a senior academic who has been involved in research, teaching and professional service in our respective

fields. We have been involved in curriculum review, development and accreditation, and each of us has served on university human research ethics committees. We have been involved for most of our professional lives in clinical and professional practice in the fields of sport and exercise.

David's reply gave us pause. We looked at each other and said: 'Well, here we are trying to do evidence-based practice — why don't we write the opening chapter? We don't consider ourselves experts but if, as David suggests, evidence-based practice is the application of principles in clinical decision making, then surely we can write about how we do that in the clinical use of exercise.'

We are committed to best practice, which we believe involves evidence and principled judgment. Perhaps to be an expert is to be a reflective practitioner who can ground professional practice in evidence and conduct practice in an ethically sensitive and socially responsible manner. Expertise requires more than simply an awareness of evidence and principles, with the hope that somehow the practitioner will automatically be able to apply them effectively in concrete situations. This book is designed to provide the principles and evidence in context, within the often messy day-to-day detail of practice. It is here that we 'do' practice, with all its challenges, frustrations and joys. It is in clinical cases that the evidence and principles are shown to be wanting, or come alive.

The authors of case studies were not invited as seasoned experts, but as practitioners with varying levels of expertise and experience who could put a human face on evidence-based practice. We are pleased and grateful that so many experts (in their own right) have accepted invitations to contribute to the book. It is hoped that the book provides a wide enough range of cases so that practitioners across a number of disciplines might be able to identify in some way with them. We hope readers will empathise with, and learn from, those who sometimes get it wrong, and share the satisfaction of getting it right.

DOING EVIDENCE-BASED CLINICAL PRACTICE: REASONING SKILLS

Clinical practice requires the application of reasoning skills to determine what constitutes 'evidence'. Practitioners must be able to identify premises, and weigh the evidence (usually numerical data), to decide whether conclusions, and the implications for practice, are supported. A good deal of undergraduate education of healthcare practitioners is devoted to the development of reasoning skills, and the application of these skills in judging the quality of clinical research. Examples of applied reasoning skills, based upon Copi (1979) and Haskins (2006), are presented in Box 1.1 below.

What is evidence? We usually expect colleagues, managers and others to produce evidence, case precedent(s), principle(s) or other forms of

---

Box 1.1 Reasoning skills for clinical practitioners

THE USE OF ARGUMENT

Argument: a statement (premise) or group of statements (premises), which are claimed to provide support for another (the conclusion).
Statement: a sentence that is either true or false.
  Broccoli is a good source of Vitamin A.
Statements can be distinguished from **questions** (eg: What is the difference between the origin and insertion of a muscle?), **proposals** (eg: Let's go skiing this weekend), **suggestions** (eg: I suggest that you reduce your caloric intake), **commands** (eg: Don't arch your back when you do that exercise), and **exclamations** (eg: Crap!), which cannot be said to be true or false.
Premise: the statements that set out reasons or evidence.
Premise indicators: since, because, follows from, as shown by, as indicated by…
Conclusion: the statement that is claimed to follow from the reasons or evidence.
Conclusion indicators: therefore, hence, thus, so, accordingly, as a result, it follows that, which implies that …

EXERCISES

Identify (using square brackets) the premises and conclusions, and *italicise* the premise and conclusion indicators in the following passages:

1 Sport physiotherapists are natural allies of their superiors (eg: medical practitioners), regardless of how ridiculous some of their decisions seem. This is the case because most people in the rehabilitation clinic feel that their chances for promotion will be jeopardised by supporting a subordinate's controversial decision.
Premise: [Most people in the rehabilitation clinic feel that their chances for promotion will be jeopardised by supporting a subordinate's controversial decision.] Premise indicator: … *because*,
Conclusion: [sport physiotherapists are natural allies of their superiors (eg: medical practitioners), regardless of how ridiculous some of their decisions seem to be.]

2 Punishing illegal drug use in sport may suppress undesirable behaviour, but it cannot teach or encourage desirable alternatives. Therefore, it is crucial to use positive techniques to model and reinforce appropriate behaviour for athletes considering performance enhancement methods.
Premise: [punishing illegal drug use in sport may suppress undesirable behaviour, but it cannot teach or encourage desirable alternatives.]
Conclusion indicator: *therefore*
Conclusion: [it is crucial to use positive techniques to model and reinforce appropriate behaviour for athletes considering performance enhancement methods.]

RECOGNISING ARGUMENTS

In addition to questions and proposals, suggestions, commands and exclamations, arguments need to be distinguished from statements of belief or opinion, descriptions, reports, illustrations and explanations.
Statements of belief or opinion: an expression of what someone happens to believe at a certain time.
  Drugs in sport should be banned.

Descriptions: one or more statements that create a certain image or picture for the reader.

> *Evda is a gregarious woman, with a wide waist and warm heart.*

Report: similar to a description, it is a group of statements that convey information about some situation or event.

> *Roger Federer, the 2006 Australian Tennis Open champion, took the crown in 2007 without losing a set throughout the whole tournament.*

Illustration: a statement about a certain subject combined with a reference to one or more specific instances of it.

> *Aerobics classes employ a variety of 'peak' formats: single peak, reverse single peak and multi-peak.*

Explanation: statement intended to show *why* something is the case.

> *Doing sit-ups with bent knees reduces the pull of the hip flexors on the spine.*

DEDUCTIVE AND INDUCTIVE ARGUMENTS

Deductive: an argument where the conclusion follows *necessarily* (ie: certainly, definitely) from the premises. Sometimes referred to as 'true by definition'.

> *All accredited physiotherapists have studied physiology. Khushboo is an accredited physiotherapist. It is the case, therefore, that Khushboo has studied physiology.*

Inductive: an argument where the conclusion follows *probably* (ie: likely, plausibly) from the premises.

> *Because the Reserve Bank raised the prime interest rate on Friday, it is likely that the major banks will increase their home loan interest rates this week.*

In science, inductive reasoning is used to generate a possible explanation (ie: hypothesis) of an observed event. Deductive reasoning is then used to generate predictions from the hypothesis. Testing follows to verify or falsify the predictions.

---

support in order to back up their judgments, policies and views. In biomedical disciplines, evidence is the substance of clinical research, and some types of research are considered more robust, and consequently, more highly valued, than other forms of research. There is no single, agreed hierarchy for evidence — debate abounds as to the value of rigorous randomised controlled trials (RCTs), because highly controlled research environments appear quite unlike the uncontrolled (frankly messy) environs of clinical practice. There is, however, broad agreement that the scientific import of randomised controlled clinical trials ranks above observational and retrospective research designs, as well as expert opinion and the insights from practical experience. See Box 1.2 for a hierarchy of evidence.

As well as evidence, there are other techniques that can, on the surface, appear convincing but, upon closer inspection, lack substance. Reasoning may be flawed and, in many cases, it may simply disguise certain personal biases, preferences or longstanding beliefs, myths and superstitions. See Box 1.3 for examples of common reasoning flaws.

A little more complicated

Evidence-based practice is not simply an academic understanding of research designs and the application of results. Sharing a catch-cry with Ben Goldacre (2009), 'I think you'll find it's a little more complicated than that …', evidence-based practice is the ongoing integration of clinical experience, client preferences, and the best available external evidence. This notion of the inter-relationship of research evidence and practical experience has some appeal. It means that research is valued for its useful contribution to clinical work, as are the insights derived from engaged and reflective practice.

Much of the rhetoric around evidence-based practice suggests that it is a process that clarifies clinical thinking, rendering decision making easier, but we have found that sometimes the opposite is true. Sometimes evidence is lacking, or of poor quality, or ambiguous. Explaining unclear research results can be taxing for practitioners, and clients sometimes prefer to believe a clean-cut sales pitch rather than the complexity of technical explanations. Further, practitioners aren't perfect. Despite the high quality of our clinical education, we and our clients come into clinical relationships

Box 1.2 Hierarchy of evidence

Systematic review: review of research studies on a specific topic that uses explicit methods to locate primary studies, and explicit criteria to assess study quality. Many systematic reviews include meta-analyses.

Meta-analysis: statistical analysis that pools the results of two or more independent research studies (usually clinical trials) through combining and re-analysing the original data, with some weighting to account for the sizes of the original studies.

Randomised controlled trials (RCTs): clinical trials in which participants are randomly allocated to either a control group or a group who receive an intervention. The two groups are similar enough as to be considered identical for any significant variables (eg: age, sex, disease status). Both groups are followed over time for specific end points.

Cohort studies: groups of people are selected on the basis of their exposure to a particular agent (eg: disease, intervention) and followed over time for specific outcomes.

Case-control studies: 'cases' with the condition are matched with 'controls' without, and a retrospective analysis used to look for differences between the two groups.

Cross-sectional survey: survey or interview of a sample of a population at one point in time.

Case report and/or case series: a report based on a single person, sometimes collected together into a short series.

Expert opinion: a consensus of professional judgment, based on the experiences of experts.

Anecdotal evidence: a stand-alone example from experience to back up a point of view.

Personal opinion: a personal belief or interpretation unsupported by evidence.

Box 1.3 Reasoning errors

Ad populum, or the Bandwagon fallacy: this involves an appeal to some popular sentiment as the reason for accepting a judgment.

That ab blaster machine is the best; everyone's buying it!

Slippery slope fallacy: this technique is often used to reject a claim or request on the basis of some catastrophic chain of events that will supposedly follow from it.

The secretaries in the rehab clinic have asked us to provide a lounge area for coffee breaks. There is no way we can fall for this. If we give them lounge areas, next they'll be asking for spas and swimming pools. We will go broke if we say yes to this request!

Ad hominem fallacy: this is a ploy to avoid having to deal with the substance of a claim by simply attacking the person.

We should reject the players' union demand for greater player safety. After all, the union boss was just arrested for drink driving as well as leaving the scene of an accident.

Inconsistency: this error involves a failure to see that a series of statements or judgments do not follow; that is, that they are contradictory.

The company policy is to provide equal pay for equal work, but only for full-time staff members.

Hasty generalisation: jumping to a general conclusion based on a single incident or a small, unrepresentative sample.

Both of my female interns fainted while watching the biopsy: the OR is no place for women!

Judging by an article in this month's Good Science magazine, super-dooper techogizmos are going to be the next big thing.

Begging the question: this means assuming the truth of the very thing you are trying to prove.

Indigenous athletes must have a 'sixth sense'; otherwise, how can we explain their seemingly supernatural talent.

Evading the issue, or **red herring**: this ruse, intentional or not, involves diverting attention away from the issue at hand to something irrelevant.

What do you mean that my rehab would be quicker if I attended all the sessions? Just look at Sam over there; he's hardly ever here.

Personal prejudice: our life experiences bias our expectations and judgments.

You know, those Italians are the worst clients; they're emotional and cannot handle painful manipulations.

Missing the point: this error involves drawing an unexpectedly wrong conclusion.

The decisions of the Sport Tribunal have been shown to be regularly inconsistent and unfair. It's about time the tribunal is abolished.

Appeal to tradition: the ploy to encourage acceptance of a claim based solely on longstanding habit.

Of course, static stretching is the best way to warm-up; it's the way we've always done it at this club.

Poisoning the well: this tactic attempts to create a prejudicial atmosphere in order to discourage opposition to a point of view.

Any Australian who questions the anti-doping code cannot possibly be a true, sport-loving Aussie.

Superstition: this is a mistaken connection thought to exist between unrelated events.

It is important that I repeat the same ritual before each game: right sock before left sock, right shoe before left shoe; otherwise my performance will suffer.

Pragmatic fallacy: this occurs when something is claimed to be true because 'it works', even though there is no demonstrable causal link.

Since I've started doing 50 sit-ups each day, I have lost weight. I am now going to do 100 sit-ups per day.

---

as complex people, with often diverse personal, cultural, and social histories that may bias reasoning and shape expectations in ways that are not always congruent (see personal prejudice in Box 1.3).

For example, many Indonesians may have difficulty accepting that some Australians can hold agnostic or atheistic views. Belief in a higher power, a god, is an important attribute that cements Indonesian social relations. The room for individual difference of belief is only around which god you recognised, and the nature of associated religious worship and holidays. To not believe in a god at all, or to be uncertain whether there is a god, is regarded as quite strange. Consider then the disconnection that could occur in clinical practice between a client who believes that his illness is a punishment from a higher power and a clinician who is an atheist.

Understanding that expert opinion is of low rank in the hierarchy of evidence, and case reports are ranked only a little higher, in this book we strive to use case studies in Section 2 in three ways: (1) to show case-by-case support for the results of rigorous clinical trials and systematic reviews; (2) to demonstrate the application of higher ranked evidence (eg: RCT results) in making clinical decisions; and (3) to highlight some of the difficulties and limitations of applying highly ranked evidence in clinical settings.

We have deliberately not 'cleaned up' the case studies in order to make neat educational points. Rather, we have quite purposefully kept them as 'true-to-life' as possible, with the sometimes messy, and other times insightful, decision making that occurs within day-to-day clinical work.

EVIDENCE-BASED CLINICAL PRACTICE: ETHICAL REASONING

Ethics is the branch of philosophy that addresses questions of right and wrong, justice and injustice, fairness and discrimination, virtue and vice. Ethical reasoning is the process of arguing from ethical principles and standards to particular conclusions and implications. It is the type of reasoning at work when someone argues, for example, that employment practices are fair when applicants are judged on relevant knowledge and ability alone.

When applied to clinical exercise practice, ethical reasoning can be used to judge the appropriateness of professional practices and relationships. Ethical reasoning will often generate or clarify value principles to help guide behaviour and improve the care of clients.

There are a number of ethical issues in clinical exercise practice, many of which centre on the practitioner–client relationship. These include informed consent, privacy, confidentiality, and role boundaries. Other issues include client autonomy and empowerment.

Risk management and ethical reasoning

Risk management is a growing concern for most organisations and businesses, including those related to clinical exercise practice. The reasoning involved in risk management is largely *self-directed*; that is, aimed at protecting a practitioner's interests or those of an organisation (usually to prevent being sued for negligence).

Ethical reasoning tends to be *other-directed*; that is, aimed at protecting the interests (eg: welfare, integrity, wellbeing) of others, in this case, clients. The two types of reasoning, risk management and ethical, can be seen as complimentary.

How much training does it take?

Ethical reasoning, just like any form of judgment, requires familiarity with principles and their application, which can improve with experience. However, principles alone are not always the best guide. Concrete examples can help, and so too can complex case studies, where you can see the principle and its application in context.

The inclusion of ethical reasoning into a book on clinical exercise practice is not intended to produce ethicists. The aim is more modest; the intention is to encourage the development of exercise clinicians as reflective practitioners, who are able to recognise and deal with ethical issues that may arise in professional practice. The ethics toolkit in Box 1.4 provides some practical examples of ethical reasoning.

Box 1.4   Ethics toolkit

The ethics toolkit provides some handy concepts, principles and standards by which to judge and deal with certain situations in clinical exercise practice, teaching, coaching and counselling.

Personhood

Personhood can be thought of as the distinctive attributes of being a person. It includes the capacity to be self-determining; that is, to contemplate alternative futures, weigh up pros and cons of choices, make choices, and accept responsibility (Downey & Telfer 1969). In popular terms, it means the ability to 'stand on your own feet' or 'make up your own mind'.

Respect for persons

Respect for persons means supporting others to be more self-determining. It may mean providing opportunities for choice, pointing out options and consequences so that the choice is a better informed one, and instilling a sense of responsibility for the consequences of the choices.

Conversely, disrespect undermines the ability of a person to be self-determining. It can occur if someone helps too little when there is a duty of care to prevent harm. For example, experience is not always the best teacher if it means that inexperienced or unfit athletes are thrown into dangerous playing conditions. Disrespect can also occur if someone helps too much, as in the case of over-protective parents who never give their children an opportunity to make decisions for themselves.

Personhood and children

Children can be thought of as not-quite-full persons, as they tend to lack the knowledge, skills and experience to make informed, responsible decisions.

Paternalism

Paternalism refers to an overly protective attitude and behaviour toward others. It can mean forcing others to do something or preventing others from doing something on the grounds that we (ie: parent, teacher, coach, therapist) know what's best for them.

'Soft' paternalism

The interference with the self-determination of others may be justifiable in cases where the person (eg: child, person with advanced Alzheimer's disease) may not be capable of informed choice. In cases like these, the practitioner provides the information to the parents or guardians so that they can make an informed decision for the person in their care.

Harm to others

This refers to the restriction of a person's liberty on the grounds that the consequences of certain behaviours harm others. For example, the ban on smoking in public places was based largely on the demonstrated harm produced by passive (ie: involuntary) inhalation.

Equality

Equality is the principle that someone should not be treated differently regardless of age, disability, ethnicity, gender, marital status, physical features, race, religion, or sexual orientation. It is often invoked to ensure that clients have equal access to services and other resources.

RESPECT FOR PERSONS — PRACTICAL APPLICATIONS

Informed consent

- **Fitness testing**

  A participant is informed of: (1) the aims of the test; (2) the benefits, risks and safeguards; and (3) the right to withdraw consent prior to the commencement of a fitness test, especially if the tests involve 'hands-on' techniques.

- **Health behaviour surveys or interviews**

  A participant is informed of: (1) the aims of the survey/interview; (2) the benefits, risks (eg: disclosure of potentially sensitive or prejudicial information) and safeguards (eg: alpha-numeric coding to protect identity); and (3) the right to withdraw consent prior to the commencement of the survey or interview.

Privacy

Conduct fitness and health screenings in a private, secure setting, especially if the procedure involves the client disrobing.

Parental consent and supervision

Ensure that the parent or guardian provides informed consent for children, and is present for any screening, testing or exercise by the children.

Confidentiality of records

Personal and health particulars can be released to outside agencies or used by other professionals only with prior written consent of the client.

Client self-care — exercise programming

A participant is given exercise options to choose from, as well as being provided with knowledge and skills (eg: taking pulse) to self-monitor and adjust exercise intensity.

Setting role boundaries

- Provide advice only within the limits of one's qualifications; otherwise, refer client to appropriate professional.

- Recognise and manage power differentials between practitioner–client (based on age, gender, physical size) in order to avoid client-dependency, vulnerability and potential abuse.

KEEPING ON DOING

Practitioners are people: we change and grow over time. Skovholt and Ronnestad (1992) mapped therapists' development over their clinical education and working life. Although Skovholt and Ronnestad interviewed counselling therapists, their model holds promise for clinical practitioners in other therapeutic disciplines. They found that the view therapists have of themselves, their confidence, and their working role and style varied with years of education and clinical experience. In this model, expert status is not a fixed point one reaches, a place of arrival, but rather an ongoing process of self-reflection, integration of learning, and increasing confidence. Because being a practicing therapist is not static, the way in which you 'do' evidence-based practice will change as you change.

Summary of key lessons

- To be an expert is to be a reflective practitioner who can ground professional practice in evidence and conduct practice in an ethically sensitive and socially responsible manner.

- The application of principles and evidence needs to be understood and applied in the context of often 'messy' everyday human relations.

- Reasoning skills are required in clinical practice to sort out what counts and is valued as evidence.

- Ethical reasoning will often generate or clarify value principles to help guide behaviour and improve the care of clients.

- Expert status is not a fixed point one reaches, a place of arrival, but rather an ongoing process of self-reflection, integration of learning, and increasing confidence.

REFERENCES

Copi, IM (1979) *Introduction to Logic*. New York: Macmillan Pub Co

Downey RS, Telfer E (1969) *Respect for Persons*, London: George, Allen and Unwin Ltd

Goldacre B (2009) *Bad science* (2nd ed). London: Fourth Estate

Haskins G (2006) *A Practical Guide to Critical Thinking*. Online. Available: http://www.skepdic.com/essays/haskins. pdf (accessed 31 May 2010)

Sackett DL (2000) The sins of expertness and a proposal for redemption. *BMJ*, 320:1283

Skovholt TM, Ronnestad MH (1992) *The Evolving Professional Self: Stages and Themes in Therapist and Counselor Development*. Chichester, England: Wiley

Chapter 2

Exercise as therapy in musculoskeletal conditions

Melainie Cameron and Christian Lorenzen

Assumed concepts

The musculoskeletal system has been described as 'the primary machinery of life', for it is the musculoskeletal system that allows us to move and act, and in action, function, and behaviour we 'live life' (Korr 1976, 1979). An operational understanding of the structure (anatomy) and function (physiology) of the musculoskeletal system is essential knowledge for clinical exercise practitioners.

INTRODUCTION

Exercise has profound effects on the musculoskeletal system. Bone and skeletal muscle respond to exercise by creating more bone and muscle. Muscle exercise responses are measured as changes in muscle girth (cross-sectional size, due to hypertrophy) and increases in strength, endurance, and speed of contraction, as well as corresponding increases in power (work over time). Bone responds to exercise training by increasing in mass, laying down new trabeculae, and increasing mineral density. Ligaments increase in tensile strength when trained under load. These effects of exercise on the musculoskeletal system have been well explored in both healthy and diseased individuals, and the results persist, albeit with some variance, across ages, genders, clinical and non-clinical populations.

Musculoskeletal conditions divide into three types: conditions of localised mechanical failure; systemic diseases with effects in the musculoskeletal system; and widespread conditions of musculoskeletally perceived pain. Conditions in this first category are easily comprehensible by most practitioners, and there are many excellent texts on the identification, diagnosis, management, and use of exercise for rehabilitation of these conditions. Consequently, we give these conditions cursory coverage in this chapter, and direct readers to other substantive sources. Systemic diseases affecting the musculoskeletal system include arthritides, and metabolic disorders of bone and muscle. Some of these conditions are covered in other chapters and cross-references are provided to avoid repetition throughout this text. Pain that is perceived as derived from the

Note: parts of this chapter are based on the literature review from Melanie Cameron's PhD thesis and on a Cochrane review currently being undertaken by both authors (Lorenzen et al 2010).

musculoskeletal system, but cannot be identified as caused by either an underlying systemic disease or localised musculoskeletal tissue failure, causes consternation for practitioners and considerable distress for clients. A large section of this chapter is devoted to this topic because vast resources may be expended on unnecessary investigations and unhelpful treatments unless practitioners have a sound appreciation of non-specific pain.

MECHANICAL MUSCULOSKELETAL CONDITIONS

Mechanical musculoskeletal conditions occur when requirements for use of musculoskeletal tissues exceed the load-bearing capacity of those tissues. Load-bearing failure may occur acutely, particularly when tissues are exposed to external trauma, or more gradually over time resulting in chronic tissue weakening and eventual failure (see Table 2.1).

Most of the tissues of the musculoskeletal system are endowed with nociceptors, thus loading these tissues near or beyond mechanical failure sends electrical signals to the brain that are interpreted as pain. Typically it is pain, rather than the functional effects of mechanical failure, that lead clients to seek treatment. Pain is far from straightforward (see further discussion on pain later in this chapter), but in most mechanical musculoskeletal conditions, pain is perceived as well localised, interpreted as arising directly from the tissues that have failed. Some musculoskeletal tissues do not appear to contain nociceptors (eg: medullary bone, central avascular regions of intervertebral discs and menisci of the knee; Mine et al 2000) and therefore cannot be identified as sources of pain.

Notwithstanding these caveats regarding the diagnostic value of pain, most assessment of clients with mechanical musculoskeletal complaints is intuitively logical. Tissues are examined individually, stressed as they would be under normal operational loads, and responses to stresses considered. For example, a client with an acute lateral ankle sprain will commonly report a history of rolling the ankle joint into excessive inversion, followed by pain localised to the lateral aspect of the ankle, tenderness when the lateral tendons are palpated, stress pain when the lateral tendons are made taut (inversion), and increased stress pain when additional load is applied to taut tendons: a clinical history and examination

findings consistent with an incomplete tear of the anterior talofibular ligament. Trainee practitioners spend considerable time learning physical examination and orthopaedic testing procedures to allow them to make assessments of mechanical musculoskeletal conditions. Rather than repeat this extensive content here, readers are directed to any of the excellent texts devoted to musculoskeletal examination (eg: Magee 2008).

Exercise for rehabilitation of mechanical musculoskeletal conditions

Exercise is a key modality for rehabilitation from mechanical musculoskeletal conditions. Principles for using exercise to induce changes in musculoskeletal tissues are outlined in Table 2.2. In making decisions regarding clinical exercise prescription, practitioners give due regard to the desired tissue level changes. In particular, practitioners take account of the mechanical function of damaged tissue, and select exercises to restore function to that tissue, or substitute that function through the increased function of another tissue. For example, in a client with a ligament rupture, clinical decisions must include whether the ligament will be surgically repaired or not. Exercise prescription to progressively increase tensile strength in a ligament with ruptured ends stitched together differs from an exercise program designed to substitute the stabilising function of a ligament through increased strength and endurance of nearby muscles.

Specificity and precision are important in exercise selection and execution. Some muscles are prime movers of joints while other muscles are stabilisers of joints, and stabilisation functions do not always recover automatically with resolution of pain or return to activities of daily living (Hides et al 1996). Current best practice includes recommending exercises to restore the stabilisation functions of local muscles concurrent with exercises to restore strength, power, and flexibility of motion producing larger (global) muscles in clients with mechanical musculoskeletal conditions.

SYSTEMIC DISEASES WITH MUSCULOSKELETAL EFFECTS

Systemic diseases with effects on the musculoskeletal system include arthritides and osteopenias. Arthritides are diseases that cause *arthritis* (joint

Table 2.1 Results of acute and chronic load failure of musculoskeletal tissues

Tissue	Acute	Chronic
Bone	Fractures Periosteal bruising Enthesitis	Stress fractures Osteitis Periostitis Enthesopathy Apophysitis
Epiphyseal plate (physis)	Salter-Harris fractures in children and teenagers	Apophysitis
Hyaline cartilage	Osteochondral fractures	Chondropathy (softening, dessication, fissuring, chronic inflammation)
Fibrocartilage	Incomplete tears Ruptures Herniation of nucleus pulposus from intervertebral disc	Chondropathy (softening, dessication, fissuring, chronic inflammation) Herniation of nucleus pulposus from intervertebral disc
Ligament (may be contiguous with joint capsule)	Sprains (incomplete tears) Ruptures (complete tears)	Chronic inflammation Joint instability
Skeletal muscle	Strains (incomplete tears) Contusions (incomplete tears with haematomata) Ruptures (complete tears) Avulsions (complete tears with small bony fragment attached)	Chronic inflammation Muscle weakness Myositis ossificans (following haematomata) Muscle atrophy (following ruptures and avulsions)
Tendon	Tendinitis (incomplete tears with acute inflammation) Enthesitis Ruptures (complete tears) Avulsions (complete tears with small bony fragment attached)	Tendinosis (chronic inflammation) Calcific tendiopathy Enthesopathy Tendon shrinkage (following ruptures and avulsions)
Bursa	Bursitis	Chronic inflammation

inflammation) and other symptoms including joint pain and swelling, reduced range of motion, and malaise. Joint damage, usually heralded by pain and progressive decline in function, is the hallmark of most types of arthritis. There are over 100 forms of arthritis, causes are often unknown, and clinical presentations vary substantially both between and within forms (Klippel et al 2008).

Osteoarthritis (OA) and rheumatoid arthritis (RA) are the two most common forms of arthritic

Table 2.2 Application of exercise to musculoskeletal tissue for specific outcomes

Tissue	Desired outcomes	Exercise selection and progression	Expected responses, cautions, and caveats
Skeletal muscle	Increase strength of contraction	Concentric and eccentric[*] contractions of muscle under load Increase load to progress training [*]Eccentric contraction can be isotonic (fixed load) or isokinetic (fixed speed). Isotonic training tends to lead to greater strength gains than does isokinetic training (Guilhem et al 2010)	Hypertrophy (increased cross-sectional area of muscle) Total load-bearing capacity increases (eg: 1RM, 3RM, 5RM) Single sets of exercises may be as effective as multiple sets in some populations (eg: untrained women; Cannon & Marino 2010)
	Increase speed of contraction	Concentric contractions (acceleration) Interval training: alternate high speed contractions with slower contractions Increase speed (reduce time taken for each contraction) and number of intervals to progress training	Hypertrophy, particularly of muscles with predominantly fast twitch (white) fibres Speed of contraction increases Same day steady state (endurance) training may compromise interval training performance (Yeo et al 2008)
	Increase endurance of contraction	Repeated concentric and eccentric contractions Increase repetitions to progress training Steady state training to maintain endurance	Hypertrophy, particularly of muscles with predominantly slow twitch (red) fibres Time to fatigue increases Same day interval training may enhance muscle adaptation, but does not appear to offer any benefits for increasing time to fatigue (Yeo et al 2008)
	Stability: contraction to maintain a stable position of a joint, or protect a joint throughout range of motion	Isometric contractions Eccentric contractions, including contractions under load (deceleration) Increase repetitions, or increase time taken for each repetition, to progress training	Hypertrophy, particularly of muscles with predominantly slow twitch (red) fibres Stabilisation training has become a popular alternative to endurance training for abdominal musculature, but the two training types recruit different muscles (Childs et al 2010)
	Increase flexibility (muscle lengthening)	Static stretching Passive stretching (assisted by another person)	Total range of motion increases Resting tone of muscle may decrease Acute decreases in contraction strength, endurance, and power may following static stretching (Yamaguchi & Ishii 2005)

(Continued)

Table 2.2 Application of exercise to musculoskeletal tissue for specific outcomes—cont'd

Tissue	Desired outcomes	Exercise selection and progression	Expected responses, cautions, and caveats
	Increase range of motion during activity (dynamic lengthening)	Dynamic stretching Contract-relax stretching	Total range of motion increases Resting tone of muscle may decrease Limited evidence that pre-sport stretching (any type) reduces injury (Fradkin et al 2006) or post exercise muscle soreness (Herbert & de Noronha 2007)
Bone	Increase bone mineral density	Weight-bearing exercises in upright posture (eg: walking, running, aerobic dance; Bonaiuti et al 2002)	Cortical thickness increases Number and thickness of trabeculae increases
Tendon and ligament	Increase strength	Concentric and eccentric contractions of muscle under load Increase load to progress training	Tensile strength increases Entheses (bony attachments) hypertrophy

disease. OA may be considered part of the normal aging process that affects most humans if they live long enough, but some people develop OA in middle age or earlier, or experience considerable pain and disability with OA and seek the assistance of medical practitioners to manage their OA (Klippel 2008).

RA is clearly identified as a disease process. The clinical presentation and symptom picture of this disease have been well documented (Arnett 1988), but its aetiology is not clear. RA is a multi-system disease that may cause dysfunction, destruction, and eventual failure in organs far removed from the musculoskeletal system. People living with RA may experience loss of functional capacity and diminished quality of life (QoL; Centres for Disease Control and Prevention [CDCP] 2000), not only due to joint and bone damage, but also due to pathology of the heart, lungs, kidneys, or gastrointestinal system (Ferrari et al 1996).

Rheumatology is a complex and specialist area of medical practice and research. The American College of Rheumatology (ACR) and American Rheumatism Association, in conjunction with other experts in the field, developed explicit diagnostic criteria for most arthritides (eg: Arnett et al 1988). Most people with arthritis experience a gradual onset of symptoms, although acute symptom onset can occur. Early arthritis symptoms may be vague, with radiographs and serology negative or indistinguishable from other diseases, and the diagnosis unclear. Diagnostic uncertainty in early arthritic disease may give way to two equally unfortunate scenarios: people with early arthritic symptoms may be told that they have a range of relatively innocuous mechanical musculoskeletal conditions (eg: bursitis, tendonitis), or they may be subject to extensive, but often inconclusive and relatively unhelpful, tests to investigate for arthritis. As arthritides progress, clinical markers (symptoms, radiography, serology) become clearer and the diagnosis apparent. Refer to Chapter 10 case study 1, and Chapter 12 case study 1, for further discussion of diagnostic delay and the application of classification criteria in arthritides.

Osteopenia is reduced bone mineral density (BMD). Precise definitions of osteopenia vary (eg: BMD one or more standard deviations below an age and sex determined mean). When osteopenia progresses to a pathological level, such that there is high risk of bone fracturing with minimal trauma or collapsing under its own weight (insufficiency fractures), it is referred to as osteoporosis. Osteopenia occurs with diseases that alter hormonal control, including hyperthyroidism, hyperparathyroidism, and Cushing's syndrome, and as a not uncommon side-effect of corticosteroid medications. Some reduction in BMD is age-related: this loss is more obvious in people of slight skeletal frame (typically women) because their peak BMD was never particularly high, and after menopause women lose the somewhat protective effect of oestrogen on bone turnover, further increasing osteopenia. Also, osteopenia occurs with bone disuse during part and whole-body rest. Exercise treatment for osteopenia in the absence of underlying disease provides a model for the exercise treatment of osteopenia secondary to metabolic disease.

Osteoporosis is a systemic skeletal disease characterised by low bone mass (osteopenia) and micro-architectural deterioration of bone tissue; thus osteoporosis may be considered the pathological advancement of osteopenia. Osteoporosis results in increased bone fragility and susceptibility to fracture (Kanis et al 2008). Hip fractures linked to osteoporosis are a global health problem (Alvarez-Nebreda et al 2008; Dawson-Hughes 2001; Liu et al 2007; Lofthus et al 2001; Siqueira et al 2005). Worldwide, the incidence of hip fractures is predicted to be 6.3 million by 2050, 3.7 times the incidence recorded in 1990. Hip fractures have significant effects on individuals because they can result in hospitalisation, disability, and are linked, albeit indirectly, to increased mortality (Center et al 1999; Sambrook & Cooper 2006).

BMD is measured as the amount of bone mass per unit volume (volumetric density, g/cm^3), or per unit area (areal density, g/cm^2; Kanis et al 2008). Several techniques are reported to determine BMD including dual-energy X-ray absorptiometry (DXA), quantitative ultrasound (QUS), magnetic resonance imaging (MRI), quantitative computed tomography (QCT) and peripheral quantitative computed tomography (pQCT). Although DXA is considered the current 'gold standard' for the clinical diagnosis of osteoporosis (Kanis

et al 2008; Royal Australian College of General Practitioners [RACGP] 2010), there are strengths and weaknesses of each method of analysis. For example, DXA provides the most available measure of fracture risk at the hip, but it is not particularly sensitive for monitoring treatment response at this site (Kanis et al 2008).

BMD values are expressed in reference to healthy young Caucasian women aged 20 to 29 years, in standard deviation units (Z scores) and reported as a T-score (Kanis et al 2008). Where population-specific databases are not available, normative data from the US National Health and Nutrition Examination Survey (NHANES III; Looker et al 1997, 1998) are used. In Australia, T-scores for fracture risk in women have been calculated from an Australian database. In men, a normative database does not exist and NHANES data are used instead. Using DXA measurements at the femoral neck, the following categorical classifications have been proposed for postmenopausal women and adult men aged 50 years and older: (1) normal = a T-score greater than or equal to -1 SD; (2) osteopenia (low bone mass) = a T-score less than -1 and greater than, but not more than, -2.5 SD; (3) osteoporosis = T-score less than or equal to -2.5 SD (Kanis et al 2008).

Because arthritides can lead to reduced physical activity, and inactivity can lead to osteopenia, arthritis and osteoporosis can co-exist. Arthritides and osteopenias are not, as frequently assumed, exclusively diseases of the elderly. The symptoms of many arthritides (eg: joint pain, muscle pain, weight loss) may commence in early adulthood, and continue through life. Juvenile and adolescent onset forms also occur, but are less common than the adult onset diseases (see Chapter 7 for juvenile arthritis). People of all ages with chronic conditions that compromise independent weight-bearing activity (eg: cerebral palsy, Huang et al 2006; osteogenesis imperfect, Leet et al 2006; coeliac disease, Ludvigsson et al 2007), are susceptible to fractures associated with low BMD and risk of fracture is amplified if the underlying disease process alters bone metabolism. Some arthritides are progressively destructive, worsening with increasing age (eg: OA, RA). In other types, symptoms are somewhat static but may be persistent (eg: post-infectious arthropathies, such as Lyme disease and Ross River fever). Regardless of the type, extent, or location of arthritis, the resultant pain, tissue atrophy, and tissue damage may reduce QoL and contribute to the development of disability (CDCP 2000). Social and psychological sequelae may include social withdrawal, loss and grief, anxiety, depression, and reduced wellbeing.

Because the causes of many arthritides are unclear, specific, targeted treatments are unavailable, and clients may try many therapies in attempts to reduce joint pain, improve function, and delay or prevent joint damage. Typically, outpatient (non-hospitalised) medical care for people with arthritides comprises an array of medications, usually provided under the care of a rheumatologist (Klippel 2008). Medications for arthritis can be grouped into four classes, each with a different therapeutic purpose: (1) analgesics, to reduce or limit pain; (2) non-steroidal anti-inflammatory drugs (NSAIDs), to reduce inflammation in joints and surrounding tissues; (3) corticosteroids, to reduce severe inflammation; and (4) disease modifying anti-rheumatic drugs (DMARDs), to modify the course of the disease by preventing joint and tissue damage. Several varieties of each drug type are available, and advances in drug treatment are ongoing.

Medications used in the management of osteopenia and osteoporosis include dietary supplementation of bone minerals (ie: calcium, magnesium) and vitamin D (Cranney et al 2000; Homik et al 1998), bisphosphonates to reduce rate of bone turnover (Homik et al 1999; Ward et al 2007), and hormonal treatments (Cranney & Wells 2003). Underlying diseases may be treated independently. Strategies for reducing the risk of hip fractures from osteoporosis include: hip protectors to reduce the force of falls (Parker et al 2005), antiresorptive therapy (calcium, phosphorous, and vitamin D supplementation, hormone replacement therapy, bisphosphonates, selective oestrogen-receptor modulators, and calcitonin) and anabolic therapy (parathyroid hormone; Sambrook & Cooper 2006; Vestergaard et al 2007).

In arthritides, surgical procedures may be used to repair or replace damaged joints when joint deterioration has not been arrested by drug therapies. Similarly, surgical repair is used for osteoporotic fractures. Because surgery induces mechanical stress on tissues, the application of exercise for post-surgical rehabilitation is essentially an extension of exercise for mechanical musculoskeletal conditions. Refer to Table 2.2 for a summary of the variations of exercise types commonly used in managing and treating mechanical musculoskeletal conditions, and the expected effects of these exercises on muscle, bone, and ligament.

Exercise as therapy for osteoporosis

Wolff's law that bone adapts and remodels according to load placed upon it is demonstrated in the application of exercise to osteopenic bone (Wolff 1986). The most substantial evidence for exercise treatment of osteoporosis is for the use of regular, moderate intensity, weight-bearing exercise to load the skeleton. A Cochrane review and meta-analysis of 18 clinical trials of exercise for osteoporosis prevention and treatment in postmenopausal women showed aerobic exercise, resistance training, and walking to be effective non-pharmacological alternatives to attenuate bone loss (Bonaiuti et al 2002). Not all exercises were equally effective at all skeletal sites. Although all exercise approaches increased BMD to some extent in the spine, walking appeared to be most effective at the hip, and a program of resisted back extension exercises appeared to increase spine BMD only. Studies of aerobic dance exercises (comprising upper limb, lower limb, and trunk exercises, a mixture of calisthenics, stretching, strengthening, and walking exercises) appeared promising, increasing BMD at the spine, hip and wrist, but comparisons between these studies were unclear because the exercise programs varied.

Paradoxically, acts of exercise such as walking (Rubin et al 2003) and aerobic dancing expose these individuals to the risk of falling, which may in turn lead to fracture. Although yet to be substantiated, whole-body vibration exercise may offer a safer alternative for reducing bone loss in people highly susceptible to hip fracture. Whole-body vibration exercise consists of standing statically or performing dynamic movements on an oscillating platform. Cited benefits include: improved muscular strength (Delecluse et al 2003; Roelants et al 2004) and flexibility (Cochrane & Stannard 2005), improved postural control in older adults (Bogaerts et al 2007) and people with neuromuscular diseases such as multiple sclerosis (Schuhfried et al 2005), reduced back pain (Rittweger et al 2002), and enhanced skeletal health of individuals susceptible to osteoporosis (Rubin et al 2004; Ward et al 2004).

The intensity of whole-body vibration exercise can be manipulated by the frequency of oscillations, measured in Hertz (Hz); and the amplitude of the oscillations, defined as the displacement of the platform from horizontal. The product of the frequency and amplitude of vibration is acceleration which has been reported in metres per second per second ($m.s^{-2}$) or in g-forces relative to the earth's gravitational force (g). Variations of exercises, such as dynamic and static squatting, can also be used to alter muscle activation during whole-body vibration exercise (Abercromby et al 2007).

Mechanisms explaining human musculoskeletal responses to whole-body vibration exercise are unclear. Several explanations have been proposed, including, but not limited to: (a) a tonic vibration reflex, that is mechanical vibration induced reflexive action of agonist and antagonist muscles (Cardinale & Bosco 2003; Russo et al 2003; Torvinen et al 2002); (b) fluid flow and intramedullary pressure produced by bone loading and deformation (Ward et al 2004); and (c) stochastic resonance, where a weak input signal, sensed by bone cell mechanoreceptor, is enhanced by 'noise' generated by vibration (Tanaka et al 2003).

Various combinations of frequency and amplitude, as well as static and dynamic exercise have been used by researchers. Inconsistent prescription of whole-body vibration makes it difficult for clinicians to determine the safest and most effective whole-body vibration exercise program. The high accelerations used by some researchers have been suggested by others to be dangerous for musculoskeletal health (Rubin et al 2003). The most effective combinations of exercise session duration and number of sessions per week are unclear.

Exercise as therapy for the arthritides

For almost 30 years, client-driven therapies, including exercise, have been used to improve the health-related QoL of people with arthritis (Fries et al 2003). Lorig's work helped initiate the widespread acceptance of client-driven interventions as therapies for people with arthritis through Arthritis Self-Management Programs (ASMP; Lorig et al 1993; see Chapter 9 for further discussion of self-management). Lorig and colleagues particularly encouraged people with arthritis to learn about arthritis, engage in regular physical activity such as warm-water exercise, and enter into partnerships with healthcare providers in order to plan and manage their arthritis. Lorig and Fries (2000) recommended many exercise programs for arthritis management, including land, water, and chair-based aerobic exercises, bicycling, flexibility and strengthening exercises for use in the home, and weight training. Movement-based programs promoted as beneficial for people with arthritides include various forms of tai chi and qigong, Feldenkrais therapy, and the Alexander technique (Lam & Horstman 2002).

Kerns and Rosenberg (2000) suggested that client-driven therapies (such as structured exercise) may not engage some people, and are associated with high drop-out rates. Keefe et al (2000) followed up this observation in a group of people with OA or RA, and found that 55% of participants identified themselves at psychological stages associated with failure to complete a course of therapy. Despite this shortcoming of structured programs, arthritis associations the world over recommend exercise and movement as self-management strategies for arthritis as part of the ASMP that stem from Lorig's work.

The evidence for exercise programs as specific therapies for altering the pathological features of arthritis (such as joint deformity and joint space loss) is somewhat lacking, but people with arthritis are not exempt from the training-related benefits of exercise (Cyarto et al 2004). Regardless of arthritis, people who do resistance training become stronger (Maurer et al 1999), and people who do aerobic exercise on a regular basis improve their cardiorespiratory capacity (de Jong et al 2003). Philbin et al (1995) demonstrated that even in elderly people with very advanced and severe OA, regular tailored training programs led to improvements in cardiovascular fitness and muscle strength without exacerbation of arthritic symptoms.

Thomas et al (2002) demonstrated in a clinical trial of 786 people, aged over 45 years, with self-reported knee pain, that home-based exercise was consistently better than no exercise in controlling pain over 6, 12, and 18-month follow-ups. Thomas and colleagues did not distinguish between OA and other causes of knee pain, and did not require that participants meet the ACR criteria for the diagnosis of OA of the knee at recruitment. OA of the knee is the most common cause of knee pain in adults aged over 45 years, but there is room to question whether the gains of exercise reported in this study showed a direct influence of exercise on OA, or a more generalised effect of exercise on pain (see Chapter 7).

Song et al (2003) conducted a randomised clinical trial (RCT) of tai chi exercises versus an attention control (telephone contact) in women aged over 55 years with ACR classified OA in any joint. Drop-out rate from this study was large (41%, recruitment n = 72, completion n = 43), raising (again) the possibility that the psychological stage of behaviour change is an important variable in taking up and keeping on with exercise, but women who persisted with tai chi exercise for 12 weeks reported statistically significantly lower levels of pain (p = 0.034), stiffness (p = 0.039), and difficulty in physical functioning (p = 0.008), as well as improvements in balance (p = 0.002) and abdominal muscle strength (p = 0.009). Despite the obvious limitation of the study being unblinded, these results are striking in a small sample, and suggest large effect sizes of tai chi on each of these variables.

The American Geriatrics Society (AGS) Panel on Exercise and Osteoarthritis (2001) reviewed RCTs of exercise interventions for people with OA. Generally, results indicated that 'increased physical activity does not produce or exacerbate joint symptoms and, in fact, confers significant health benefits' (p 810). On the basis of these data, the AGS panel recommended moderate physical activities, including flexibility, strength, and endurance training, 3–7 times per week for adults aged 65 years and older with OA (AGS 2001).

van den Ende et al (1998) completed a systematic review of the evidence for structured, aerobic exercise in treating RA. This review was updated a decade later (Hurkmans et al 2009); two new studies were added, but the conclusions altered little. van den Ende et al (1998) and Hurkmans et al (2009) concluded that dynamic exercise at 55–60% of maximal heart rate for 20 minutes, twice per week, for at least 6 weeks, was effective in increasing aerobic capacity and muscle strength in people with RA. Furthermore, this level of training produced no detrimental effects

on RA progression. The evidence was inadequate for van den Ende et al to conclude whether such exercise programs had any detrimental effects on joint stability or radiological markers of RA progression, or produced any improvements in functional ability. It is possible that people with RA who undertake regular, dynamic exercise may become physically fitter, but not necessarily demonstrate increased physical function.

de Jong et al (2003) conducted a randomised, controlled clinical trial of the efficacy and safety of 2 years of high-intensity exercise training in 309 adults with RA. The 1.25 hour-long exercise program, undertaken twice each week, comprised warm-up and cool-down exercises as well as 20 minutes of stationary bicycle training, 20 minutes of circuit training, and 20 minutes of games such as badminton, volleyball, indoor soccer, or basketball. Participants in both the exercise and control groups were assessed at baseline and 6-monthly intervals for functional ability (measured using the McMaster Toronto Arthritis Patient Preference Disability Questionnaire [MACTAR; Tugwell et al 1987] and the Health Assessment Questionnaire [HAQ; Fries et al 1980]), physical capacity (aerobic fitness, muscle strength), emotional status (measured using the Hospital Anxiety and Depression Scale [HADS; Zigmond & Snaith 1983]), radiographic progression of disease (measured using the Larsen score for large joints), and disease activity (measured using the Disease Activity Score [DAS; van Gestel et al 1996, 1998] with four variables).

After 2 years 281 people remained in the study. The exercise group (n = 136) reported significantly better functional ability than the control group (n = 145) using the MACTAR (p < .02) but not on the HAQ. This discrepancy between measures was attributed by the authors to the 'HAQ's lack of sensitivity to change in exercise trials' (p 2421). Significant improvements in aerobic fitness (p < .01) and emotional status (p < .01) were also demonstrated in the exercise group, but declines in these variables in the control group contributed to these results. Muscle strength increased, and DAS decreased gradually, in both groups over time, and the groups did not differ significantly on these measures at the end of the study.

Participants with more radiographic evidence of joint damage at baseline showed more progression in joint damage over time, and this trend was more obvious in the exercise group, but the differences between groups were not statistically significant. The authors considered that this non-significant finding demonstrated the safety of the exercise program, arguing that progression over time is the natural and expected course of RA. Because only participants without prosthetic joints were recruited for this study, it is likely that the sample represented people with RA with relatively low levels of joint damage. Recognising this limitation of their study, de Jong et al (2003) offered a caution that until further research supported their findings clinicians might prefer to tailor for clients exercise programs that spare damaged joints.

de Jong et al (2003) reported their study as a comparison of high-intensity exercise against physical therapy, but this description is inaccurate. Participants in both the exercise and control groups sought physical therapy treatment during the trial period. Participants in the control (usual care) group were restricted in their capacity to seek physical therapy care: 'Patients assigned to the UC [usual care] group were treated by a physical therapist only if this was regarded as necessary by their attending physician.' (de Jong et al: 2416). Furthermore, the precise type of physical therapy was not defined in the study, and included any combination of 'hydrotherapy [exercise in water], and different types of physical therapy (active, passive, or applications)' (de Jong et al: 2419). A physical therapy consultation might be sought because a participant is injured, because a participant has experienced a disease flare, or for an issue unrelated to the trial or indeed to RA. In de Jong et al's study, the distinction between groups was that the exercise group undertook a structured program of high-intensity weight-bearing exercise twice per week whereas the control group did not. It is not reasonable to draw conclusions regarding water exercise or physical therapy from the de Jong et al study.

Possible mechanisms of action for exercise in arthritides

We have incomplete knowledge of the cellular level effects of exercise on healthy joints, let alone joints altered by arthritic disease. Vilensky argued (1998), consistent with Melzack and Wall's (1965) gate control theory of pain, that 'physical stimuli such as … range-of-motion exercise reduce pain because cutaneous afferent impulses inhibit transmission of articular nociceptive impulses in the spinal cord' (p 180). Vilensky applied the gate control theory to OA, but there appear to have been no studies specifically investigating pain inhibition in OA. Logically, spinal interneuronal inhibition of pain transmission should occur following the stimulation of healthy and diseased joints alike. It seems unlikely that any particular type of arthritis would dampen or enhance the inhibitory process, provided that that joint sensation remains intact (eg: not neuropathic osteoarthropathy).

Synovial fluid of healthy joints contains high concentrations of hyaluronan (hyaluronic acid), which for over 5 decades has been understood to be important for joint lubrication and maintaining the viscosity of joint fluid (Ogston & Stanier 1953). Hyaluronan concentrations are lower in the synovial fluid of joints affected by RA than in healthy joints (Balazs et al 1967), and may be increased by the intra-articular injection of corticosteroids (Pitsillides et al 1993).

Pitsillides et al (1999) demonstrated the importance of movement and loading on joint function in mammals. Left hock (tibiotalar) joints of five female Welsh mountain sheep were surgically immobilised using internal fixation that prevented both loading and articulation of the joints. After 12 weeks the sheep were euthenased by phenobarbitone injection. Synovial fluid samples aspirated from both the left (immobilised) and right (control) hock joints, and samples of synovial tissue (membrane) were dissected from the anterior and posterior compartments of all joints. Synovial fluid samples were assayed to determine concentrations of hyaluronan, and synovial tissue samples were analysed, using cellular staining and microdensitometry scanning, for evidence of enzyme activity (non-specific esterase and uridine diphosphoglucose dyhydrogenase) essential for hyaluronan formation. In the immobilised joints, hyaluronan concentrations were significantly decreased, and cellular evidence of enzyme activity was also lower, than in their corresponding controls. Pitsillides et al (1999) suggested that joint homeostatic mechanisms for the production of hyaluronan are controlled by mechanoreceptors. Despite the obvious limitations of applying a study on the healthy joints of animals to humans with arthritis, it is plausible that exercises that move joints (eg: walking, tai chi) may contribute to improved joint function through the production of hyaluronan.

NON-SPECIFIC MUSCULOSKELETAL PAIN DIAGNOSES

Modern musculoskeletal rehabilitation is complicated by non-specific pain diagnoses. It is a considerable challenge for clinical exercise practitioners that, quite simply, not all musculoskeletal pain can be explained.

Traditionally, musculoskeletal therapists, including physiotherapists, osteopaths, and chiropractors, have sought to explain clients' pain presentations, and their own work, using idiosyncratic musculoskeletal labels. For example, chronic low back pain has variously been attributed to facet joint dysfunction, vertebral subluxation, somatic dysfunction, sacroiliac joint dysfunction, muscle spasm, muscle imbalance, and muscle trigger points, to name but a few of the descriptors. Some disciplines have gone further still, describing joint dysfunctions in terms of bony position or motion restriction.

These musculoskeletal labels have appealed to generations of practitioners because they are supposedly based on an understanding of anatomy and physiology (first principles). Sometimes this assumption is a leap of faith. Unfortunately, much of this labelling has not stood up to ongoing scientific scrutiny including advances in understanding of anatomy and physiology through to diagnostic and clinical testing.

Bogduk (1997: 191–2) reviewed several commonly posited explanations for chronic low back pain in light of the following four postulates:

For any structure to be deemed a cause of back pain:

1 The structure should have a nerve supply, for without access to the nervous system, it could not evoke pain [see earlier note on first principles].

2 The structure should be capable of causing pain similar to that seen clinically. Ideally, this should be demonstrated in normal volunteers, for inferences drawn from clinical studies may be compromised by observer bias or poor patient reliability.

3 The structure should be susceptible to diseases or injuries that are known to be painful. Ideally, such disorders should be evidence upon investigation of the patient, but this may not always be possible.

4 The structure should have been shown to be a source of pain in patients, using diagnostic techniques of known reliability and validity.

Bogduk constructed a matrix to correlate possible diagnoses of chronic low back pain against these postulates, and reported that zygapophyseal joint pain, sacroiliac joint pain, and internal disc disruption were the diagnoses supported by the greatest amount of scientific data including controlled studies, identifiable valid, reliable, provocative diagnostic or imaging procedures. Conversely, 'office' diagnoses such as trigger points, muscle imbalance, or joint dysfunction that do not require invasive tests were found to be both unsupported by controlled studies and unverified by reliable, valid diagnostic procedures. In more recent years disciplines that previously favoured these diagnostic labels have experienced considerable professional angst, and in some cases, paradigm shift, as they have tried to reconcile years of clinical experience and practice with seemingly unsubstantiated diagnoses and diagnostic practices (see Mirtz et al 2009 for such a discussion pertaining to chiropractic).

Zygapophyseal joint pain, sacroiliac joint pain, and internal disc disruption combined account for slightly more than 60% of patients with chronic low back pain (Bogduk 1997). Although these diagnoses are prevalent, it is clear that almost 40% of chronic low back pain is not so readily explained.

Further, zygapophyseal joint pain, sacroiliac joint pain, and internal disc disruption are, in themselves, somewhat poorly specified diagnostic labels. To be able to identify that pain is perceived as originating from a zygapophyseal (facet) joint is simply localisation. This diagnosis does not explain the cause of pain at a structural or physiological level.

Historically we have relied on Rene Descartes' 17th century descriptions to inform our understanding of pain: 'Fast moving particles of fire … the disturbance passes along the nerve filament until it reaches the brain …' (Descartes

1647). Descartes thought of the human body in structural terms, a radical view in his day, which gave rise to the belief that the body and the mind were distinct (body–mind split). Although Descartes' ideas were part of an important trend towards a more scientific understanding of pathologies, Cartesian thinking fails to explain a large portion of human pain. Sometimes it holds sufficiently well: when I place my hand into a fire, I display a protective withdrawal response to acute traumatic tissue damage and I feel pain that I can localise to the site of the burn. But in many cases, including prolonged pain and pain associated with emotionally and socially charged situations, Descartes' explanation is inadequate: Why do amputated limbs hurt? Why does my back ache weeks, months, or years after the initial injury? Why does one woman scream in the pain of childbirth and another woman make no sound? Why do soldiers not feel the pain of wounds until after the battle? Why do athletes train through injuries? Pain, it seems, is a construct of the brain, a response to actual or anticipated tissue damage (Butler & Mosely 2003), and that response may be amplified or dampened by social and cultural environment, expectations, beliefs, and attitudes. See Chapter 10, case study 2 (Mark), for further exploration of the unity of body and mind.

Recognising that our current knowledge is limited, both in our capacity to explain a large proportion of the pain presentations in clinical practice, and in the depth of explanations that can be offered for other pain syndromes, is a source of discontent for practitioners and clients alike. We want to be able to answer our clients' questions about their pain. We want to be knowledgeable, and to be confident that our knowledge is of the solid and unshakable kind. Unfortunately the state of the science in musculoskeletal pain is such that we cannot explain the origin of a substantial proportion of musculoskeletal pain. There is little else for it — clinical exercise practitioners need to become comfortable with broad diagnostic labels such as 'non-specific low back pain' and with admitting to clients that the precise cause of such pain is unknown.

Something other than pain?

Pain is by far the most common reason why clients seek musculoskeletal care, but some clients present with concerns other than pain, or in adjunct to pain. For example, a client with a sprained ankle may be concerned about a sense that the ankle feels unstable, and worried about the possibility of repeating the injury. Clients' fears, avoidance of some behaviours, and confidence in action (self-efficacy) are key issues in the clinical use of musculoskeletal exercise. See Chapter 7 for further discussion of chronic pain, pain behaviour, and pain beliefs.

FURTHER ROLES FOR EXERCISE

Exercise makes many valuable contributions in the management of musculoskeletal conditions. The physiological effects of exercise on bone, muscle, and ligament are largely preserved in people with musculoskeletal diseases and non-specific pain syndromes, although expected gains may be somewhat slower than in apparently healthy clients. Moreover, clients with musculoskeletal conditions (mechanical, systemic, and non-specific pain syndromes alike) who exercise regularly and safely report effects in reducing or controlling pain, improving balance, increasing self-efficacy and self-confidence, improved sleeping, less general fatigue, and improved perceived health and wellbeing (see Table 2.3). Although some of these effects are non-specific, they are valuable and meaningful to clients, and should not be dismissed.

Although the general effects of exercise appear to persist across the range of musculoskeletal conditions, diseases, and pain presentations, the reverse is not so: there is limited evidence that specific exercises afford benefit in the management of non-specific musculoskeletal pain. For example, the Australian Acute Musculoskeletal Pain Guidelines Group (2003) recommended general exercise and staying active, as opposed to specific back strengthening or stretching exercises, as strategies for managing acute non-specific low back pain. Refer to Chapter 18 case study 3, and Chapter 19 case study 1 for further discussion of evidence-based management of spinal pain.

Despite the inclusion of advice to stay active as part of modern low back pain management, there have been few head-to-head comparisons of staying active and bed-rest (previous common wisdom for low back pain). Dahm et al (2010) updated a Cochrane review (Hilde et al 2006) of such comparative studies, found no new

Table 2.3 Examples of evidence of diverse exercise effects in clients with musculoskeletal conditions or diseases

Population	Effect/s	Summary of evidence	
Adults with mechanical (non-specific) neck pain, or neck disorder with headache, including whiplash associated disorders	• Reduce pain • Improve function • Improve overall perceived effectiveness of treatment	Kay et al (2005): Systematic review of 31 randomised clinical trials	
		Stretching and strengthening of neck and shoulder musculature	Moderate evidence for pain in chronic neck pain (pooled SMD -0.42 [95% CI: -0.83 to -0.01]), and neck pain with headache, in the short and long term
		Eye-fixation and proprioception exercises as part of a larger exercise program	Moderate evidence for pain, function, and global perceived effect in chronic neck pain short term, and for pain and function for acute and sub-acute whiplash associated disorders, with or without headache, in the long term
Adults with non-specific low back pain: acute, sub-acute, or chronic	• Reduction in pain severity measured on a 100 point pain scale • Improvement in condition specific physical functioning • Perceived global improvement • Return to work and/or absenteeism	Hayden et al (2005): Systematic review of 61 randomised controlled trials	
		Specific exercises as part or only treatment for acute low back pain	No evidence of differences in short-term pain relief between exercises and no treatment (-0.59/100; 95% CI: -12.69 to 11.51) Also, no difference in pain relief when exercise is compared to other conservative treatments (0.31/100; 95% CI: -0.10 to 0.72) Similarly, no evidence of significant effect of exercise on functional outcomes
		Sub-acute low back pain	Insufficient evidence to support or refute the effectiveness of exercise in sub-acute low back pain for reducing pain severity or improving function Some evidence that graded exercise (ie: work hardening) reduces absenteeism
		Strengthening and stabilising exercises for chronic low back pain	Strong evidence that exercise is as effective as other conservative treatments Significant but small improvements in pain (7/100) and physical function (< 3/100) in exercise groups over control groups Larger effect sizes (eg: pain 13.3/100) are found with individually designed programs delivered in healthcare settings rather than programs for the general population

(Continued)

Table 2.3 Examples of evidence of diverse exercise effects in clients with musculoskeletal conditions or diseases—cont'd

Population	Effect/s	Summary of evidence	
Adults with previous episodes of non-specific low back pain	• Reduction in and/or prevention of recurrent episodes of low back pain • Reduction in sick leave due to low back pain	Choi et al (2010): Systemic review of 9 clinical trials of 9 exercise based interventions for low back pain prevention	
		Exercises commenced as part of treatment for low back pain	Conflicting evidence as to prevention of recurrence
		Exercises commenced post-treatment (ie: when pain-free) for prevention of future episodes of low back pain	Moderate evidence of reduction in number of future episodes of low back pain over 1.5 to 2 years follow-up Very low quality evidence of reduction in the number of sick leave days taken due to low back pain over 1.5 to 2 years follow-up

studies, and re-analysed the 10 studies worthy of inclusion in the original review. Some studies had multiple components (ie: addressed more than one question). In conducting this systematic review, composite studies were divided into component parts and data re-analysed according to research questions. In people with acute non-specific low back pain, or low back pain with sciatica, six studies included comparisons of advice to rest in bed with advice to stay active, four studies compared advice to rest in bed with other treatments, two studies compared different lengths of bed rest, and two studies compared advice to stay active with other treatments. No studies compared different ways of delivering advice to stay active, and studies were of low to moderate quality. Moderate quality evidence demonstrated that people with acute low back pain without neurological deficits (ie: non-specific spinal pain) experience small improvements in pain relief and ability to perform everyday activities if they receive and follow advice to stay active compared with resting in bed, but people with sciatica (demonstrated by hard neurological signs) experience little or no difference between the two approaches. Further, three RCTs (n = 931) showed little or no difference between advice for specific exercises, rest in bed, or staying active for people with acute non-specific low back pain. Although these studies were considered low

quality evidence, they confirmed the assertion of existing management guidelines that specific exercise programs appear to offer no benefits over general exercise (routine physical activity and incidental activity) for people with acute non-specific low back pain.

CAUTIONS AND CLOSING REMARKS

Caveats are necessary at this point: the adage 'No pain, no gain' has little place here. Exercising to produce pain appears to be of no real value, and can be harmful in some cases. As a general rule, musculoskeletal clients are advised to exercise within their pain-free thresholds, and in time, with graduated training, these thresholds will probably increase. Similar cautions apply to fatigue, increasing training loads (weight, speed, resistance, or repetitions), and challenges to balance. Although, there is value in using exercise to extend clients' functional capacity, progressions of exercise should be graduated and monitored because each of these progressions risks injury if excessive.

Further, musculoskeletal exercise rehabilitation is a realm inhabited by many fads. Clinicians and clients alike are cautioned to seek out reliable, valid, scientific evidence of the efficacy of any exercise or program rather than listening to the appraisal of proponents. Consider as an example Trees et al's (2007) Cochrane review of five clinical trials using several different exercise programs (including hydrotherapy, strength training, balance and proprioceptive training, accelerated exercise rehabilitation, and exercise as a part of usual conservative care) for treating anterior cruciate ligament (knee) injuries in combination with collateral ligament and meniscal damage in adults. Although methodological differences between these studies meant that data could not be pooled, and no studies compared exercise with no exercise, Trees et al (2007) were unable to identify support to favour one type of exercise program over any other.

Similarly, in a systemic review of 12 clinical trials of exercise for the management of patellofemoral pain syndrome in adolescents and young adults, Heintjes et al (2003) identified limited evidence to support exercise therapy as more effective than no exercise with respect to pain reduction, and conflicting evidence with respect to functional improvement. Moreover, there is strong evidence that open and closed kinetic chain exercises are equally effective for managing this condition.

Stretching to reduce delayed onset muscle soreness is a long held dogma of exercise practitioners. Herbert and de Noronha (2007) conducted a Cochrane review meta-analysis of trials of stretching exercises to prevent or reduce muscle soreness after exercise. They identified highly consistent results across 10 studies — three studies in which stretching was undertaken before vigorous exercise and seven studies in which stretching was performed after other exercise — to conclude that stretching has minimal or no effect on muscle soreness from one-half to 3 days post exercise. Robust evidence such as this Cochrane review may challenge practitioners' and clients' long-held beliefs and reshape aspects of musculoskeletal clinical exercise practice. Although we hold to the view that exercise, generally, is good for most people most of the time, further research is required to substantiate the efficacy of some exercise treatments and to determine the most effective forms of exercise.

Summary of key lessons

- Exercise shows some benefits for most musculoskeletal conditions, including mechanical conditions, systemic diseases with musculoskeletal effects, and non-specific musculoskeletal pain syndromes, but the application of exercise and the possible mechanisms of action differ between conditions.

- In mechanical musculoskeletal conditions, exercises are selected to effect physiological changes in specific tissues.

- In osteopenias, exercises used to increase BMD include skeletal load-bearing such as walking and aerobic dance, resistance training, and whole-body vibration.

- In arthritides, exercise is used to maintain joint ranges of motion, prevent inactivity, and promote self-management.

- In non-specific pain syndromes the effects of exercise are more generalised, including reduction in pain and maintenance of physical function and activities of daily living.

REFERENCES

Abercromby AF, Amonette WE, Layne CS, et al (2007) Variation in neuromuscular responses during acute whole-body vibration exercise. *Medicine and Science in Sports and Exercise*, 39,1642–50

Alvarez-Nebreda ML, Jiménez AB, Rodríguez P, et al (2008) Epidemiology of hip fracture in the elderly in Spain. *Bone*, 42, 278–85

American Geriatrics Society (AGS) Panel on Exercise and Osteoarthritis (2001) Exercise prescription for older adults with osteoarthritis pain: consensus practice recommendations. A supplement to the AGS Clinical Practice Guidelines on the management of chronic pain in older adults. *Journal of the American Geriatrics Society*, 49, 808–23

Arnett FC, Edworthy SM, Bloch DA, et al (1988) The American Rheumatism Association 1987 revised criteria for the classification of rheumatoid arthritis. *Arthritis and Rheumatism*, 31, 315–24

Australian Acute Musculoskeletal Pain Guidelines Group (2003) *Evidence-based Management of Acute Musculoskeletal Pain*. Bowen Hills, Australia: Australian Academic Press

Balazs EA, Watson D, Duff IF, et al (1967) Hyaluronic acid in synovial fluid. I. Molecular parameters of hyaluronic acid in normal and arthritis human fluids. *Arthritis and Rheumatism*, 10, 357–76

Bogaerts A, Verschueren S, Delecluse C, et al (2007) Effects of whole-body vibration training on postural control in older individuals: a 1 year randomized controlled trial. *Gait & Posture*, 26, 309–16

Bogduk N (1997) *Clinical Anatomy of the Lumbar Spine and Sacrum*. Edinburgh: Churchill Livingstone

Bonaiuti D, Shea B, Iovine R, et al (2002) Exercise for preventing and treating osteoporosis in postmenopausal women. *Cochrane Database of Systematic Reviews*, Issue 2. Art No: DOI: 10.1002/14651858.CD000333

Butler D, Moseley GL (2003) *Explain Pain*. UK: NOIgroup Publications

Cannon J, Marino FE (2010) Early-phase neuromuscular adaptations to high- and low-volume resistance training in untrained young and older women. *Journal of Sports Science*, Nov 3:1–10. [Epub ahead of print]

Cardinale M, Bosco C (2003) The use of vibration as an exercise intervention. *Exercise and Sport Sciences Reviews*, 31, 3–7

Center JR, Nguyen TV, Schneider D, et al (1999) Mortality after all major types of osteoporotic fracture in men and women: an observational study. *Lancet*, 353, 878–82

Centers for Disease Control and Prevention (CDCP) (2000) Health-related quality of life among adults with arthritis: Behavioral Risk Factor Surveillance System, 11 states, 1996–1998. *Morbidity and Mortality Weekly*, Report 49, 366

Childs JD, Teyhen DS, Casey PR, et al (2010) Effects of traditional sit-up training versus core stabilization exercises on short-term musculoskeletal injuries in US Army soldiers: a cluster randomized trial. *Physical Therapy*, 90, 1404–12

Choi BKL, Verbeek JH, Tam WWS, et al (2010) Exercises for prevention of recurrences of low-back pain. *Cochrane Database of Systematic Reviews*, Issue 1. DOI: 10.1002/14651858.CD006555.pub2

Cochrane DJ, Stannard SR (2005) Acute whole-body vibration training increases vertical jump and flexibility performance in elite female field hockey players. *British Journal of Sports Medicine*, 39, 860–5

Cranney A, Welch V, Adachi J, et al (2000) Calcitonin for preventing and treating corticosteroid-induced osteoporosis. *Cochrane Database of Systematic Reviews*, Issue 1. DOI: 10.1002/14651858.CD001983

Cranney A, Wells GA (2003) Hormone replacement therapy for postmenopausal osteoporosis. *Clinics in Geriatric Medicine*, 19, 361–70

Cyarto EV, Moorhead GE, Brown WJ (2004) Updating the evidence relating to physical activity intervention studies in older people. *Journal of Science and Medicine in Sport*, 7(Suppl 1): 30–8

Dahm KT, Brurberg KG, Jamtvedt G, et al (2010) Advice to rest in bed versus advice to stay active for acute low-back pain and sciatica. *Cochrane Database of Systematic Reviews*, Issue 6. DOI: 10.1002/14651858.CD007612.pub2

Dawson-Hughes B (2001) Epidemiology of osteoporotic fractures in the United States. *Bone*, 29(3): 298–9

de Jong Z, Munneke M, Zwinderman AH, et al (2003) Is a long-term high-intensity exercise program effective and safe in patients with rheumatoid arthritis? *Arthritis and Rheumatism*, 48, 2415–24

Delecluse C, Roelants M, Verschueren S (2003) Strength increase after whole-body vibration compared with resistance training. *Medicine and Science in Sports and Exercise*, 35, 1033–41

Descartes R (1647) *The description of the human body* (incomplete). Published posthumously, circa 1664

Ferrari R, Cash J, Maddison P (1996) *Rheumatology guidebook: A step-by-step guide to diagnosis and treatment*. Oxford, England: Bios Scientific

Fradkin AJ, Gabbe BJ, Cameron PA (2006) Does warming up prevent injury in sport? The evidence from randomised controlled trials. *Journal of Science and Medicine in Sport*, 9: 214–20

Fries J F, Lorig K, Holman HR (2003) Patient self-management in arthritis? Yes! *The Journal of Rheumatology*, 30, 1130–2

Fries JF, Spitz PW, Kraines RG, et al (1980) Measurement of patient outcome in arthritis. *Arthritis and Rheumatism*, 23, 137–45

Guilhem G, Cornu C, Guével (2010) A Neuromuscular and muscle-tendon adaptations to isotonic and isokinetic eccentric exercise. *Annals of Physical and Rehabilitation Medicine*, 53: 319–41

Hayden J, van Tulder MW, Malmivaara A, et al (2005) Exercise therapy for treatment of non-specific low back pain. *Cochrane Database of Systematic Reviews*, Issue 3. Art No: CD000335. DOI: 10.1002/14651858.CD000335.pub2

Heintjes E, Berger MY, Bierma-Zeinstra SMA, et al (2003) Exercise therapy for patellofemoral pain syndrome. *Cochrane Database of Systematic Reviews*, Issue 4. DOI: 10.1002/14651858.CD003472

Herbert RD, de Noronha M (2007) Stretching to prevent or reduce muscle soreness after exercise. *Cochrane Database of Systematic Reviews*, Issue 4. DOI: 10.1002/14651858.CD004577.pub2

Hides JA, Richardson CA, Jull GA (1996) Multifidus muscle recovery is not automatic following resolution of acute first episode low back pain. *Spine*, 21: 2763–9

Hilde G, Hagen KB, Jamtvedt G, et al (2006) Advice to stay active as a single treatment for low-back and sciatica. *Cochrane Database of Systematic Reviews*, Issue 2. DOI: 10.1002/14651858.CD003632.pub2

Homik J, Cranney A, Shea B, et al (1999) Bisphosphonates for treating osteoporosis caused by the use of steroids. *Cochrane Database of Systematic Reviews*, Issue 1. DOI: 10.1002/14651858.CD001347

Homik J, Suarez-Almazor ME, Shea B, et al (1998) Calcium and vitamin D for corticosteroid-induced osteoporosis. *Cochrane Database of Systematic Reviews*, Issue 2. DOI: 10.1002/14651858.CD000952

Huang RP, Ambrose CG, Sullivan E, et al (2006) Functional significance of bone density measurements in children with osteogenesis imperfecta. *The Journal of Bone and Joint Surgery*, 88, 1324–30

Hurkmans E, van der Giesen FJ, Vliet Vlieland TPM, et al (2009) Dynamic exercise programs (aerobic capacity and/or muscle strength training) in patients with rheumatoid arthritis. *Cochrane Database of Systematic Reviews*, Issue 4. DOI: 10.1002/14651858.CD006853.pub2

Kanis JA, McCloskey EV, Johansson H, et al (2008) A reference standard for the description of osteoporosis. *Bone*, 42, 467–75

Kay TM, Gross A, Goldsmith C, et al (2005) Cervical Overview Group. Exercises for mechanical neck disorders. *Cochrane Database of Systematic Reviews*, Issue 3. DOI: 10.1002/14651858.CD004250.pub3

Keefe FJ, Lefebvre JC, Kerns RD, et al (2000) Understanding the adoption of arthritis self-management: Stages of change profiles among arthritis patients. *Pain*, 87, 303–13

Kerns RD, Rosenberg R (2000) Predicting responses to self-management treatments for chronic pain: Application of the pain stages of change model. *Pain*, 84, 49–55

Keysor JJ (2003) Does late-life physical activity or exercise prevent or minimize disablement? A critical review of the scientific evidence. *American Journal of Preventative Medicine*, 25(Suppl 2), 129–36

Klippel JH, Stone JH, Crofford LJ, et al (eds) (2008) *Primer on the Rheumatic Diseases* (13th ed). New York: Springer

Korr IM (1976) The spinal cord as organizer of disease processes: some preliminary perspectives. *Journal of the American Osteopathic Association*, 76, 35–45

—— (1979) The spinal cord as organizer of disease processes: II The peripheral autonomic nervous system. *Journal of the American Osteopathic Association*, 79, 82–90

Lam P, Horstman J (2002) *Overcoming Arthritis*. Melbourne, Australia: Dorling Kindersley

Leet AI, Mesfin A, Pichard C, et al (2006) Fractures in children with cerebral palsy. *Journal of Pediatric Orthopedics*, 26, 624–7

Liu JM, Ning G, Chen JL (2007) Osteoporotic fractures in Asia: risk factors and strategies for prevention. *Journal of Bone Mineral Metabolism*, 25, 1–5

Lofthus C, Osnes E, Falch J, et al (2001) Epidemiology of hip fractures in Oslo, Norway. *Bone*, 29, 413–18

Looker AC, Orwoll ES, Johnston CC, et al (1997) Prevalence of low femoral bone density in older US adults from NHANES III. *Journal of Bone and Mineral Research*, 12: 1761–8

Looker AC, Wahner HW, Dunn WL, et al (1998) Updated data on proximal femur bone mineral levels of US adults. *Osteoporosis International*, 8: 468–86

Lorenzen C, Naughton G, Cameron M, et al (2010) Whole body vibration for preventing and treating osteoporosis (Protocol). Cochrane Database of Systemic Reviews, Issue 3. DOI: 10.1002/14651858.CD008417

Lorig K, Fries JF (2000) *The Arthritis Helpbook* (5th ed). Cambridge, MA: Perseus Books

Lorig K, Mazonson P, Holman H (1993) Evidence suggesting that health education for self-management in patients with chronic arthritis has sustained health benefits while reducing health care costs. *Arthritis and Rheumatism*, 36, 439–46

Ludvigsson JF, Michaelsson K, Ekbom A, et al (2007) Coeliac disease and the risk of fractures — a general population-based cohort study. *Alimentary Pharmacology & Therapeutics*, 25, 273–85

Magee DJ (2008) *Orthopedic Physical Assessment* (5th ed). St Louis, Missouri: Elsevier

Maurer BT, Stern AG, Kinossian B, et al (1999) Osteoarthritis of the knee: Isokinetic quadriceps exercise versus an educational intervention. *Archives of Physical Medicine and Rehabilitation*, 80, 1293–9

Melzack R, Wall PD (1965) Pain mechanisms: a new theory. *Science*, 150, 971–9

Mine T, Kimura M, Sakka A, et al (2000) Innervation of nociceptors in the menisci of the knee joint: an immunohistochemical study. *Archives of Orthopaedic Trauma and Surgery*. 120: 201–4

Mirtz TA, Morgan L, Wyatt LH, et al (2009) An epidemiological examination of the subluxation construct using Hill's criteria of causation. *Chiropractic & Osteopathy*, 17:13 DOI:10.1186/1746-1340-17-13

Ogston AG, Stanier JE (1953) The physiological functions of hyaluronic acid in synovial fluid; viscous, elastic and lubricant properties. *Journal of Physiology*, 199, 244–52

Parker MJ, Gillespie WJ, Gillespie LD (2005) Hip protectors for preventing hip fractures in older people. *Cochrane Database of Systematic Reviews*, Issue 3. DOI: 10.1002/14651858.CD001255.pub3

Philbin EF, Groff GD, Ries MD, et al (1995) Cardiovascular fitness and health in patients with end-stage osteoarthritis. *Arthritis and Rheumatism*, 38, 799–805

Pitsillides AA, Skerry TM, Edwards JCW (1999) Joint immobilization reduces synovial fluid hyaluronan concentration and is accompanied by changes in synovial intimal cell populations. *Rheumatology*, 38, 1108–12

Pitsillides AA, Will RK, Bayliss MT, et al (1993) Circulating and synovial fluid hyaluronan levels: effects of intra-articular corticosteroid on the concentration and rate of turnover. *Arthritis and Rheumatism*, 37, 1030–8

Royal Australian College of General Practitioners (RACGP) (2010) Guideline for the prevention and treatment of osteoporosis in postmenopausal women and older men. RACGP: Melbourne

Rejeski WJ, Ettinger WH Jr, Martin K, et al (1998) Treating disability in knee osteoarthritis with exercise therapy: A central role for self-efficacy and pain. *Arthritis Care and Research*, 11, 94–101

Rittweger J, Just K, Kautzsch K, et al (2002) Treatment of chronic lower back pain with lumbar extension and whole-body vibration exercise: a randomized controlled trial. *Spine*, 27, 1829–34

Roelants M, Delecluse C, Verschueren SM. (2004) Whole-body-vibration training increases knee-extension strength and speed of movement in older women. *Journal of the American Geriatrics Society*, 52, 901–8

Rubin C, Pope M, Fritton JC, et al (2003) Transmissibility of 15-hertz to 35-hertz vibrations to the human hip and lumbar spine: determining the physiologic feasibility of delivering low-level anabolic mechanical stimuli to skeletal regions at greatest risk of fracture because of osteoporosis. *Spine*, 28, 2621–7

Rubin C, Recker R, Cullen D, et al (2004) Prevention of postmenopausal bone loss by a low-magnitude, high-frequency mechanical stimuli: a clinical trial assessing compliance, efficacy, and safety. *Journal of Bone and Mineral Research*, 19, 343–51

Russo CR, Lauretani F, Bandinelli S, et al (2003) High-frequency vibration training increases muscle power in postmenopausal women. *Archives of Physical Medicine and Rehabilitation*, 84, 1854–7

Sambrook P, Cooper C (2006) Osteoporosis. *Lancet*, 367, 2010–18

Schuhfried O, Mittermaier C, Jovanovic T, et al (2005) Effects of whole-body vibration in patients with multiple sclerosis: a pilot study. *Clinical Rehabilitation*, 19, 834–42

Siqueira F, Facchini L, Hallal P (2005) The burden of fractures in Brazil: a population-based study. *Bone*, 37, 261–6

Song R, Lee E-O, Lam P, et al (2003) Effects of Tai Chi exercise on pain, balance, muscle strength, and perceived difficulties in physical functioning in older women with osteoarthritis: a randomized clinical trial. *The Journal of Rheumatology*, 30, 2039–44

Tanaka SM, Alam IM, Turner CH (2003) Stochastic resonance in osteogenic response to mechanical loading. *FASEB Journal*, 17, 313–14

Thomas KS, Muir KR, Doherty M, et al (2002) Home based exercise programme for knee pain and knee osteoarthritis: Randomised controlled trial. *British Medical Journal*, 325, 752–7

Torvinen S, Kannu P, Sievanen H, et al (2002) Effect of a vibration exposure on muscular performance and body balance. Randomized cross-over study. *Clinical Physiology and Functional Imaging*, 22, 145–52

Trees AH, Howe TE, Grant M, et al (2007) Exercise for treating anterior cruciate ligament injuries in combination with collateral ligament and meniscal damage of the knee in adults. *Cochrane Database of Systematic Reviews*, Issue 3. DOI: 10.1002/14651858. CD005961.pub2

Tugwell P, Bombardier C, Buchanan WW, et al (1987) The MACTAR Patient Preference Disability Questionnaire-an individualized functional priority approach for assessing improvement in physical disability in clinical trials in rheumatoid arthritis. *The Journal of Rheumatology*, 14, 446–51

van den Ende CHM, Vleit Vleiland TPM, Munneke M, et al (1998) Dynamic exercise therapy for treating rheumatoid arthritis. *Cochrane Database of Systematic Reviews*, Issue 4. DOI: 10.1002/14651858.CD000322.pub2

van Gestel AM, Haagsma CJ, van Riel PL (1998) Validation of rheumatoid arthritis improvement criteria that include simplified joint counts. *Arthritis and Rheumatism*, 41, 1845–50

van Gestel AM, Prevoo MLL, Van't Hof MA, et al (1996) Development and validation of the European League Against Rheumatism response criteria for rheumatoid arthritis. Comparison with the preliminary American College of Rheumatology and the World Health Organization/International League Against Rheumatism criteria. *Arthritis and Rheumatism*, 39, 34–40

Vestergaard P, Jorgensen NR, Mosekilde L, et al (2007) Effects of parathyroid hormone alone or in combination with antiresorptive therapy on bone mineral density and fracture risk - a meta-analysis. *Osteoporosis International*, 18, 45–57

Vilensky JA. (1998) Innervation of the joint and its role in osteoarthritis. In: KD Brandt, M Doherty, LS Lohmander (eds), *Osteoarthritis*. Oxford, UK: Oxford University Press, pp 176–88

Ward K, Alsop C, Caulton J, et al (2004) Low magnitude mechanical loading is osteogenic in children with disabling conditions. *Journal of Bone and Mineral Research,* 19, 360–69

Ward L, Tricco A, Phuong PN, et al (2007) Bisphosphonate therapy for children and adolescents with secondary osteoporosis. *Cochrane Database of Systematic Reviews*, Issue 4. DOI: 10.1002/14651858. CD005324.pub2

Wolff J (1986) The Law of Bone Remodeling (translation of the German 1892 edition). Springer: Berlin Heidelberg New York

Yamaguchi T, Ishii K (2005) Effects of static stretching for 30 seconds and dynamic stretching on leg extension power. *Journal of Strength and Conditioning Research*, 19: 677–83

Yeo WK, Paton CD, Graham AP, et al (2008) Skeletal muscle adaptation and performance responses to once a day versus twice every second day endurance training regimens. *Journal of Applied Physiology*, 105: 1462–70

Zigmond AS, Snaith RP (1983) The hospital anxiety and depression scale. *Acta Psychiatrica Scandanvia*, 67, 361–70

Chapter 3

Exercise as therapy in cardiovascular disease

Steve Selig, Itamar Levinger and Suzanne Broadbent

Assumed concepts

The following is assumed knowledge for readers of this chapter:

- cardiac cycle: timing of key events including valvular movements, pressures, volumes, flows, and their relationships with electrical events (electrocardiogram)
- Starling Law of the heart: relationship between diastolic filling and systolic function
- La Place Law of the heart: relationship between myocardial oxygen consumption, left ventricular dimensions (size and wall thickness) and intra-cardiac pressures
- risk factors for coronary artery disease
- basic understanding of the range of congenital and acquired cardiovascular disease.

INTRODUCTION

Cardiovascular disease (CVD) is a term encompassing the diseases of the cardiovascular system (eg: myocardium, heart valves, pericardium, pacemaker and conduction tissues, and the coronary, cerebral and peripheral circulations) (Gersh 2000). Although the incidence and prevalence of cardiovascular disease has been falling in Australia for decades, it remains a leading cause of mortality at 35%, as recently as 2005, second only to cancer (Tong & Stevenson 2007). Approximately 24% of Australian adults who live independently have CVD (Tong & Stevenson 2007), whilst the prevalence is much higher (56%) in adults living in institutionalised facilities such as nursing homes. Surprisingly, the female contribution to the overall burden of CVD is 10% higher than for males, even after adjusting for female longevity. The economic impact of CVD on the Australian health system is enormous, with an estimated direct cost of $5.5 billion annually, representing 11% of the national health budget (Australian Institute of Health and Welfare [AIHW] 2004). In contrast to Australia and the developed world, the rates of CVD in the developing world are accelerating as lifestyles shift from traditional to Western in many regions.

The chain of events from risk factors to acute coronary events and heart failure is summarised in Figure 3.1. Risk factors can be classified as: metabolic that include obesity, insulin resistance and/or type 2 diabetes mellitus and dyslipidaemias

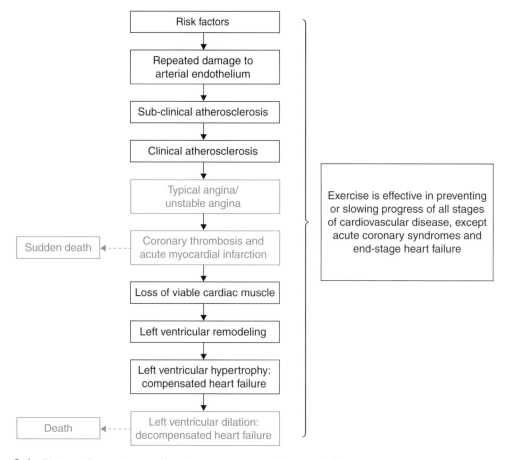

Figure 3.1 Chain of events leading to cardiovascular mortality

(see Chapter 6); cardiovascular that include hypertension, auto-immune and inflammatory over-activity; behavioural factors such as diet, sedentary living, smoking and substance abuse; and hereditary factors. Physical inactivity is the second most important risk factor for CVD mortality, after smoking (Gersh 2000; Tong & Stevenson 2007). Individuals who develop coronary artery disease (CAD) are at greatly elevated risk of suffering acute coronary events such as myocardial infarction or unstable angina, and approximately 50% of these events are associated with a high risk of sudden death (Gersh 2000). Many individuals who survive a myocardial infarction will be left with impaired cardiac structure and function, exposing them to future risk of chronic heart failure and high risk of cardiovascular mortality. Similarly, those with cerebrovascular disease are exposed to increased risk of suffering a stroke.

PHYSICAL INACTIVITY AND CARDIOVASCULAR DISEASE

Physical inactivity has been recognised as one of the major risk factors threatening global health (Murray & Lopez 1996) and is an important risk factor for CVD (Fletcher et al 1996; Haskel 1984; Smith et al 1995). A landmark statement by the US Surgeon General in 1996 (Fletcher et al 1996) proposed that there is clear evidence that sedentary living is as important as traditional cardiovascular risk factors such as smoking and hypertension in predicting cardiovascular morbidity and mortality.

When evaluating the evidence concerning the cardiovascular health benefits of exercise and physical activity, it is important to segregate the literature according to the following factors:

1 Exercise capacity (ie: single measure of fitness, usually cross-sectional studies)

and prediction of cardiovascular health outcomes in:

(a) people free from cardiovascular risk factors or disease
(b) people with cardiovascular risk factors
(c) people with current cardiovascular disease.

2 Exercise training (ie: gains in exercise capacity, usually longitudinal studies) and prediction of cardiovascular health outcomes in:

(a) people free from cardiovascular risk factors or disease (primary prevention)
(b) people with cardiovascular disease (secondary prevention and rehabilitation).

Evidence in support of exercise and physical activity for reducing cardiovascular morbidity and mortality lies in studies that have shown that regular exercise and physical activity ('training') can prevent illness in the first place (primary prevention) or prevent new occurrence, relapse or further progression of cardiovascular conditions (secondary prevention and rehabilitation). This chapter will address all of these relationships, but particularly those related to secondary prevention and rehabilitation.

The influence of exercise capacity as a single observation on all-cause mortality is illustrated by the studies of Blair and colleagues who showed in 25 341 men that mortality was higher in low-fit non-smoking individuals compared to high-fit individuals who smoke (Blair et al 1996). This data does not support a recommendation to smoke, but rather underlines the strong positive influences of fitness on mortality. They reported similar observations for the impact of physical fitness in reducing the impacts of hypertension and hypercholesterolaemia on mortality. When the same group conducted longitudinal exercise intervention studies on 9777 men, they showed that improvements in aerobic power were strongly associated with reduced mortality outcomes for each of 4 decades of life from 45–54 years to 75–84 years (Blair et al 1995).

Improvements in physical fitness have also been linked to reductions in all-cause and cardiovascular mortality in other longitudinal studies (Smith et al 1995; Georgiou et al 2001). In a study spanning 22 years with an initial cohort of 2014 healthy men aged 40–60 years, it was reported that increases in physical fitness were a strong predictor of all-cause

and cardiovascular mortality, greater than smoking, triglyceride levels, systolic blood pressure (SBP), and exercise ECG abnormalities (Erikssen et al 1998). Even moderate improvements in physical fitness can improve health status (Erissen et al 1998; Shiroma & Lee 2010), functional capacity and quality of life (QoL) and decrease rates of hospitalisation and mortality (Belardinelli et al 1999; Piepoli & Capucci 2000; Smart & Marwick 2004; Whellan et al 2001). Regular physical activity may reduce cardiac re-hospitalisation costs by up to 38% (Georgiou et al 2001; Ades et al 1992) and it may benefit all patients with heart disease even those with severe chronic heart failure (CHF) (Murtagh et al 2010).

There are many diseases of the cardiovascular system, including hypertension, CAD, ischaemic heart disease (IHD), peripheral arterial disease (PAD), valvular disease and CHF. This chapter will highlight the therapeutic roles that exercise can play for conditions that represent early, mid and late progressions of cardiovascular disease: hypertension, CAD and/or IHD, CHF, peripherd artery disease, and valvular disease. These diseases have been selected because: (a) they are common; (b) there is strong evidence that exercise is therapeutic for these conditions; and (c) clinical exercise practitioners work with clients with these conditions.

HYPERTENSION

Hypertension is clinically defined as systolic blood pressure (SBP) above 140 mmHg and/or diastolic blood pressure (DBP) above 90 mmHg (Egan et al 2010). Hypertension is the most common cause of CHF (Nicholls 1996; Gheorghiade & Bonow 1998; Levi et al 1996) and has serious negative chronic influences on diastolic structure and function. Increases in renin-angiotensin-aldosterone activity and increase in norepinephrine levels can cause peripheral vasoconstriction, increase fluid retention and cause increases in both pressure preloads and afterloads (Canobbio 1990). That, in turn, may lead to LV hypertrophy, contractile dysfunction and myocardial infarction (Cleland 1999; Ogino et al 2004; Unger 2002).

Drugs to treat hypertension (Ernsberger & Koletsky 2006) include:

- angiotensin-converting enzyme (ACE) inhibitors that block the renin-angiotensin-aldosterone (RAS) system

- angiotensin II receptor blockers (ARBs) to specifically inhibit the vasoconstrictor and pro-atherogenic properties of angiotensin II
- diuretics to reduce the fluid and sodium loads on the cardiovascular system
- beta-blockers to inhibit the sympathetic influences on both blood vessels and the heart
- calcium channel blockers to inhibit calcium facilitation of vascular and myocardial contractile activity.

Approximately two-thirds of patients with hypertension will be treated with two or more anti-hypertensive medications (Chobanian et al 2003). The most commonly prescribed classes of drugs for the treatment of hypertension are angiotensin converting enzyme inhibitors (ACE-inhibitors) and beta-blockers (Sarafidis & Bakris 2006). Reductions in SBP of 10 mmHg has been shown to reduce mortality by 15%, the risk of myocardial infarction by 11% and microvascular complications (retinopathy or nephropathy) by 13% (Adler et al 2000).

ACE-inhibitors work partly through their vasodilatory actions (Gersh 2000; Cohn 1993). ACE-inhibitors cause direct smooth muscle relaxation and dilatation of arteries by preventing the conversion from angiotensin I to angiotensin II in the lungs (Gheorghiade et al 2000). ACE-inhibitors are widely used in the treatment of hypertensive individuals who also have type 2 diabetes melitis (T2DM) as they reduce BP with no effect or even small benefits on insulin sensitivity and lipid metabolism (Lithell 1991; Hauf-Zachariou et al 1993; Giordano et al 1995). In addition, ACE-inhibitors enhance endothelial function in patients with T2DM (O'Driscoll et al 1999).

Beta-blockers inhibit the effects of over-activation of the sympathetic nervous system and reduce cardiovascular morbidity and mortality (Gersh 2000; Packer et al 2001; Poole-Wilson et al 2003; UK Prospective Diabetes Study Group 1998; Sharpe & Doughty 1998). Previously, beta-blockers were not the drug of choice for hypertensive individuals who also had insulin resistance or T2DM, as they had adverse effects on glycaemic control, insulin resistance and lipoprotein metabolism (Sarafidis & Bakris 2006; Lithell 1991; Jacob et al 1996; Jacob et al 1998; Giugliano et al 1997; Bell 2004). Some of the more recent beta-blockers also block alpha-1 receptors (eg: carvedilol and labetalol). These promote vasodilatation and also may have favourable metabolic effects on insulin resistance and lipid metabolism (Sarafidis & Bakris 2006; Jacob et al 1998). Carvedilol, a non-selective beta-blocker with alpha-1 blocking properties, exerts no adverse influences on metabolism (Uzunlulu et al 2006) and may even improve insulin resistance (Jacob et al 1996; Bakris et al 2004) and glucose (Jacob et al 1996; Giugliano et al 1997; Bakris et al 2004) and lipid metabolism; the latter by increasing high density lipoprotein (HDL) cholesterol and decreasing total cholesterol, low density lipoprotein (LDL) and triglycerides in hypertensive individuals with and without T2DM (Hauf-Zachariou et al 1993; Jacob et al 1996; Giugliano et al 1997; Seguchi et al 1990) . Despite the wide availability of pharmacological treatment options, it has been reported that up to 77% of people with hypertension do not receive optimal drug regimes. In addition, these medications do have some side-effects that affect their applicability (see Table 3.1).

Exercise training and hypertension

Aerobic training inhibits and reduces the incidence of hypertension (Pescatello et al 2004) by lowering SBP and DBP (Hagberg et al 2000; Sciacqua et al 2003; Schneider et al 1992). Aerobic training also lowers resting and sub-maximal heart rates (Schneider et al 1992; Schneider et al 1984; Krotkiewski et al 1985), and increases stroke volume and cardiac output (ACSM 2010). In a meta-analysis of 44 randomised controlled trials (RCTs), Kesaniemi et al (2001) reported that aerobic training significantly reduced SBP in normotensive and hypertensive (-2.6 and -7.7 mmHg, respectively) individuals and DBP (-1.8 and -5.8 mmHg, respectively). Similarly, meta-analyses by Fagard (1999) calculated that the average reduction of SBP after RT is ~3.2 mmHg and DBP by ~2.5 mmHg. Although these changes appear to be small, falls of similar magnitudes appear to be clinically significant by reducing the risks for CAD and stroke (Collins et al 1990).

Most hypertensive individuals are overweight or obese and there is strong association between obesity and fitness levels (see Figure 3.2). There are also associations between fitness, fatness and blood pressure. Although higher fitness levels are

Table 3.1 Medications used in cardiovascular disease

Class of drug (generic)	Main use	Mechanism of actions	Effects on exercise capacity
Angiotensin Converting Enzyme Inhibitors (ACEI) (Captopril, Enalapril, Ramipril)	IHD, CHF, HT, PAD	↓ BP; vasodilator in congestive heart failure; ↓ heart failure and ventricular remodelling	↑ for CHF and perhaps HT; ↔ for others
Angiotensin II receptor blockers (ARB) (Ibesartan, Losartan)	IHD, CHF, HT	Similar to above; also ↓ atherogenesis and ↓ thrombosis	↑ for CHF and perhaps HT; ↔ for others
Endothelin blockers	IHD, CHF, HT	↑ healthy endothelium; ↓ BP; ↓ atherogenesis ⇒ ↓ smooth muscle cell proliferation; ↓ heart failure	↑ for CHF and perhaps HT; ↔ for others
Ca++ channel blockers	HT, CHF	↓ blood vessel tone; ↑ 02 to heart; ↓ work of heart	↑ for angina; ↓ or ↔ for others
Beta-blockers (atenolol, sotalol)	CHF	↓ arrhythmias; ↓ BP; ↓ HR; ↓ angina; ↓ AMI risk and used acutely in AMI; ↓ anxiety; ↓ tremors	↑ for angina; ↓ HR during maximal and sub-maximal exercise; ↓ or ↔ for others
Statins (HMG-CoA reductase inhibitors)	Lipids	↓cholesterol production and stabilise lesion	↔
Thiazide Diuretics (Benzothiadiazine)	CHF, HT	↑ NaCl excretion ⇒ ↑ urine ⇒ ↓ BP; ↓ fluid loads and cardiac work in HF, but ↓ K+	↑ for CHF and perhaps HT; ↔ for others
Loop Diuretics (Ethacrynic Acid; Furosemide)	CHF, HT	↑ Urine ⇒ ↓ BP; ↓ fluid loads and cardiac work in HF, but ↓ K+	↑ for CHF and perhaps HT; ↔ for others
Potassium-sparing diuretics (Spironolactone)	CHF, HT	As above, but does not ↓ K+	↑ for CHF and perhaps HT; ↔ for others
Digoxin (digitoxin)	CHF, aF	↑ cardiac contractility in HF, treat arrhythmias (aF)	↑ for angina or aF; ↓ or ↔ for others
Nitrates (nitroglycerin, glyceryl trinitrate)	IHD, PAD	vasodilator including coronary arteries ⇒ ↑ 02 to heart and other tissues; ↓ ischaemic pain in angina and PAD	↑ for angina or CHF; ↓ or ↔ for others
Anti-thrombogenics (aspirin, warfarin)	IHD, CHF, HT, aF, PAD	↓ platelet reactivity ⇒ ↓ risk of thromboses; warfarin is used for aF	↔ except exercise is safer for aF, IHD, CHF

Note: HT = hypertension; IHD = ischaemic heart disease associated with coronary artery disease (CAD); PAD = peripheral arterial disease; CHF = chronic heart failure; aF = atrial fibrillation.

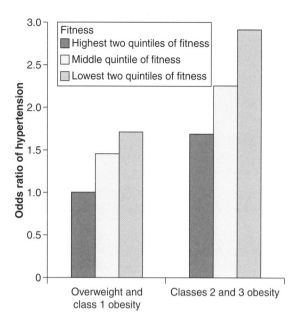

Figure 3.2 **Fitness and obesity both predict the risk of hypertension, with lower levels of obesity and higher levels of fitness being associated with lower risks of hypertension**
[Source: adapted from Wing et al 2007]

associated with lower glycosylated haemoglobin (HbA1C) and blood pressure, it is important to acknowledge that it is uncommon to find obese people who are also fit (Wing et al 2007). Nevertheless, there is good evidence that people who are fit whilst obese have lower blood pressures than those that are unfit and obese, but if they also lose weight, then blood pressure will be even lower (Wing et al 2007). In that sense, the benefits of fitness and leanness on blood pressure appear to be somewhat independent and so gaining fitness is a healthy strategy for obese individuals even if they do not lose weight.

CORONARY ARTERY DISEASE

The common cause of CHF has shifted from hypertension to coronary artery disease (CAD) (Gheorghiade & Bonow 1998; Gheorghiade et al 2000), partly attributed to improved survival rates from acute myocardial infarction. Gheorghiade and Bonow (1998) reviewed 10 years of CHF treatment trials (more than 20 000 patients) and found that nearly 70% of the patients suffered first from CAD. CAD is defined as a disease that

obstructs blood supply, oxygen and nutrients from the heart (Meltzer et al 1983; Gersh 2000). The aetiology of CAD is multifactorial, and includes smoking, increased blood lipids, a sedentary lifestyle, family history of CAD, hypertension and obesity.

Atherosclerosis is a progressive disease describing the accumulation of cholesterol, fats, platelets, smooth muscle cells and cellular debris (fibromuscular plaque) in the intima of blood vessels (Gersh 2000) that may lead to acute coronary thrombosis and acute myocardial infarction (AMI) (Gersh 2000). Sequelae to AMI include loss of viable myocardium, myocardial scarring and remodeling that lead to impaired LV contractility or chronic heart failure (Antman & Braunwald 2001; Meltzer et al 1983), cardiac tachy-arrhythmias due to up-regulation of sympathetic influences on cardiac pacemaker tissues and disruptions to normal His-Purkinje conduction that may lead to ventricular de-synchronisation. Changes to cardiac rhythms may also be associated with elevations in extracellular potassium concentrations in ischemic zones and in borders between ischemic and non-ischaemic zones (Antman & Braunwald 2001).

Exercise and CAD

There is an abundance of evidence suggesting that exercise training, particularly aerobic training, can positively influence a wide array of risk factors for CAD. This section addresses the evidence concerning the efficacy of exercise conditioning for those already with CAD, including those with current typical angina. Regular exercise not only reduces the risk of CAD, but also benefits those who have been diagnosed. In particular, aerobic exercise is associated with many positive structural and functional myocardial and peripheral vascular adaptations (Franklin et al 2002). The sympathetic nervous response which increases heart rate (through the binding of catecholamines to beta receptors in cardiac tissue) and blood pressure (through vasoconstriction) at rest and during sub-maximal exercise, is reduced with regular exercise and the parasympathetic or vagal response is increased (Malfatto et al 2000; Malfatto et al 2002; Legramante et al 2006). Exercise-induced improvements in autonomic neural regulation of the sinoatrial node, such as increased R-R variance and enhanced spontaneous baroreflex, are associated with decreased morbidity and mortality (Lucini et al 2002). Aerobic exercise training reduces both heart rate and systolic blood pressure at given sub-maximal workloads, and so rate-pressure product (RPP) is reduced and this helps to explain lower myocardial oxygen demand at these workloads. On the supply side, lower heart rates at sub-maximal workloads means that the ventricle spends a greater percentage of time in diastole, and coronary artery flow (myocardial oxygen supply) is higher in diastole compared to systole. Together, the lower RPP and heart rates as a result of aerobic training create greater myocardial oxygen reserves and are anti-anginal.

There is considerable evidence that exercise improves functional and morphological aspects of cardiac microvasculature (Gielen et al 2001). For example, cardiac endothelial function and arteriolar dilation are improved through increased endothelium-relaxing factor or nitric oxide (NO), nitric oxide synthase, and adenosine, thus increasing cardiac capacity (Kemi & Wisloff 2010; Gielen et al 2001; Hambrecht et al 2003; Duncker & Bache 2008; Meka et al 2008). Coronary artery smooth muscle becomes more sensitive to vasodilators and more permeable (Gielen et al 2001). Exercise will also stimulate the growth of collateral blood vessels in ischaemic patients that serve to modulate blood flow in the myocardium (Duncker & Bache 2008), and will improve perfusion by increasing the total vascular bed cross-sectional area (Gielen et al 2001).

There is considerable evidence to show that aerobic training results in increased cardiac output, stroke volume, plasma volume and cardiac contractility, thus improving exercise capacity in the normal and CAD populations (Libonati et al 1999; Yu et al 2004). Structural changes to the heart found post-MI and in CHF, notably left ventricular remodelling, are affected by regular exercise. Ventricular hypertrophy may be partially reversed with aerobic exercise training, ejection fraction and ventricular filling rates increased, and both end diastolic volume and atrial filling rates may be decreased (Yu et al 2004; Haykowski et al 2000).

In cardiac patients, especially CHF, ultra-structural analysis of muscle biopsies have shown a decrease in oxidative capacity of the muscles as seen by a reduced volume density and surface area of the cristae of mitochondria (Drexler et al 1992). The decreased mitochondrial volume correlates with the aerobic capacity of the patient (including reduced oxidative enzymes) suggesting a large contribution of altered oxidative metabolism to exercise intolerance (Drexler et al 1992).

Peripheral adaptations to endurance or aerobic-type training have been well documented (Seals et al 1984; Hagberg et al 1989; Meredith et al 1989), and include increased local vasodilation of blood vessels in skeletal muscle due to increased NO and adenosine (Giallauria et al 2006); increased a-vO_2 difference (Seals et al 1984); increased capillary density and oxygen extraction into muscle tissue; increased mitochondrial density and activity of oxidative enzymes such as citrate synthase and cytochrome-c oxidase (Tyni-Lenné et al 1998); and increases in type 1 oxidative muscle fibres (Haykowski et al 2005). Skeletal muscle biopsies in CHF patients show moderate atrophy and biochemical alterations, including a shift in fibre type distribution towards type 2 fibres (Lipkin et al 1988; Mancini et al 1992).

Peripheral adaptations are a major factor contributing to increased VO_{2peak} in healthy individuals and those with CAD. There are two reasons for measuring VO_{2peak} in cardiac patients. Firstly, oxygen consumption less than 14 ml/kg/min is one of the guidelines used for determining the need for heart transplantation (Mancini et al 1991; Aaronson & Mancini 1995). Secondly, VO_{2peak} may assist in prognostic assessment. For example, CHF patients with a reduced capacity of exercising muscle to utilise oxygen (Drexler & Coats 1996), and with a VO_{2peak} of less than 14 ml/kg/min, have a poor prognosis (Roul et al 1994). In addition, VO_{2peak} is a major independent predictor of death in the general population (Blair et al 1995) and those with CVD (Cohn et al 1993; Roul et al 1994; Blair et al 1996; Myers & Gullestad 1998; Kavanagh et al 2002). Blair et al (1995) have shown that over a 5-year period men who improved from unfit to fit reduced their mortality risk by 44%, compared to men who remained unfit. For people with CHF, it has been reported that exercise training improved fitness and reduced mortality compared to non-exercise controls (18% versus 40.8% respectively, p = 0.01), cardiac events (34% versus 75.5% respectively, p = 0.006), hospitalisation related to CHF (10% versus

28.6% respectively, p = 0.02), and improved QoL (Belardinelli et al 2000).

Regular aerobic and resistance exercise training also reduce the risk of CAD, and further cardiac events, by changing body composition and having a significant effect on blood lipid profiles (Franklin et al 2002; Tambalis et al 2009). Muscle mass is increased with regular exercise while body fat is reduced. Total cholesterol, LDL and triglycerides are decreased, thus reducing the risk of vascular inflammation, atherosclerotic plaques, strokes and hypertension (Jollife et al 2001; Franklin et al 2002). HDL will increase with exercise, especially weight-bearing exercise, also contributing to the removal of coronary blockages (Tikkanen et al 1999). The sympathetic catecholamine response to exercise increases lipolysis in both adipose tissue and skeletal muscle (Horowitz & Klein 2000). While the sympathetic drive may be blunted by chronic endurance training, regular moderate intensity aerobic exercise of a duration longer than 60 minutes increases fat oxidation of adipose lipid stores in preference to carbohydrate stores (Horowitz & Klein 2000). Research suggests that most of the fatty acids oxidised during exercise originate in subcutaneous adipose stores and intramuscular triglycerides rather than intra-abdominal adipose tissue (Horowitz & Klein 2000). The transport and metabolism of intramuscular triglycerides and free fatty acids is enhanced with aerobic exercise, with evidence suggesting that muscle contractions increase the activity of long chain fatty acid and triglyceride transporter molecules (Tikkanen et al 1999; Horowitz & Klein 2000).

There is still some debate as to the most effective intensity of exercise training for CAD patients, especially with regard to the lowering of blood lipids. Historically, research suggests that low to moderate intensity aerobic exercise increases aerobic capacity in de-conditioned and symptom-limited patients without risk of adverse cardiac events (Izawa et al 2004; Nelson et al 2007). Low to moderate intensity exercise should also increase fat oxidation, because peak fat oxidation occurs at 65% of VO_{2max} (Horowitz & Klein 2000), and decreases with higher exercise intensity that increasingly relies on carbohydrate metabolism. However, a systematic review of the responses of blood lipids to aerobic, resistance and combined aerobic-resistance training, by

Tambalis et al (2009) found that higher intensity aerobic exercise programs (>65% VO_{2max}) showed significantly greater effects on HDL-C, total cholesterol, triglycerides and LDL-C than low to moderate intensity programs. The authors noted that resistance training programs had a significant reduction on LDL-C, with less effect on HDL-C and total cholesterol, while combined aerobic and resistance training programs also showed significant reductions in LDL-C and increases in HDL-C. Both frequency and intensity of exercise sessions may affect the lipid response, and exercise capacity (Peschel et al 2007). Peschel et al (2007) found that 4 weeks of high frequency (daily) sub-maximal exercise significantly improved lipid profiles, work capacity, blood pressure, fasting blood glucose and body mass index (BMI) in CAD patients but most significantly, reduced the expression of atherogenic and inflammatory adhesion molecules (MAC-1 and VLA-4), thus reducing the risk of atherosclerosis.

The effect of higher intensity exercise on CAD patients is less clear. Studies by Ehsani et al (1986), Rognmo et al (2004), and Wisløff et al (2007) found significantly greater physiological and psychological improvements for CAD patients undertaking higher intensity interval training than those undertaking traditionally prescribed moderate intensity exercise, or controls. Significantly increased maximal oxygen consumption, increased time to fatigue, increased ischaemic threshold, increased anaerobic threshold, improved work economy, improved left ventricular size and function and improved HDL cholesterol have been reported with higher intensity interval training, in the absence of adverse cardiac events, but the authors clearly state that patients must be hemodynamically stable and stratified as 'low risk' before participating in such higher intensity exercise.

PERIPHERAL ARTERY DISEASE

Peripheral artery disease (PAD) describes arterial occlusions of the lower extremities caused by atherosclerosis and the disease may progress from asymptomatic to the hallmark symptom of exercise-induced claudication pain, and finally to tissue necrosis that may require limb amputation (Aronow 2007). A simple method for preliminary diagnosis is the ankle-brachial blood pressure index (Sontheimer 2006). Various methods of arteriography may be used for more definitive diagnosis (Sontheimer 2006). Treatment options include medical (anti-thrombogenic, anti-hypertensive and anti-atherogenic medications), lifestyle (exercise, diet and smoking cessation) and surgical interventions (stents, angioplasty, arterectomies and bypass grafts) (Sontheimer 2006). Cilostazol, an anti-thrombogenic and vasodilator, is used for relief of exercise-induced claudication pain (Aronow 2007).

Exercise training and PAD

The goals of exercise interventions for people with PAD are to increase the pain-free walking distance and speeds, to improve peripheral circulation via vascular regeneration and collateralisation, and to improve overall fitness and VO_{2peak} (Duprez 2007). For people with symptomatic ischaemic heart disease exercise interventions should focus on load-bearing aerobic exercise, such as walking at speeds that exceed the claudication pain threshold, but are below the angina pain threshold. Walking with lower pain cannot be tolerated for long, so interval training is a useful alternative or adjunct to continuous exercise.

CHRONIC HEART FAILURE

Changes to the heart structure and/or function may cause an inability of the left ventricle (LV) to pump blood as required to satisfy the body's metabolic needs. Chronic reduction in LV pumping capacity is known as chronic heart failure (CHF; Gersh 2000; AIHW 2001).

In order to maintain adequate cardiac output and arterial pressure, the sympathetic nervous system is activated and endocrine glands secrete hormones and enzymes, resulting in vasoconstriction of peripheral arteries, water and sodium retention, dilation of the heart and myocardial hypertrophy (Green et al 1989). Pharmacological treatments for CHF focus on improving LV contractile function, reducing the effects of catecholamines on the heart, decreasing fluid and sodium retention, inhibiting over-active sympathetic and rennin-angiotensin-aldosterone systems and aggressive attention to cardiovascular risk factors (Gersh 2000; Way 2002; Leblance 2000). Anti-remodelling of the myocardium is also an important therapeutic goal.

Fatigue, dyspnoea and a reduction in skeletal muscle strength are hallmark characteristics of patients with CHF (Drexler & Coats 1996; Harrington et al 1997; Mancini et al 1992; Magnusson et al 1994). Alterations in the periphery, rather than central and cardiac abnormalities, are major contributors to these characteristics and may also limit exercise capacity in these patients. Peripheral deficits include increased peripheral vascular resistance, reductions in blood flow to skeletal muscles and skeletal muscle structural and metabolic abnormalities (Coats 1993; Tavazzi & Gianuzzi 2001; Piepoli et al 1996; Peters et al 1997; Perreault et al 1993; Williams & Ward 1998). It has been speculated that abnormalities intrinsic to skeletal muscle limit exercise capacity for patients with CHF. There are two main reasons for this assumption. First, despite improvements in LV function and central hemodynamics with pharmacological management, exercise capacity and VO_{2peak} do not consistently improve (Bristow et al 1994; Fowler 1998). Second, there is no correlation between cardiac function (ejection fraction) and exercise intolerance or VO_{2peak} (Keteyian et al 1999; Higginbotham et al 1983; Szlachcic et al 1985; Massie 1988; Franciosa et al 1981). A reduction in maximal oxygen consumption and exercise intolerance is part of the ageing process and is a hallmark of patients with CHF (Fletcher et al 2001; Piepoli et al 2001).

There are two main reasons for measuring VO_{2peak} for patients with CHF. First, oxygen consumption less than 14 ml/kg/min is used as a clinical input into decision making regarding the need for heart transplantation (Aaronson & Mancini 1995; Mancini et al 1991). Second, VO_{2peak} seems be a strong prognostic indicator in CHF with patients with VO_{2peak} of less than 14 ml/kg/min having a poor prognosis (Roul et al 1994).

The mortality outcomes associated with exercise training for CHF patients remain contentious. The early mortality outcome study of Belardinelli and colleagues (2000) reported a halving of mortality for their active CHF participants in an exercise intervention trial lasting 14 months, compared to their inactive control participants (18% versus 41%, p = 0.01) (Belardinelli et al 2000). They also reported lower hospitalisation related to CHF (10% versus 28.6% respectively, p = 0.02), acute cardiac events (34% versus 75.5% respectively, p = 0.006) and improved QoL. However, since this frequently cited study, the large randomised HF-ACTION trial of 2331 participants was equivocal on mortality outcomes (O'Connor et al 2009); it was only after the investigators adjusted for highly prognostic but pre-selected characteristics that a mortality benefit was ascribed to the exercise training group. These findings need to be interpreted in light of the very small intervention effect on VO_{2peak} of just 4% in the HF-ACTION trial, well below what most investigators would advocate as needed for both functional and clinical benefits. The training intervention was sound, but the data may have been affected by lower than expected adherence rates amongst the active participants.

Before the late 1990s, physicians commonly recommended bed rest and avoidance of activity for patients with CHF (McKelvie et al 1995; McDonald et al 1972). Gradually, rehabilitation programs were developed to include low and then moderate intensity aerobic exercise such as walking, cycling and swimming that involve large muscle groups (Coats 1993; King 2001; Pollock et al 2000). This type of exercise has been shown to help prevent heart disease (Fletcher et al 1996; Haskel 1984) and decrease symptoms (Piepoli & Capucci 2000; Piepoli et al 2001). The benefits of aerobic training are well documented and include: improved central hemodynamics (Fletcher et al 1996) and myocardial function (decreased oxygen demands, prevention of myocardial ischemia and increase oxygen supply) (Haskel 1984; Letac et al 1977; Stolen et al 2003); decreased HR at rest or any given sub-maximal exercise (Haskel 1984; Letac et al 1977; Hambrecht et al 2000); decreased sympathetic tone and increased vagal activity (Fletcher et al 1996; Belardinelli et al 1999); and decreased afterload and peripheral resistance (Hambrecht et al 2000). Aerobic exercise also improves endothelial function and blood flow (Hambrecht et al 1997, 1998; Berdeaux et al 1994; Vita & Keaney 2000; Kobayashi et al 2003; Hosokawa et al 2003), increases capillary diameter of working muscles in order to decrease the diffusion distance, delays anaerobic metabolism (Belardinelli et al 1999) and improves exercise capacity and VO_{2peak} (Fletcher et al 1996; Stolen et al 2003; Hagberg et al 1984). In addition, aerobic training assists in maintaining normal body mass (Smith et al 1995).

Until the mid-1990s, resistance training (RT) was not recommended for people with cardiac disease in general and patients with CHF in particular. RT was not recommended because of a concern for increases in wall tension and rate pressure product (RPP) due to increased blood pressure and after-load which may cause acute myocardial insufficiency and/or accelerate the chronic LV remodelling process (Painter & Hanson 1984; Mitchell & Wildenthal 1974). The RPP (HR × SBP/100) is a measurement that represents the oxygen demand by the myocardium. An increase in oxygen demand by the myocardium may cause a negative imbalance between oxygen demands and oxygen supply which, in turn, may expose the patients to myocardial ischemia (King 2001; Stewart 1989). In addition, results from a study that was conducted by Elkayam and colleagues (1985) raised a concern that isometric exercise significantly deteriorates cardiac performance in some patients with advanced CHF. They reported that during isometric exercise systemic vascular resistance increased while cardiac index and stroke volume index decreased (Elkayam et al 1985). This study however, examined the patients response to 5–7 minutes of isometric exercise at 30% of maximal voluntary contraction which is not recommended for any population (Pollock et al 2000; Feigenbaum & Pollock 1999). Levinger et al have shown that RT has a limited effect on LV structure and function as no significant changes were found for end-diastolic diameter (EDD), end-systolic diameter (ESD), ejection fraction (EF), fractional shortening (FS), and stroke volume (SV) within each group and/or when the data was analysed with the effect of time between the groups (pre-post) (Levinger et al 2005a). However, post-training (training versus control) comparisons revealed a significantly higher EF (by 26%) and FS (by 32%) in the training group, which was due to a combination of training and detraining effects on the trained and control group respectively. The positive aspect is that even though RT had no significant effect on the LV structure and/or function it may have inhibited the reduction in LV contractile function, as measured by EF and FS, which is a hallmark of patients with CHF. Others also reported no changes in LV structure and function or an improvement in LV function in young, elderly and cardiac populations after

RT (Haykowski et al 2000; Haennel et al 1991; Delagardelle et al 1999; Kanakis & Hickson 1980). Pu et al (2001) reported that 10 weeks high intensity RT had no significant effect on LV EF or any other LV measurements (E/A ratio and LV diameter) in older women with CHF. As such, RT is recommended for inclusion in regular rehabilitation programs for these patients (Fletcher et al 2001; Pollock et al 2000; ACSM 2010).

There are four main training guidelines that may assist in prevention of undesired increases in RPP during RT: (1) the use of moderate weights (usually between 10–15 repetitions); (2) training in correct lifting and breathing techniques which assists the avoidance of a Valsalva manoeuvre; (3) a range of rate perceived exertion of 11 to 14 (Borg scale between 6–20); and (4) the use of isotonic resistance exercises rather than isometric resistance exercises (Pollock et al 2000; ACSM 2010; Selig et al 2010). It has been shown that RT improves both endurance and strength of patients with CHF (Maiorana et al 2000; Selig et al 2004; Hare et al 1999; Levinger et al 2005b), and is a safe method of training even 6 weeks after MI (Stewart et al 1998). It is well documented that cardiac patients who undergo RT that includes 10–12 exercises, 3 days/week through 8–12 weeks increased their strength by 18–90% (Levinger et al 2005b; Stewart et al 1998; Maiorana et al 1997; McCartney et al 1991; Sparling et al 1990; Keleman 1986; Wilk et al 1991; Beniamini 1999) and exercise endurance by 10–15% (Maiorana et al 2000; Stewart et al 1998; McCartney et al 1991; Kelemen et al 1986). Studies have shown the important role muscle strength and endurance play in improving the functional ability and QoL of cardiac patients (Selig et al 2004; Levinger et al 2005b; Stewart et al 1998; Delagardelle et al 1999; Ades et al 2003). Moreover, it has been shown that physical activity may improve mental health and self efficacy (Taylor et al 1985; Ewart et al 1986) which in turn may increase QoL (Swank et al 2002; Tyni-Lenné et al 2001). Also it has been shown that an increase in aerobic capacity is associated with an increase in QoL parameters such as social competence emotional function and self perceived control (Quittan et al 1999; Oka et al 2000). These data emphasises the importance of combining RT in a regular exercise cardiac rehabilitation program.

AORTIC STENOSIS

Aortic stenosis (AS) describes a condition where the aortic valve fails to open completely on systole, often due to calcification of an ageing valve. Predisposing factors included congenital bicuspid valve and include acute rheumatic fever and these result in earlier calcification of the valve. In order to maintain cardiac output in AS, the left ventricle needs to generate higher systolic pressures and this can eventually lead to LV hypertrophy, a cause of heart failure. The LV-aorta pressure gradient defines the severity of AS: mild ≤ 20 mmHg, moderate 20–50 mmHg, severe ≥ 50 mmHg. Severity is also indicated by aortic valve area. AS is often accompanied by aortic incompetence, although at lesser severity than the AS. Severe AS is an absolute contraindication to exercise (ACSM 2010) and care needs to be taken with moderate AS (ACSM 2010). See Chapter 13, case study 2, for an exploration of safe exercise therapy for a client with moderate AS. To our knowledge, there are no randomised clinical trials on the effects of exercise training for people living with moderate AS and almost no published evidence on this topic.

HYPERTROPHIC OBSTRUCTIVE CARDIOMYOPATHY

Hypertrophic obstructive cardiomyopathy (HOCM) is an important cause of sudden cardiac death in young individuals, including young athletes, and is the prototypic form of pathological cardiac hypertrophy. HOCM is also a major cause of morbidity in older individuals (Marian 2010). The disease is primarily one of cardiac myocytes, and is characterised morphologically by concentric and often asymmetric cardiac hypertrophy, unexplained left ventricular hypertrophy, usually involving the interventricular septum (Seggewiss & Rigopoulos 2003) or a non-dilated left ventricle and preserved systolic function (Marian 2010). Pathologically, HOCM is characterised by gross cardiac hypertrophy, hypertrophy and disarray of myocytes, hypertrophy/hyperplasia of tissue or the coronary arteries interstitial fibrosis, and mitral valve leaflet abnormalities (Franklin et al 1997; Marian 2010). The terms HOCM and hypertrophic cardiomyotheraphy (HCM) are used somewhat interchangeably, but in this chapter we focus on the obstructive (and more dangerous) form of cardiomyopathy.

Most HOCM patients are asymptomatic or mildly symptomatic, with sudden exercise-induced chest pain due to increased oxygen demand and myocardial hypoperfusion. Palpitations, dyspnea with exertion, syncope and dizziness are fairly common (Seggewiss & Rigopoulos 2003; Cirino & Ho 2008). However, HOCM-related structural cardiovascular abnormalities are the major cause of sudden death in young athletes, and there is currently a medical consensus on the need for cardiovascular screening (12-lead ECG, medical examination, clinical exercise testing) to identify such abnormalities in young athletes (Franklin et al 1997; Corrado et al 1998; Corrado et al 2005). There are no randomised clinical studies on the effects of exercise training for individuals with HOCM but management guidelines suggest: (1) medical, pharmaceutical and surgical treatment of diastolic dysfunction, thromboembolisms, ventricular outflow obstruction, atrial fibrillation and other arythmias; (2) implantable cardioverter defibrillators for those at high risk of cardiac arrest; and (3) the avoidance of competitive endurance training, high-intensity exercise (eg: sprinting), intense isometric exercise (eg: heavy resistance training), dehydration, hypovolemia (eg: constant use of diuretics), and medications that decrease after-load (eg: ACE-inhibitors, angiotensin receptor blockers, direct vasodilators) (Seggewiss & Rigopoulos 2003;

Cirino & Ho 2008). Clinical exercise practitioners are advised to follow ACSM clinical guidelines for heart failure, in prescribing exercise for clients with HOCM. See Chapter 13, case study 3, for an account of newly diagnosed cardiomyopathy in an athlete (possible HOCM).

Cardiac rehabilitation exercise

ACSM and the American Heart Association (AHA) (ACSM 2010) recommend moderate intensity (40–60% HR reserve) exercise, including aerobic, resistance and flexibility exercise, at least 3 days per week, and preferably daily, for older adults, those with CAD, hypertension, hypercholesterolemia and type 2 diabetes (Franklin et al 2002; Nelson et al 2007). The recommendations include cardiac rehabilitation exercise programs. Standard cardiac rehabilitation programs have four recognised phases (see Table 3.2).

Phase 1 rehabilitation involves short-term patient care within the hospital, and usually consists of improving the patient's strength for activities for daily living (ADL), under medical supervision, together with lifestyle, dietary and exercise advice. Phase 2 rehabilitation exercise is considered to be outpatient and may last 8–12 weeks depending upon the severity of the cardiac procedure undergone, and the risk stratification of the patient (low-, moderate-, high-risk). Risk status may be determined by the onset of ST-segment depression, angina, serious arrhythmias and reduced ejection fraction (Franklin et al 2002).

Table 3.2 Phases of cardiac rehabilitation

Phase	Time	Therapy
Phase 1	Inpatient (3–5 days)	Lifestyle advice; behaviour modification; activities for daily living (ADL), direct hospital supervision
Phase 2	Outpatient (8–12 weeks) Patients may be stratified according to risk	Hospital or physical therapist-supervised; clinical rehabilitation exercise programs; may be supervised
Phase 3	Community programs — initial, 12 weeks plus	Community-based exercise programs; clinical rehabilitation programs; non-supervised
Phase 4	Community programs — maintenance	Non-supervised

Research has consistently shown that regular exercise combined with lifestyle advice and appropriate medication successfully reduces the risk of secondary cardiac events. Phase 2 cardiac rehabilitation programs are associated with reduced coronary risk factors, significant improvements in exercise tolerance and functional capacity, reduced depression and improved QoL (Franklin et al 2002; Jollife et al 2001; Rees et al 2004; Nelson et al 2007). Yet formal cardiac rehabilitation exercise programs are under-utilised worldwide (Franklin et al 2002). Exercise-based rehabilitation for CAD and CHF has been systematically reviewed by Jollife et al (2001) and Rees et al (2004) for the Cochrane Collaboration. Jollife et al (2001) reported that a pooled analysis of 7683 CAD patients showed that an exercise only rehabilitation intervention reduced all-cause mortality by 27%, while comprehensive cardiac rehabilitation (exercise as part of a broader re-education cardiac program) reduced all-cause mortality to a lesser degree. Furthermore, total cardiac mortality was reduced by 31% with an exercise only rehabilitation program, and by 26% with the comprehensive cardiac program. Total and LDL cholesterol was also significantly reduced with a comprehensive cardiac program. The evidence for reduced mortality with exercise-based rehabilitation for CHF patients is also substantial (Rees et al 2004). Exercise training improved QoL and significantly increased exercise capacity (VO_{2max}, incremental test time, 6-minute walk distance, work capacity). While the findings of both reviews are based on studies involving primarily male, middle-aged and moderate to low-risk patients, the evidence in support of cardiac rehabilitation exercise as a means of reducing all-cause and cardiac mortality, is overwhelming. Moderate-intensity cardiac rehabilitation exercise for 3–6 months increased patient VO_{2peak} by 11 to 36%, with the greatest improvement in the most de-conditioned individuals (Leon et al 2005). Research shows improved physiological and psychological measures from cardiac rehabilitation, including neural control (Radaelli 1996; Keteyian et al 1997), QoL (Kavanagh et al 1996; Willenheimer et al 1998; Izawa et al 2004), exercise tolerance (Demopoulos et al 1997; Tyni-Lenné et al 1998), left ventricular function (Goebbels 1998; Rinder et al 1999; Giannuzzi et al 2003), skeletal muscle physiology (Cider et al 1997; Hambrecht et al 1997), peripheral blood flow, and endothelial function (Katz et al 1997; Callaerts-Végh et al 1998; Hambrecht et al 1998).

Ideally Phase 2 rehabilitation exercise programs should be supervised by a health professional, and ECG and blood pressures should be monitored (ACSM 2010). Exercise guidelines suggest that low to moderate intensity aerobic and resistance training should be included, initially for at least 30 minutes per session, for a minimum of three sessions per week. Moderate intensity exercise has been recommended at 40–60% of $VO_{2reserve}$ or heart rate reserve, with more vigorous (higher-intensity) exercise as tolerated recommended at 60–85% of HR reserve (Nelson et al 2007). Intermittent aerobic training is recommended for de-conditioned patients or those with symptom-limits such as angina or severe hypertension. Steady-state or constant-load aerobic exercise may be more suitable for patients who are lower risk. As cardiac patients may be taking beta-blockers to reduce heart rate, cardiac output and hypertension, the 10 point Borg Scale can be used to set exercise intensity limits (eg: moderate intensity, 5–6 Borg Scale; higher intensity, 7–8 Borg Scale). METS may also be used (eg: 3–6 METS, moderate intensity; >6 METS, higher intensity). The duration and frequency of exercise sessions can be increased during the 12 weeks of Phase 2 rehabilitation, providing adverse symptoms do not occur. Phase 3 and 4 cardiac rehabilitation exercise is considered to be low-risk and for patients who are hemodynamically stable, and able to participate in community exercise or unsupervised exercise programs. Daily exercise is recommended by ACSM, with intensities ranging 50–85% $VO_{2reserve}$, 5–8 Borg Scale and 6–10 METS (Nelson et al 2007). Both aerobic and resistance training exercise are recommended, with aerobic sessions 3–7 times per week, and resistance training suggested 2–3 times per week. Flexibility exercises and exercises specifically to reduce the risk of falls in older people, are also recommended.

Exercise training before cardiac surgery

There is growing interest in the recommendation of pre-surgical exercise training to prepare CAD and CHF patients for heart surgery and achieve better postoperative outcomes (Hadj et al 2006; Hulzebos et al 2006; Herdy et al 2008). Hulzebos et al (2006) and Herdy et al (2008) found that preoperative daily sessions of respiratory exercises (intramuscular therapy) significantly reduced pulmonary and cardiac complications, and the length of postoperative hospital stay, even in patients who underwent the normal postoperative Phase 1 cardiac rehabilitation. Whole-body preoperative exercise training twice a week, twice daily, in combination with antioxidant metabolic therapy, and mental/relaxation therapy, (Hadj et al 2006) also significantly improved postoperative recovery (length of hospital stay, time in intensive care, QoL, systolic blood pressure, oxidative stress). This area of exercise prescription needs to be explored further as preoperative training combined with Phase 1 and Phase 2 cardiac rehabilitation has the potential to reduce post-surgical complications,

length of hospital stay and cardiac mortality, and to improve QoL.

SUMMARY

Meta-analyses have substantiated that lifestyle interventions that include exercise reduce all-cause and cardiovascular mortality (Thompson et al 2003). Part of the benefit may lie in the retardation of disease progression or even plaque regression, whilst those who did not undertake lifestyle interventions continued to develop coronary artery stenoses (Ornish et al 1998). This may be particularly helpful for those with diffuse coronary artery disease for which standard revascularisation treatments (angioplasty, stents and bypass grafts) are not available (see Table 3.3).

Table 3.3 Principles of exercise prescription for cardiovascular disease

Exercise prescription for cardiovascular diseases	HT	AS	HOCM	IHD/CAD	PAD	CHF
Peak intensity: aerobic:% of VO_{2peak}	$\leq 70\%$ $VO_{2\ peak}$; $BP_{brachial} \leq$ 220/110 mmHg	$\leq 70\%$ $VO_{2\ peak}$; $BP_{brachial}$ + aortic valve pressure gradient $\leq$ 220/110 mmHg	$< 70\%$ $VO_{2\ peak}$	$\leq$ angina threshold	$\geq$ claudication threshold and $\leq$ angina threshold	$\leq 70\%\ VO_{2peak}$, but also depends on fatigue and breathlessness
Duration	≥ 45 min per day; ≥ 60 min per day if needing to lose weight; add bursts of physical activity to interrupt sedentary behaviour			As for HT, AS and HOCM, but also limited by pain		As for HT and AS, but depends on fatigue
Frequency	Most (5–7) days of the week					
Mode	Should align with exercise likes. Should conform to precautions					
Volume	≥ 4000 kJ per week ≥ 8000 kJ per week if needing to lose weight					
Peak intensity: resistance % of 1RM	$\leq 70\%$ of 1RM					

Table 3.3 Principles of exercise prescription for cardiovascular disease—cont'd

General precautions	Check clients for any adverse signs or symptoms since their last exercise session and record these. Check clients for compliance to all prescribed medications. Check breathing (rate and subjective depth), pulse (rate and rhythm), BP and HbO$_2$sat% (if oximeter is available) at start of each session, during peak exercise if possible and again before the client leaves the facility. Use RPE in preference to HR to determine exercise intensity for most situations. Clients with cardiovascular disease are susceptible to vaso-vagal episodes including syncope and strategies to prevent and manage this are needed. Chest pain typical of angina, unexpected breathlessness or unexplained fatigue are reasons to stop exercise or not start exercise. Clients with comorbid diabetes may not experience ischaemic pain and need to be monitored for other signs and symptoms. Avoid exercise in extreme environmental conditions. BCLS equipment and staff trained in BCLS must be available at all sessions. Staff must also be conversant with the procedures for calling for ACLS.					
Exercise prescription for cardiovascular diseases	HT	AS	HOCM	IHD/CAD	PAD	CHF
Specific precautions	Avoid exercise that involves: straining; breath holding; exercise in deep water	Be aware of the severity of AS, particularly in relation to the LV-Aorta pressure gradient at systole	Monitor for arrhythmias and ischaemia	Anginine should be available Refer for worsening ischaemic pain	Anginine should be available Refer for worsening ischaemic pain	Weight gain since last session ≥ 2kg may indicate fluid retention Many patients are on beta blockers with blunted heart rate responses to exercise For severe breathlessness or unexpected fatigue during exercise, stop, reassure and possibly refer

Note: HT = hypertension; AS = aortic stenosis; HOCM = hypertrophic obstructive cardiomyopathy; IHD = ischaemic heart disease associated with coronary artery disease (CAD); PAD= peripheral arterial disease; CHF = chronic heart failure; VO$_{2peak}$ = peak aerobic power; BP$_{brachial}$ = blood pressure measured by sphygmomanometry at the brachial artery; BCLS = basis cardiac cardiopulmonary life support; ACLS = advanced cardiac cardiopulmonary life support; LV = left ventricle; RPE = rating of perceived exertion, HbO$_2$sat% = oxygen saturation level in blood (oxyhaemoglobin) .

Summary of key lessons

- The incidence and prevalence of cardiovascular disease has been falling in the developed world, but remains a leading cause of morbidity and mortality.

- A wide range of congenital and acquired cardiovascular diseases respond to exercise training.

- Exercise should be used in conjunction with, not as a replacement for, medical interventions for people living with cardiovascular diseases.

- Exercise can be effectively used as an intervention during most stages of progression of ischaemic heart disease (IHD), except during acute coronary events and end-stage heart failure. Exercise improves both morbidity and mortality outcomes for most cardiovascular disease and is effective for both primary and secondary prevention. More evidence is needed to determine the value of exercise for people with valvular disease, and the mortality outcome data for exercise in CHF is equivocal.

- Although there are many precautions that need to be taken for exercise interventions for people with cardiovascular diseases, these can normally be managed by clinical exercise practitioners and the benefits outweigh the risks.

REFERENCES

Aaronson KD, Mancini DM (1995) Is percentage of predicted maximal exercise oxygen consumption a better predictor of survival than peak exercise oxygen consumption for patients with severe heart failure. *Journal of Heart and Lung Transplantation*, 14:981–9

Adamopoulos S, Parissis J, Kremastinos D (2003) New aspects for the role of physical training in the management of patients with chronic heart failure. *International Journal of Cardiology*, 90(1):1–14

Ades PA, Huang D, Weaver SO, et al (1992) Cardiac rehabilitation participation predicts lower rehospitalization costs. *American Heart Journal*, 123:916–21

Adler AI, Stratton IM, Neil HA, et al (2000) Association of systolic blood pressure with macrovascular and microvascular complications of type 2 diabetes (UKPDS 36): prospective observational study. *British Medical Journal*, 321(7258):412–19

American College of Sports Medicine (ACSM) (2000) Exercise and type 2 diabetes: position stand of the American College of Sports Medicine. *Medicine and Science in Sports and Exercise*, 32(7):1345–60

—— (2010) *ACSM's Resource Manual for Guidelines for Exercise Testing and Prescription* (6th ed). Philadelphia: Wolters Kluwer: Lippincott Williams & Wilkins

Antman EM, Braunwald E (2001) Acute myocardial infarction. In: Braunwald E, Zipes D, Libby P (eds) *Heart Disease* (vol 2). Philadelphia: WB Saunders Company, pp 1114–219

Aronow WS (2007) Peripheral arterial disease. *Geriatrics*, 62(1):19–25

Australian Institute of Health and Welfare (2001) *Heart, Stroke and Vascular Diseases*. Canberra: AIHW, pp 14

—— (2004) *Health System Expenditure on Disease and Injury in Australia, 2000-01* Health and Welfare Expenditure Series No.19 Cat. no. HWE 26. Canberra: AIHW

Bakris GL, Fonseca V, Katholi RE, McGill JB, Messerli FH, Phillips RA, et al (2004) Metabolic effects of carvedilol vs metoprolol in patients with type 2 diabetes mellitus and hypertension: a randomized controlled trial. *The Journal of the American Medical Association*, 292(18):2227–36

Belardinelli R, Georgiou D, Gianci G, et al (2000) Exercise training for patients with chronic heart failure reduced mortality and cardiac events and improved quality of life. *The Western Journal of Medicine*, 172(1):28

Belardinelli R, Georgiou D, Cianci G, et al (1999) Randomized, controlled trail of long-term moderate exercise training in chronic heart failure: effects on functional capacity, quality of life and clinical outcome. *Circulation*, 99:1173–82

Bell DS (2004) Advantages of a third-generation beta-blocker in patients with diabetes mellitus. *American Journal of Cardiology*, 93(9A):49B–52B

Beniamini Y, Rubenstein JJ, Faigenbaum AD, Lichtenstein AH, Crim MC (1999) High-intensity strength training of patients enrolled in an outpatient cardiac rehabilitation program. *Journal of Cardiopulmonary Rehabilitation*, 19:8–17

Berdeaux A, Ghaleh B, Dubosi-Rande JL, et al (1994) Role of vascular endothelium in exercise-induced dilation of large epicardial coronary arteries in conscious dogs. *Circulation*, 89:2799–808

Blair SN, Kampert JB, Paffenbarger RS, et al (1996) Influences of cardiorespiratory fitness and other precursors on cardiovascular disease and all-cause mortality in men and women. *The Journal of the American Medical Association*, 276(3):205–10

Blair SN, Kohl HW 3rd, Barlow CE, et al (1995) Changes in physical fitness and all-cause mortality. A prospective study of healthy and unhealthy men. *The Journal of the American Medical Association*, 273(14):1093–8

Bristow MR, O'Connell JB, Gilbert EM, et al (1994) Dose-response of chronic ß-blocker treatment in heart failure from either idiopathic dilated or ischemic cardiomyopathy. *Circulation*, 891632–42

Callaerts-Végh Z, Wenk M (1998) Influence of intensive physical training on urinary nitrate elimination and plasma endothelin-1 levels in patients with congestive heart failure. *Journal of Cardiopulmonary Rehabilitation and Prevention* 18(6):450–7

Canobbio MM (1990) *Cardiovascular disorders*. St Louis, Missoury: CV Mosby Company

Chobanian A.V, Bakris GL, Black HR, et al (2003) Seventh report of the joint national committee on prevention, detection, evaluation, and treatment of high blood pressure. *Hypertension*, 421206

Cider A, Tygesson H, Hedberg M, et al (1997) Peripheral muscle training in patients with clinical signs of heart failure. *Scandinavian journal of rehabilitation medicine*, 29(2):121–7

Cirino AL, Ho C (2008) Familial hypertrophic cardiomyopathy overview. In: Pagon R, Bird T, Dolan C, Stephens K (eds) *Gene Reviews*. Seattle WA: University of Seattle

Cleland JGL (1999) Progression from hypertension to heart failure. *Cardiology*, 92(Suppl 1):10–19

Coats AJS (1993) Exercise rehabilitation in chronic heart failure. *Journal of the American College of Cardiology*, 22(Suppl A):172A–177A

Cohn JN, Johnson GR, Shabetav R, et al (1993) Ejection fraction, peak exercise oxygen consumption, cardiothoracic ratio, ventricular arrhythmias, and plasma norepinephrine as determinants of prognosis in heart failure. *Circulation*, 87(Suppl VI):VI5–VI16

Collins R, Peto R, MacMahon S, et al (1990) Blood pressure, stroke, and coronary heart disease. Part 2, Short-term reductions in blood pressure: overview of randomised drug trials in their epidemiological context. *Lancet*, 335(8693):827–38

Corrado D, Basso C, Schiavon M, et al (1998) Screening for hypertrophic cardiomyopathy in young athletes. *New England Journal of Medicine*, 339(6):364–9

Corrado D, Pelliccia A, Bjornstad H, et al (2005) Cardiovascular pre-participation screening of young competitive athletes for prevention of sudden death: proposal for a common European protocol. Consensus statement of the study group of Sports Cardiology of the Working Group of Cardiac Rehabilitation and Exercise Physiology and the Working Group of Myocardial and Pericardial Diseases of the European Society of Cardiology. *European Heart Journal*, 26(5):516–24

Delagardelle C, Feiereisen P, Krecke R, et al (1999) Objective effects of a 6 months' endurance and strength training program in outpatients with congestive heart failure. *Medicine and Science in Sports and Exercise*, 31(8):1102–7

Demopoulos L, Bijou R, Fergus J, et al (1997) Exercise training in patients with severe congestive heart failure:Enhancing peak aerobic capacity while minimizing the increase in ventricular wall stress. *Journal of the American College of Cardiology*, 29(3):597–603

Drexler H, Riede U, Munzel T, et al (1992) Alterations of skeletal muscle in chronic heart failure. *Circulation*, 85(5):1751–9

Drexler MDH, Coats MDA (1996) Explaining fatigue in congestive heart failure. *Annual Reviews in Medicine*, 47(1):241–56

Duncker D, Bache R (2008) Regulation of coronary blood flow during exercise. *Physiological Reviews*, 88(3), 1009–1086

Duprez DA (2007) Pharmacological interventions for peripheral artery disease. *Expert Opin Pharmacother*, 8(10):1465–77

Egan BM, Zhao Y, Axon RN (2010) US trends in prevalence, awareness, treatment, and control of hypertension, 1988–2008. *JAMA*, 303: 2043–50

Ehsani A.A, Biello DR, Schultz J, et al (1986) Improvement of left ventricular contractile function by exercise training in patients with coronary artery disease. *Circulation*, 74(2):350–8

Elkayam U, Roth A, Weber L, et al (1985) Isometric exercise in patients with chronic advanced heart failure: hemodynamic and neurohumoral evaluation. *Circulation*, 72(5):975–81

Erikssen G, Liestol K, Bjornholt J, et al (1998) Changes in physical fitness and changes in mortality. *Lancet*, 352:759–62

Ernsberger P, Koletsky RJ (2006) Metabolic effects of antihypertensive agents: role of sympathoadrenal and renin-angiotensin systems. *Naunyn-Schmiedeberg's Archives of Pharmacology*, 373(4):245–58

Fagard RH (1999) Physical activity in the prevention and treatment of hypertension in the obese. *Medicine and Science in Sports and Exercise*, 31(11):S624–S630

Feigenbaum MS, Pollock ML (1999) Prescription of resistance training for heath and disease. *Medicine and Science in Sports and Exercise*, 31(1):38–45

Fletcher GF, Balady G, Blair SN, et al (1996) Statement on exercise: benefits and recommendations for physical activity programs for all Americans. *Circulation*, 94:857-862

Fowler MB (1998) ß-blockers in heart failure: do they improve the quality as well as the quantity of life? *European Heart Journal*, 19 (Suppl P):P17–P25

Franciosa JA, Park M, Levine TB (1981) Lack of correlation between exercise capacity and indexes of resting left ventricular performance in heart failure. *The American Journal of Cardiology*, 47:33–9

Franklin B, Bonzheim K, Warren J, et al (2002) Effects of a contemporary, exercise-based rehabilitation and cardiovascular risk-reduction program on coronary patients with abnormal baseline risk factors. *Chest*, 122:338–43

Franklin BA, Fletcher GF, Gordon N, et al (1997) Cardiovascular evaluation of the athlete. Issues regarding performance, screening and sudden cardiac death. *Sports Med*, 24(2):97–119

Georgiou D, Chen Y, Appadoo S, et al (2001) Cost-effectiveness analysis of long-term moderate exercise training in chronic heart failure. *The American Journal of Cardiology*, 87–984–8

Gersh BJ (2000) *Mayo Clinical Heart Book*. New York: William Morrow & Co

Gheorghiade M, Bonow RO (1998) Chronic heart failure in the United States: a manifestation of coronary artery disease. *Circulation*, 97:282–9

Gheorghiade M, Cody RJ, Francis GS, et al (2000) Current medical therapy for advanced heart failure. *Heart and Lung*, 29(1):16–32

Giallauria F, De lorenzo A, Pilerci F, et al (2006) Long-term effects of cardiac rehabilitation on end-exercise heart rate recovery after myocardial infarction. *European Journal of Cardiovascular Prevention and Rehabilitation*, 13(4):544–50

Giannuzzi P, Temporelli PL, Corrà U, et al (2003) Antiremodeling effect of long-term exercise training in patients with stable chronic heart failure results of the exercise in left ventricular dysfunction and chronic heart failure (ELVD-CHF) trial. *Circulation*, 108(5):554–9

Gielen S, Schuler G, Hambrecht R (2001) Exercise training in coronary artery disease and coronary vasomotion. *Circulation*, 103, 1–6

Giordano M, Matsuda M, Sanders L, et al (1995) Effects of angiotensin-converting enzyme inhibitors, Ca2+ channel antagonists, and alpha-adrenergic blockers on glucose and lipid metabolism in NIDDM patients with hypertension. *Diabetes*, 44(6):665–71

Giugliano D, Acampora R, Marfella R, et al (1997) Metabolic and cardiovascular effects of carvedilol and atenolol in non-insulin-dependent diabetes mellitus and hypertension. A randomized, controlled trial. *Annals of Internal Medicine*, 126(12):955–9

Goebbels U (1998) A randomized comparison of exercise training in patients with normal vs reduced ventricular function. *Chest*, 113(5):1387–93

Green HJ, Sutton J, Young P, Cymerman A, Houston CS (1989) Operation Everest II: muscle energetics during maximal exhaustive exercise. *Journal of Applied Physiology*, 66(1):142–50

Hadj A, Esmore D, Rowland M, et al (2006) Pre-operative preparation for cardiac surgery utilising a combination of metabolic, physical and mental therapy. *Heart Lung Circular*, 15(3):172–81

Haennel RG, Quinney A, Kappagoda CT (1991) Effects of hydraulic circuit training following coronary artery bypass surgery. *Medicine and Science in Sports and Exercise*, 23(2):158–65

Hagberg JM, Ehsani AA, Goldring D, et al (1984) Effect of weight training on blood pressure and hemodynamics in hypertensive adolescents. *The Journal of Pediatrics*, 104:147–51

Hagberg JM, Park JJ, Brown MD (2000) The role of exercise training in the treatment of hypertension. *Sports Medicine*, 30(3):193–206

Hambrecht R, Adams V, Erbs S, et al (2003) Regular physical activity improves endothelial function in patients with coronary artery disease by increasing phosphorylation of endothelial nitric oxide synthase. *Circulation*, 107(25):3152–8

Hambrecht R, Fiehn E, Yu J, et al (1997) Effects of endurance training on mitochondrial ultrastructure and fiber type distribution in skeletal muscle of patients with stable chronic heart failure. *Journal of the American College of Cardiology*, 29(5):1067–73

Hambrecht R, Fiehn E, Weigl C, et al (1998) Regular physical exercise corrects endothelial dysfunction and improves exercise capacity in patients with chronic heart failure. *Circulation*, 98(24):2709–15

Hare DL, Ryan TM, Selig SE, et al (1999) Resistance exercise training increases muscle strength, endurance, and blood flow in patients with chronic heart failure. *The American Journal of Cardiology*, 83, 1674–7

Harrington D, Anker SD, Chua TP, et al (1997) Skeletal muscle function and its relation to exercise tolerance in chronic heart failure. *Journal of the American College of Cardiology*, 30(7):1758–64

Haskel WL (1984) Cardiovascular benefits and risk of exercise: the scientific evidence. In: Strauss R (ed.): *Sport Medicine*. Philadelphia: WS Saunders Company, pp 57–76

Hauf-Zachariou U, Widmann L, Zulsdorf B, et al (1993) A double-blind comparison of the effects of carvedilol and captopril on serum lipid concentrations in patients with mild to moderate essential hypertension and dyslipidaemia. *European Journal of Clinical Pharmacology*, 45(2):95–100

Haykowski M, Riess K, Figgures L, et al (2005) Exercise training improves aerobic performance and musculoskeletal fitness in female cardiac transplant recipients. *Current Controlled Trials in Cardiovascular Medicine*, 6:10–14

Haykowsky M, Humen D, Teo K, et al (2000) Effect of 16 weeks of resistance training on left ventricular morphology and systolic function in healthy men>60 years of age. *The American Journal of Cardiology*, 85:1002–6

Herdy A, Marcchi P, Vila A, (2008) Pre- and postoperative cardiopulmonary rehabilitation in hospitalised patients undergoing coronary artery bypass surgery: a randomized controlled trial. *American Journal of Physical Medicine and Rehabilitation*, 87(9):714–19

Higginbotham MB, Morris KG, Conn EH, et al (1983) Determinants of variable exercise performance among patients with severe left ventricular dysfunction. *The American Journal of Cardiology*, 51:52–60

Horowitz J, Klein S (2000) Lipid metabolism during endurance exercise. *American Journal of Clinical Nutrition*, 72:558S–563S

Hosokawa S, Hiasa Y, Takahashi T, et al (2003) Effect of regular exercise on coronary endothelial function in patients with recent myocardial infarction. *Circulation Research*, 67:221–4

Hulzebos E, Helders P, Favié N, et al (2006) Preoperative intensive inspiratory muscle training to prevent postoperative pulmonary complications in high-risk patients undergoing CABG surgery. *Journal of the American Medical Association*, 296(15):1851–7

Izawa K, Hirano Y, Yamada S, (2004) Improvement in physiological outcomes and health-related quality of life following cardiac rehabilitation in patients with acute myocardial infarction. *Circulation Journal*, 68(4):315–20

Jacob S, Rett K, Henriksen EJ (1998) Antihypertensive therapy and insulin sensitivity: do we have to redefine the role of beta-blocking agents? *American Journal of Hypertension*, 11(10):1258–65

Jacob S, Rett K, Wicklmayr M, et al (1996) Differential effect of chronic treatment with two beta-blocking agents on insulin sensitivity: the carvedilol-metoprolol study. *Journal of Hypertension*, 14(4):489–94

Jolliffe JA, Rees K, Taylor RS, et al (2001) Exercise-based rehabilitation for coronary heart disease. *Cochrane Database of Systematic Reviews*, (1):CD001800

Kanakis C, Hickson CR (1980) Left ventricular responses to a program of lower-limb strength training. *Chest*, 78(4):618–21

Kavanagh T, Mertens DJ, Hamm LF, et al (2002) Prediction of long-term prognosis in 12 169 men referred for cardiac rehabilitation. *Circulation*, 106:666–73

Kavanagh T, Myers MG, Hamm LF, et al (1996) Quality of life and cardiorespiratory function in chronic heart failure:Effects of 12 months' aerobic training. *Heart*, 76(1):42–9

Kelemen MH, Stewart KJ, Gillilan RE, et al (1986) Circuit weight training in cardiac patients. *Journal of the American College of Cardiology*, 7:38–42

Kemi OJ, Wisloff U (2010) High-intensity aerobic exercise training improves the heart in health and disease. *Journal of Cardiopulmonary Rehabilitation and Prevention*, 30:2–11

Kesaniemi YK, Danforth E Jr, Jensen MD, et al (2001) Dose-response issues concerning physical activity and health: an evidence-based symposium. *Medicine and Science in Sports and Exercise*, 33(6 Suppl):S351–S358

Keteyian SJ, Brawner CA, Schairer JR, et al (1999) Effects of exercise training on chronotropic incompetence in patients with heart failure. *American Heart Journal*, 138(2) (Part 1):233–40

Keteyian SJ, Brawner CA, Schairer JR (1997) Exercise testing and training of patients with heart failure due to left ventricular systolic dysfunction. *Journal of Cardiopulmonary Rehabilitation*, 17:19–28

King CML (2001) The effect of resistance exercise on skeletal muscle abnormalities in patients with advanced heart failure. *Progress in Cardiovascular Nursing*, 16:142–51

Kobayashi N, Tsuruya Y, Lwasawa T, et al (2003) Exercise training in patients with chronic heart failure improves endothelial function predominantly in the trained extremities. *Circulation Journal*, 67:505–10

Krotkiewski M, Lonnroth P, Mandroukas K, et al (1985) The effects of physical training on insulin secretion and effectiveness and on glucose metabolism in obesity and type 2 (non-insulin-dependent) diabetes mellitus. *Diabetologia*, 28(12):881–90

Leblance MH (2000) Current pharmacological therapy for congestive heart failure. In: Jobin J, Maltais F, LeBlanc P, Simard C (eds) *Advances in Cardiopulmonary Rehabilitation*. Champaign, IL: Human Kinetics, pp 32–7

Legramante J, Iellamo F, Massaro M, et al (2006) Effects of residential exercise training on heart rate recovery in coronary artery patients. *American Journal of Physiology*, 292(1):510–15

Leon AS, Franklin BA, Costa F, et al (2005) Cardiac rehabilitation and secondary prevention of coronary heart disease: an American Heart Association scientific statement from the Council on Clinical Cardiology (Subcommittee on Exercise, Cardiac Rehabilitation, and Prevention) and the Council on Nutrition, Physical Activity, and Metabolism (Subcommittee on Physical Activity):in collaboration with the American Association of Cardiovascular and Pulmonary Rehabilitation. *Circulation*, 111(3):369–76

Letac B, Cribier A, Desplanches JF (1977) A study of left ventricular function in coronary patients before and after physical training. *Circulation*, 56(3):375–8

Levi D, Larson MG, Vasan RS, et al (1996) The progression from hypertension to congestive heart failure. *The Journal of the American Medical Association*, 275(20):1557–62

Levinger I, Bronks R, Cody DV, et al (2005a) The effect of resistance training on left ventricular function and structure of patients with chronic heart failure. *International Journal of Cardiology*, 105:159–63

Levinger I, Bronks R, Cody DV, et al (2005b) Resistance training for chronic heart failure patients on beta blocker medications. *International Journal of Cardiology*, 102(3):493–9

Libonati J, Colby A, Caldwell T, et al (1999) Systolic and diastolic cardiac function time intervals and exercise capacity in women. *Medicine & Science in Sports & Exercise*, 31(2):258–63

Lipkin DP, Jones DA, Round JM, et al (1988) Abnormalities of skeletal muscle in patients with chronic heart failure. *International Journal of Cardiology*, 18(2):187–95

Lithell HO (1991) Effect of antihypertensive drugs on insulin, glucose, and lipid metabolism. *Diabetes Care*, 14(3):203–9

Lucini D, Milani R, Costantino G, et al (2002) Effects of cardiac rehabilitation and exercise training on autonomic regulation in patients with coronary artery disease. *American Heart Journal*, 143:977–83

Magnusson G, Isberg B, Karlberg KE, et al (1994) Skeletal muscle strength an endurance in chronic congestive heart failure secondary to idiopathic dilated cardiomyopathy. *The American Journal of Cardiology*, 73:307–9

Maiorana A, O'Driscoll G, Cheetham C, et al (2000) Combined aerobic and resistance exercise training improves functional capacity and strength in CHF. *Journal of Applied Physiology*, 88(5):1565–70

Maiorana AJ, Briffa TG, Goodman C, et al (1997) A controlled trail of circuit weight training on aerobic capacity and myocardial oxygen demand in men after coronary artery bypass surgery. *Journal of Cardiopulmonary Rehabilitation*, 17, 239–47

Malfatto G, Branzi G, Riva B, et al (2002) recovery of cardiac autonomic responsiveness with low-intensity physical training in patients with chronic heart failure. *European Journal of Heart Failure*, 4:159–66

Malfatto G, Facchini M, Sala L, et al (2000) Long-term lifestyle changes maintain the autonomic modulation induced by rehabilitation after myocardial infarction. *International Journal of Cardiology*, 74:171–6

Mancini DM, Eisen H, Kussmaul W, et al (1991) Value of peak exercise oxygen consumption for optimal timing of cardiac transplantation in ambulatory patients with heart failure. *Circulation*, 83:778–86

Mancini DM, Walter G, Reichek N, et al (1992) Contribution of skeletal muscle atrophy to exercise intolerance and altered muscle metabolism in heart failure. *Circulation*, 85(4):1364–73

Marian AJ (2010) Hypertrophic cardiomyopathy: from genetics to treatment. *European Journal Clinical Investigations*, 40(4):360–9

Massie BM (1988) Exercise tolerance in congestive heart failure. *The American Journal of Medicine*, 84 (Suppl 3A):75–82

McCartney N, McKelvie RS, Haslam, DRS, et al (1991) Usefulness of weightlifting training in improving strength and maximal power output in coronary artery disease. *The American Journal of Cardiology*, 67:939–45

McDonald CD, Burch, GE, Walsh JJ (1972) Prolonged bed rest in the treatment of idiopathic cardiomyopathy. *The American Journal of Medicine*, 52, 41–50

McKelvie RS, Teo KK, McCartney N, et al (1995) Effects of exercise training in patients with congestive heart failure: a critical review. *Journal of the American College of Cardiology*, 25(3):789–96

Meka N, Katragadda S, Cherian B, et al (2008) Endurance exercise and resistance training in cardiovascular disease. *Therapeutic Advances in Cardiovascular Disease*, 2: 115–21

Meltzer LE, Pinneo R, et al (1983) *Intensive Coronary Care:A Manual for Nurses*. Maryland: Robert Bradly Company

Meredith C, Frontera W, Fisher E, Hughes V, Herland J, Edwards J, Evans W (1989) Peripheral effects of endurance training in young and old subjects. *Journal of Applied Physiology*, 66(6):2844–9

Mitchell JH, Wildenthal K (1974) Static (isometric) exercise and the heart: physiological and clinical considerations. *Annual Review of Medicine*, 24, 369–81

Murray CJL, Lopez AD (1996) Evidence-based health policy lessons from the global burden of disease study. *Science*, 274:740–3

Murtagh EM, Murphy MH, Boone-Heinonen J (2010) Walking: the first steps in cardiovascular disease prevention. *Current Opinions in Cardiology*, 25:490–6

Myers J, Gullestad L (1998) The role of exercise testing and gas-exchange measurement in the prognostic assessment of patients with heart failure. *Current Opinion in Cardiology*, 13(3):145–55

Nelson M, Rejeski W, Blair S, et al (2007) Physical activity and public health in older adults: recommendations from the American College of Sports Medicine and the American Heart Association. *Medicine and Science in Sports and Exercise*, 39(8):1435–45

Nicholls MG (1996) Hypertension, hypertrophy, heart failure. *Heart*, 76 (Suppl 3):92–7

O'Connor CM, Whellan DJ, Lee KL (2009) Efficacy and safety of exercise training in patients with chronic heart failure: HF-ACTION randomized controlled trial. *JAMA*, 301(14):1439–50

O'Driscoll G, Green D, Maiorana A, et al (1999) Improvement in endothelial function by angiotensin-converting enzyme inhibition in non-insulin-dependent diabetes mellitus. *The Journal of the American College of Cardiology*, 33(6):1506–11

Ogino K, Ogura K, Kinugawa T, et al (2004) Neurohumoral profiles in patients with hypertrophic cardiomyopathy: differences to hypertensive left ventricular hypertrophy. *Circulation Research*, 68:444–50

Oka R, De Marco T, Haskell WL, et al (2000) Impact of home-based walking and resistance training program on quality of life in patients with heart failure. *The American Journal of Cardiology*, 85:365–9

Ornish D, Scherwitz LW, Billings JH, et al (1998) Intensive lifestyle changes for reversal of coronary heart disease. *JAMA*, 280(23)

Packer M, Coats AJS, Fowler MB, et al (2001) Effects of carvedilol on survival in severe chronic heart failure. *The New England Journal of Medicine*, 344(22):1651–8

Painter P, Hanson P (1984) Isometric exercise: implications for the cardiac patients. *Cardiovascular Review and Reports*, 5:261–79

Perreault CL, Gonzales-Serratos H, Litwin SE, et al (1993) Alterations in contractility and intracellular Ca^{2+} transients in isolated bundles of skeletal muscle fibers from rats with chronic heart failure. *Circulation Research*, 73:405–12

Pescatello LS, Franklin BA, Fagard R, et al (2004) American College of Sports Medicine. Position stand: exercise and hypertension. *Medicine and Science in Sports and Exercise*, 36(3):533–53

Peschel T, Sixt S, Beitz F, et al (2007) High, but not moderate frequency and duration of exercise training induces down-regulation of the expression of inflammatory and atherogenic adhesion molecules. *Eur J Cardiovasc Prev Rehabil*, 14(3):476–82

Peters DG, Mitchell HL, McCune SA, et al (1997) Skeletal muscle sarcoplasmic reticulum Ca^{2+}-ATPase gene expression in congestive heart failure. *Circulation Research*, 81:703–10

Piepoli M, Clark AL, Volterrani M, Adamopoulos S, et al (1996) Contribution of muscle afferents to the hemodynamic, autonomic, and ventilatory responses to exercise in patients with chronic heart failure. *Circulation*, 93:940–52

Piepoli MF, Capucci A (2000) Exercise training in heart failure: effect on morbidity and mortality. *International Journal of Cardiology*, 73:3–6

Piepoli MF, Scotte AC, Capucci A, et al (2001) Skeletal muscle training in chronic heart failure. *Acta Physiologica Scandinavica*, 171, 295–303

Pollock ML, Franklin BA, Balady GJ, et al (2000) Resistance exercise in individuals with and without cardiovascular disease: benefits, rationale, and prescription an advisory from the committee on exercise, rehabilitation, and prevention, council on clinical cardiology, American Heart Association. *Circulation*, 101, 828–33

Poole-Wilson PA, Swedberg K, Cleland JGF, et al (2003) Comparison of carvedilol and metoprolol on clinical outcomes in patients with chronic heart failure in the Carvedilol or Metoprolol European Trial (COMET): randomised controlled trial. *Lancet*, 362:7–13

Pu C, Johnson M, Forman D, Hausdorff J, (2001) Randomized trial of progressive resistance training to counteract the myopathy of chronic heart failure. *Journal Applied Physiology*, 90(6):2341–50

Quittan M, Sturm B, Wiesinger GF, et al (1999) Quality of life in patients with chronic heart failure: a randomized controlled trial of changes induced by regular exercise program. *Scandinavian Journal of Rehabilitation Medicine*, 31, 223–8

Radaelli A, Coats AJ, Leuzzi S, et al (1996) Physical training enhances sympathetic and parasympathetic control of heart rate and peripheral vessels in chronic heart failure. *Clinical Science*, 91(Suppl):92–4

Rees K, Taylor R, Singh S, et al (2004) Exercise based rehabilitation for heart failure. *Cochrane Database of Systematic Reviews*, 3:CD003331

Rinder MR, Miller TR, Ehsani AA, et al (1999) Effects of endurance exercise training on left ventricular systolic performance and ventriculoarterial coupling in patients with coronary artery disease. *American Heart Journal*, 138(1 Part 1):169–74

Rognmo Ø, Hetland E, Helgerud J, et al (2004) High intensity aerobic interval exercise is superior to moderate intensity exercise for increasing aerobic capacity in patients with coronary artery disease. *European Journal of Cardiovascular Prevention and Rehabilitation*, 11: 216–22

Roul G, Moulichon ME, Bareiss P, et al (1994) Exercise peak VO$_2$ determination in chronic heart failure: is it still of value? *European Heart Journal*, 15:495–502

Sarafidis PA, Bakris GL (2006) Antihypertensive treatment with beta-blockers and the spectrum of glycaemic control. *Quarterly Journal of Medicine*, 99(7):431–6

Schneider SH, Amorosa LF, Khachadurian AK, et al (1984) Studies on the mechanism of improved glucose control during regular exercise in type 2 (non-insulin-dependent) diabetes. *Diabetologia*, 26(5):355–60

Schneider SH, Khachadurian AK, Amorosa LF, et al (1992) Ten-year experience with an exercise-based outpatient life-style modification program in the treatment of diabetes mellitus. *Diabetes Care*, 15(11):1800–10

Sciacqua A, Candigliota M, Ceravolo R, et al (2003) Weight loss in combination with physical activity improves endothelial dysfunction in human obesity. *Diabetes Care*, 26, 1673–8

Seals D, Hagberg J, Hurley B, et al (1984) Endurance training in older men and women: cardiovascular responses to exercise. *Journal Applied Physiology*, 57(4):1024–29

Seggewiss H, Rigopoulos A (2003) Management of hypertrophic cardiomyopathy in children. *Paediatr Drugs*, 5(10):663–72

Seguchi H, Nakamura H, Aosaki N, et al (1990) Effects of carvedilol on serum lipids in hypertensive and normotensive subjects. *European Journal of Clinical Pharmacology*, 38:S139–S142

Selig SE, Carey MF, Menzies DG, et al (2004) Moderate-intensity resistance exercise training in patients with chronic heart failure improves strength, endurance, heart rate variability, and forearm blood flow. *Journal of Cardiac Failure*, 10(1):21–9

Selig S, Levinger I, Williams A, et al (2010) Exercise and Sports Science Australia Position Statement on Exercise Training and Chronic Heart Failure. *Journal of Science and Medicine in Sport*, 13:288–94

Sharpe N, Doughty, RN (1998) Left ventricular remodelling and improved long-term outcomes in chronic heart failure. *European Heart Journal*, 19(Suppl B):B36–B39

Shiroma EJ, Lee IM (2010) Physical activity and cardiovascular health: lessons learned from epidemiological studies across age, gender, and race/ethnicity. *Circulation*, 122:743–52

Smart N, Marwick TH (2004) Exercise training for patients with heart failure: a systemic review of factors that improve mortality and morbidity. *American Journal of Medicine*, 116(10):693–706

Smith SD, Blair SN, Criqui MH, et al (1995) Preventing heart attack and death in patients with coronary disease. *Circulation*, 92(1):2–4

Sontheimer DL (2006) Peripheral vascular disease: diagnosis and treatment. *American Family Physician*, 73(11):1971–6

Sparling, PB, Cantwell JD, Dolan CM, Niederman RK (1990) Strength training in a cardiac rehabilitation program: a six-month follow-up. *Archives of Physiology and Medicine Rehabilitation*, 71:148–52

Stewart KJ (1989) Resistive training effects on strength and cardiovascular endurance in cardiac and coronary prone patients. *Medicine and Science in Sports and Exercise*, 21(6):678–82

Stewart KJ, McFarland LD, Weinhofer JJ, et al (1998) Safety and efficacy of weight training soon after acute myocardial infarction. *Journal of Cardiopulmonary Rehabilitation*, 18:37–44

Stolen KQ, Kemppainen J, Ukkonen H, et al (2003) Exercise training improves biventricular oxidative metabolism and left ventricular efficiency in patients with dilated cardiomyopathy. *Journal of the American College of Cardiology*, 41(3):460–7

Swank AM, Funk DC, Barnard KL, et al (2002) Combined high intensity strength and aerobic training enhances quality of life outcomes for individuals with CHF. *Journal of Exercise Physiology*, 20502(2):36–41

Szlachcic J, Massie BM, Kramer BL, et al (1985) Correlates and prognostic implication of exercise capacity in chronic congestive heart failure. *The American Journal of Cardiology*, 55:1037–42

Tambalis K, Panagiotakos D, Kavoura S, et al (2009) Responses of blood lipids to aerobic, resistance and combined aerobic with resistance exercise training: a systematic review of current evidence. *Angiology*, 60:614–32

Tavazzi L, Giannuzzi P (2001) Physical training as a therapeutic measure in chronic heart failure: time for recommendations. *Heart*, 86:7–11

Thompson PD, Buchner D, Pina IL, et al (2003) Exercise and physical activity in the prevention and treatment of atherosclerotic cardiovascular disease: a statement from the Council on Clinical Cardiology (Subcommittee on Exercise, Rehabilitation, and Prevention) and the Council on Nutrition, Physical Activity, and Metabolism (Subcommittee on Physical Activity) *Circulation*, 107(24):3109–116

Tikkanen H, Hämäläinen E, Härkönen M (1999) Significance of skeletal muscle properties on fitness, long-term physical training and serum lipids. *Atherosclerosis*, 142(2):367–78

Tong B, Stevenson C (2007) Comorbidity of cardiovascular disease, diabetes and chronic kidney disease in Australia. *Cardiovascular Disease*, Series no.28. Cat. no. CVD 37. Canberra: Australia: Australian Institute of Health and Welfare (AIHW)

Tyni-Lenné R, Dencker K, Gordon A, et al (2001) Comprehensive local muscle training increases aerobic working capacity and quality of life and decreases neurohormonal activation in patients with chronic heart failure. *European Journal of Heart Failure*, 3:47–52

Tyni-Lenné R, Gordon A, Europe E, et al (1998) Exercise-based rehabilitation improves skeletal muscle capacity, exercise tolerance, and quality of life in both women and men with chronic heart failure. *Journal of Cardiac Failure*, 4(1):9–17

UK Prospective Diabetes Study Group (1998) Efficacy of atenolol and captopril in reducing risk of macrovascular and microvascular complications in type 2 diabetes: UKPDS 39. UK Prospective Diabetes Study Group. *British Medical Journal*, 317(7160):713–20

Unger T (2002) The role of the renin-angiotensin system in the development of cardiovascular disease. *The American Journal of Cardiology*, 89:3A–10A

Uzunlulu M, Oguz A, Yorulmaz E (2006) The effect of carvedilol on metabolic parameters in patients with metabolic syndrome. *International Heart Journal*, 47: 421–30

Vita J, Keaney J (2000) Exercise — toning up the endothelium? *The New England Journal of Medicine*, 342:503–5

Way A.C (2002) Carvedilol may be new therapeutic strategy for canine heart disease. *Doctor of Veterinary Medicine*, 33(1):1S

Whellan DJ, Shaw LK, Bart BA, et al (2001) Cardiac rehabilitation and survival in patients with left ventricular systolic dysfunction. *American Heart Journal*, 142:160–6

Wilk NA, Sheldahl LM, Levandoski SG, et al (1991) Transfer effect of upper extremity training to weight carrying in men with ischemic heart disease. *Journal of Cardiopulmonary Rehabilitation*, 11:365–72

Willenheimer R, Erhardt L, Cline C, et al (1998) Exercise training in heart failure improves quality of life and exercise capacity. *European Heart Journal* 19(5):774–81

Williams JH, Ward CW (1998) Changes in skeletal muscle sarcoplasmic reticulum function and force production following myocardial infarction in rats. *Experimental Physiology*, 83:85–94

Wing RR, Jakicic J, Neiberg R, et al (2007) Fitness, fatness, and cardiovascular risk factors in type 2 diabetes: look ahead study. *Medicine and Science in Sports and Exercise*, 39(12):2107–16

Wisløff U, Støylen A, Loennechen J, et al (2007) Superior cardiovascular effect of aerobic interval training versus moderate continuous training in heart failure patients: a randomized study. *Circulation*;115:3086–94

Yu C-M, Sheung-Wai L, Lam M-F, et al (2004) Effect of a cardiac rehabilitation program on left ventricular diastolic function and its relationship to exercise capacity in patients with coronary heart disease: Experience from a randomized, controlled study. *American Heart Journal*, 147(5):11–18

Chapter 4

Exercise as therapy in respiratory conditions

Suzanne Broadbent, Sarah-Johanna Moss and Cilas Wilders

Assumed concepts

This chapter is based on the assumption that readers already understand key concepts and have background knowledge in, and understanding of:

- human anatomy of the respiratory and circulatory systems
- the mechanics of breathing and pulmonary gas exchange
- key physiological terms such as hypocapnia, oxygen desaturation, hypercapnia and inflammatory response
- lung function testing using a spirometer.

INTRODUCTION

Respiratory diseases encompass both obstructive and restrictive pulmonary diseases and conditions. Chronic obstructive pulmonary diseases (COPDs) include chronic bronchitis, emphysema and obstructive bronchiolitis, and are characterised by airway obstruction and progressive airway limitation that is not fully reversible (Rabe et al 2007; Romer 2009). Asthma is a chronic inflammatory disorder characterised by airway hyper-responsiveness, airflow obstruction that is usually reversible, and other respiratory symptoms (wheezing, dyspnea). Restrictive pulmonary conditions include interstitial lung diseases such as asbestosis and silicosis, chronic infections, sarcoidosis, neoplastic disorders, vascular disorders, drug injury, fibrotic disorders, and skeletal restrictions to breathing (kyphosis; see Chapter 12 for case study) (Mason et al 2005; Holland & Hill 2008; Romer 2009).

Respiratory diseases have a major impact on the utilisation of healthcare resources. While the underlying pathology involves the lungs, the associated physical deconditioning and psychological responses contribute to the resulting morbidity. The Australian Institute of Health and Welfare (AIHW) presents data for chronic obstructive diseases, specifically emphysema, bronchitis and asthma, and according to the 2008 statistics, 3.3% of the Australian population suffer from COPD and 10.3% suffer from asthma (Australian Centre for Asthma Monitoring 2006). However, the prevalence of COPD is considerably higher in older age groups (8%) and women (Ries 2008), and the National Health Surveys (NHS) admitted that COPD is probably under-reported in younger age groups. The mortality rate from COPD is relatively high, representing 45.2% of all respiratory disease deaths, and 3.7% of all deaths (Australian Centre for Asthma Monitoring 2006). COPD was also listed as an associated cause of death, most often when cardiovascular disease or lung cancer was the underlying cause of death. Asthma is relatively common and the prevalence in Australia remains high by international standards. The prevalence of asthma is higher in adolescents with 11.5% of females presenting with asthma compared to 8.9% of males. Generally females between the ages of 15 and 80 years showed a higher prevalence than males. Furthermore, Aboriginal and Torres Strait Islanders show a greater prevalence of asthma compared to other Australians (16.5% versus 10.2% in 2005; Australian Centre for Asthma Monitoring 2008). Compared to international standards, death rates due to asthma are high in Australia, 0.24% of all deaths (Australian Centre for Asthma Monitoring 2008), and the risk of dying from asthma increases with age. The burden of the disease is considerably high, and is in fact the leading specific cause of disease burden in children and adolescents under 15 years (17.3%; Australian Centre for Asthma Monitoring 2008).

While the pathophysiologies of the various respiratory diseases differ substantially, the common factor associated with them is that the ability to perform physical activity is limited, with dyspnea (breathlessness), fatigue, anxiety and progressive disability reducing exercise tolerance and quality of life (QoL) (Mason et al 2005; Ries 2008). Pulmonary rehabilitation combines multidisciplinary and broad interventions which are evidence-based, and include patient assessment, disease and self-management, exercise training, pharmacological interventions and nutritional education (Lacasse et al 2006; Ries 2008). The main aims are to improve QoL, psychological wellbeing, dyspnea, functional capacity and reliance of the healthcare system. There is overwhelming evidence that pulmonary rehabilitation, including exercise, significantly improves patient wellbeing, functional capacity and disease management (Lacasse et al 2006; Ries 2008).

Risk factors for respiratory diseases include: smoking; environments with high levels of air pollution (smoke, fumes, gases); allergens such as pollens, dust mites, moulds, fungi, yeasts and animal dander; industrial dust (eg: asbestos, silicon); repeated bouts of bronchitis; inhalation of drugs (eg: cocaine); and genetic links with some autoimmune conditions (eg: asthma, cystic fibrosis) (Baroffio et al 2009). Exercise may also be a risk factor for asthma (Carlin et al 2009; Romer 2009).

CHRONIC OBSTRUCTIVE LUNG CONDITIONS

Emphysema and chronic bronchitis

The major physiological limitation in COPD is increased airway resistance due to reduced cross-sectional airway diameter, which produces entrapment of air and hyperinflation of the lungs. Chronic bronchitis results in inflammation and scarring of the large airways, with a sputum-producing cough for at least 3 months in each of 2 consecutive years (Romer 2009; Ries 2008; Newall et al 2005). Emphysema is the permanent enlargement of airspaces distal to the terminal bronchiole, including the destruction of the alveolar walls (Romer 2009). Typically there is an increased inflammatory response, with alveolar macrophages, lymphocytes and neutrophils invading lung tissue, and with the release of many inflammatory mediators (eg: cytokines, proteases, growth factors) which also damage lung tissue (Baroffio et al 2009). It is common for COPD patients to show symptoms of both chronic bronchitis and emphysema. Functional capacity and exercise tolerance are reduced by interacting factors. There are abnormalities in gas exchange, structural and functional changes in the mechanics of ventilation, cardiovascular limitations, peripheral muscle dysfunction and severe dyspnea. Severe damage to the alveolar walls and parenchymal elastin results in reduced elastic recoil and airway tethering, and the airways collapse prematurely when intrathoracic pressure is increased during breathing. The lungs do not empty completely, resulting in dynamic hyperinflation, inefficient action of the inspiratory muscles, increased loading of the lungs and chest wall, and thus a significant increase in the work of breathing. With severe COPD, the mechanical inefficiency and respiratory muscle load may lead to hypoventilation during intense exercise (Carlin et al 2009). Systemic oxygen delivery will be reduced because of hypercapnia and hypoxemia, and pH will also decrease. Hypoxia and low pH stimulate the ventilatory drive, and therefore breathing rate may be increased, peripheral skeletal muscle function may be affected, and sensations of dizziness, dyspnea and limb discomfort may occur.

Furthermore, chronic lung diseases may cause cardiovascular complications, notably 'cor pulmonale', which refers to right ventricular hypertrophy, dilation and possibly right heart failure (Sietsema 2001). Alveolar hypoxemia may cause pulmonary vasoconstriction which increases vascular resistance to blood flow. Pulmonary hyperinflation will also increase right ventricular after-load, which may lead to right heart failure (Sietsema 2001; Romer 2009).

Cystic fibrosis

Cystic fibrosis (CF) is a hereditary disease, considered to be autosomal recessive. The disease is caused by a mutation in the gene cystic fibrosis transmembrane conductance (CFTC) regulator which results in only one copy of the protein, a chloride ion channel necessary for creating sweat, digestive juices and mucous (Gruber et al 2008; Romer 2009). CF affects the exocrine glands in the lungs, liver, pancreas and intestines, resulting in abnormally thick mucous that obstructs lung function, reduced secretion of pancreatic enzymes, impaired growth and deficiency of fat soluble vitamins (Bradley & Moran 2008). Patients are prone to repeated lung infections, and although life expectancy has increased in recent years, patients usually survive only until their early thirties (Gruber et al 2008). Under-nutrition and loss of muscle function are also symptomatic of CF. Management and treatment of CF has improved in past decades, and physical training, airway clearance and conventional physiotherapy have been shown to increase QoL, exercise capacity and dyspnea (Davis et al 1996; Bradley et al 2005; Bradley & Moran 2008). More specifically, aerobic exercise and strength training can improve aerobic capacity, muscle strength and endurance, flexibility, coordination, onset of fatigue and body composition (Gruber et al 2008; Bradley & Moran 2008; Bradley et al 2005). Some studies have shown improved pulmonary function (total lung capacity [TLC]; forced expiratory volume in one second [FEV_1]) (Bradley & Moran 2008), but much of the literature shows improvements in aerobic capacity and strength rather than lung function (Bradley & Moran 2008; Cooper & Storer 2009).

Most research suggests that long-term training provides more substantial improvements in health, fitness and QoL (Bradley & Moran 2008).

Asthma

There is some debate as to whether asthma is associated with COPD or whether it is a separate disease. The symptoms of the three conditions may well overlap, but clinically asthma is considered to be a hyperreactive inflammatory condition with reversible airway limitation, and as such, will be treated here as a separate condition. Asthma also produces dyspnea, wheezing, coughing and chest tightness, and this is due to the activation of immune cells and pro inflammatory cytokines in response to an allergen or cold, dry air. Chronic airway inflammation eventually results in structural changes of the smooth muscle and epithelium of the airways, with increased deposition of collagen and proteoglycans under the basement membrane and airway walls, causing fibrosis (Anderson & Holzer 2000; Anderson & Kippelen 2008; Baroffio et al 2009). There is hypertrophy and hyperplasia of the airways, with angiogenesis. The thickening of the airway wall may result in relatively irreversible narrowing of the airways, and may be combined with mucous hypersecretion and distal airway blockage. As the production of lung surfactant is reduced, atelectasis or closure of peripheral lung units may occur, with reduced lung volume and hypoxia due to a mismatch in ventilation and perfusion.

Asthma may be induced by exercise as a consequence of evaporative water loss in inspired air (Anderson & Kippelen 2008). The bronchial mucosa and airway surfaces become cool and dehydrated, causing changes in bronchial blood flow and a release of inflammatory cells and mediators such as prostaglandins, leukotriennes and histamine, thus triggering bronchospasm (Tan & Spector 1998; Anderson & Holzer 2000). High ventilation rates during intense exercise, especially in cold, dry air, promote hyper-responsiveness and bronchoconstriction (Anderson 2006). To minimise the chances of exercise induced asthma (EIA) or exercise induced bronchoconstriction (EIB), EIA current guidelines recommend that patients exercise in warmer, humid air (e.g. swimming), undergo a longer low intensity warm up before an exercise session, and participate in a cool down session after the exercise bout (Anderson 2006; Anderson & Kippelen 2008).

Table 4.1 Interpretation of pulmonary testing for respiratory disorders

	Obstructive	Restrictive	Vascular
FEV$_1$ (L)	↓	↓	↔
FVC (L)	↓	↓	↔
FEV$_1$/FVC	↓	↔ or ↓	↔
TLC (L)	↑	↓	↔
VC (L)	↓	↓	↔
FRC (L)	↑	↓	↔
RV (L)	↑	↓	↔
Dl$_{CO}$	↔ or ↓	↔ or ↓	↓

Note: ↔, no change; ↑, increased; ↓, decreased; ↔ or ↓, no change early in disease but a decrease later ; FEV$_1$, forced expiratory volume in 1 second; FVC, forced vital capacity; TLC, total lung capacity; VC, vital capacity; FRC, functional residual capacity; RV, residual volume; Dlco, carbon monoxide diffusing capacity.

(Source: adapted from ACSM 2010)

Table 4.2 GOLD Guidelines for COPD diagnosis and staging

Stage[a]	Predicted FEV$_1$[b]	Symptom	Severity
1	≥ 80%	± symptoms	Mild
2	50–79%	± symptoms	Moderate
3	30–49%	± symptoms	Severe
4	< 30% or < 50% with chronic respiratory failure	± symptoms	Very severe

Note: FEV$_1$, forced expiratory volume in 1 second; FVC, forced vital capacity; a for stages 1 through 4, FEV$_1$/FVC ratio needs to be < 70%; b FEV$_1$ values based on post-bronchodilator measurements.

(Source: adapted from ACSM 2010)

Respiratory diagnosis and pharmacology

Clinically, respiratory disorders are diagnosed with pulmonary function testing (spirometer and/or peak flow meter), and the interpretation of respiratory disorders is outlined in Table 4.1. Forced vital capacity (FVC, expired air volume), forced expiratory volume in one second (FEV$_1$), the FEV$_1$/FVC ratio and peak expiratory flow (PEF) are commonly used to detect the extent of COPD, thus influencing the type of pulmonary rehabilitation and exercise program to be prescribed.

The American Thoracic Society (ATS), the American College of Sports Medicine (ACSM), the American Association of Cardiovascular and Pulmonary Rehabilitation (AACVPR) and the Global Initiative for COPD (GOLD) all produce guidelines for spirometric classification of COPD (see Table 4.2). However, spirometric classification does not include other aspects of COPD such as functional capacity and dyspnea, and so the multidimensional BODE index (Pauwels et al 2001) (see Table 4.3) is also useful for assessing the severity of the disease and for predicting mortality, through the use of functional assessments. COPD lung damage is irreversible but there is much evidence to show that pulmonary rehabilitation, including exercise, may improve functional capacity and QoL. Common pharmacotherapies include bronchodilators (ß2-adrenoreceptor agonists, anticholinergics, methylxanthines), inhaled corticosteroids and oxygen therapy (Carlin et al 2009). Respiratory strengthening exercises may also be beneficial (Lacasse et al 2006), and exercise as tolerated is recommended to improve functional capacity, reduce dyspnea and reduce anxiety and depression associated with COPD.

Patients with EIA or EIB may undergo pharmacological or indirect testing to confirm a diagnosis of EIA/EIB. For example, inhaled powdered mannitol, nebulised hypertonic saline or AMP appear to be effective for diagnosing EIA amongst athletes and recreational exercisers as these tests reflect the level of inflammation in the airways (Rundell & Slee 2008). Guidelines that diagnose EIA/EIB on the basis of respiratory function after an exercise challenge

Table 4.3 BODE index

Variable	Points on BODE Index			
	0	1	2	3
FEV$_1$ (% predicted)	≥ 65	50 – 64	36 – 49	≤ 35
6 min walk test (m)	≥ 350	250 – 349	150 – 249	≤ 149
MMRC dyspnea scale	0 – 1	2	3	4
BMI	> 21	≤ 21		

Note: BODE, BMI, air flow obstruction, dyspnea and exercise capacity; FEV$_1$, forced expiratory volume in 1 second; MMRC scale, Modified Medical Research Council scale; BMI, body mass index.

(Source: adapted from ACSM 2010)

are clearly defined. Post-exercise decreases in FEV$_1$ between 10–20% have been used (Rundell & Slee 2008). Both the American Thoracic Society and the European Respiratory Society recommend a >10% decrease in FEV$_1$, based on two standard deviations from the mean baseline FEV$_1$ in a healthy population, as a criterion for EIA/EIB. The ACSM recommends a fall in FEV$_1$ of > 15% (Thompson et al 2010). The usual exercise challenge is of a relatively high intensity exercise bout (80–90% maximum heart rate) of 6–8 minutes duration, in ambient conditions of 20–25 degrees Celsius with relative humidity < 50%. Spirometry is conducted pre- and post-exercise. However, this exercise intensity may not identify all EIA/EIB sufferers and some researchers have found that exercise at 95% of predicted maximum heart rate produces a greater fall in FEV$_1$ (Carlsen et al 2000). It is likely that higher V$_E$ at greater workloads affects the onset of EIA/EIB symptoms, suggesting that there should be changes to the standardisation of exercise intensities for EIA/EIB testing protocols.

Cystic fibrosis — diagnosis, treatment and pharmacology

CF patients on average make 4.7 clinic visits per year and are admitted to the hospital at least once per year (Cystic Fibrosis Foundation [CF Foundation] 2001). In 1970 only 10% of patients on the Fibrosis Foundation Patient Registry were > 18 years of age, while in 2000 38.7% of patients were > 18 years. In the USA, the Caucasian population has a CF carrier rate of 1 in 25 and an incidence of 1 in 2500 live births (CF Foundation 2001). 70% of CF patients are diagnosed by the age of 1 year (CF Foundation 2001). The most useful diagnostic test remains the sweat test, a quantitative pilocarpine iontophoresis test in which electrolytes are measured in collected sweat. Sodium chloride concentration above 50 mEq/L (children) or 60 mEq/L (adults) is regarded as a positive result for CF. Diagnosis is confirmed by the documentation of CFTR dysfunction through mutation analysis.

Treatment for patients with CF is indicated in the literature to be most successful when a multidisciplinary model approach is followed. This approach would include a physician, nurse, respiratory therapist, dietitian and a social worker (Yankaskas et al 2004). In CF patients, the pulmonary status of the patients should be regularly monitored and assessed. Spirometry, specifically FEV$_1$, and oxygen saturation should form the basis of these assessments. The treatment of patients with CF includes antibiotic therapy for pulmonary exacerbations, chronic suppressive therapy, airway clearance (inclined chest tapping or percussion) and exercise, therapy with mucolytic agents, bronchodilators and anti-inflammatory agents, supplemental oxygen, and nutritional support (Davis et al 1996; Marshall & Samuelson 1998).

A variety of airway clearance techniques are available, which include conventional chest physiotherapy (CPT), active cycle breathing, forced expiratory technique, positive expiratory pressure (PEP) devices, autogenic drainage, and high frequency chest wall oscillation systems. A meta-analysis suggests that CPT resulted in greater sputum production than no treatment, and that the addition of exercise improved FEV$_1$. No other differences between different modalities were found (Thomas et al 1995). Physical activity has been indicated to help with airway clearance by increasing sputum clearance (Zach et al 1981; Bradley & Moran 2008) and preventing a decline in pulmonary function (Schneiderman-Walker et al 2000). In order to prescribe physical activity or exercise to patients with CF, clinical exercise testing should be performed.

RESTRICTIVE LUNG CONDITIONS

Restrictive respiratory disorders are not as prevalent as COPD, and are more variable. They include interstitial lung diseases (asbestosis, silicosis, fibrosis), organic and drug inhalation injuries, kyphoscoliosic restrictions to breathing, chronic infections, neoplastic disorders, connective tissue diseases and pulmonary haemorrhagic syndromes (Romer 2009; Carlin et al 2009). The common factor among these conditions is abnormal lung mechanics, where the lung is unable to expand normally, and the lung parenchyma, pleura and thoracic cage may be affected (Romer 2009; Carlin et al 2009).

Typically the volume of air entering the lungs is restricted. Total lung capacity (TLC) is reduced, defined by forced vital capacity (FVC), and functional residual capacity (FRC) and residual volume (RV) are lower than normal. Diffusing capacity is low and exercise-induced hypoxemia occurs early in the development of restrictive lung conditions. Flow limitation is usually not a problem unless the restrictive condition is also combined with COPD, for example from cigarette smoking. Exercise-induced hypoxemia occurs from the mismatch between ventilation and perfusion, which is due to the increase in alveolar dead space ventilation. The dead-space ventilation is caused by: (1) an increase in the ventilation rate during exercise, leading to rapid shallow breathing, often in excess of 50 breaths per minute; (2) low breathing reserve, increasing the work of breathing; and (3) a reduced lung capillary bed surface area due to either tissue damage (eg: asbestosis), or reduced capillary bed recruitment (eg: pulmonary hypertension).

Interstitial lung diseases (ILD) involve pathology of the lung parenchyma, and the lung becomes stiff and non-compliant, with reduced elasticity. The lung function testing criteria for ILD is reduced TLC with a normal ration of FEV_1 to FVC (Romer 2009). The reduced diffusion capacity and hypoxemia may not be apparent unless the patient is exercising, and there is reduced pulmonary transit time for oxygen delivery (Harris-Eze et al 1996). Patients who are prescribed corticosteroids and immunosuppressants may also suffer from drug-induced myopathy, which contributes to fatigue.

In assessing the scale of breathing restriction, chest radiographs may be useful for assessing the structure of the lung wall and thorax, possible kyphoses, lung volume and the presence of abnormalities (alveolar, pleural or interstitial). High resolution CT scans may assess interstitial changes, and pulse oximetry and arterial blood gas sampling are helpful to determine the degree of gas exchange abnormality (Carlin et al 2009). Pulmonary function tests typically show decreases in FVC, FEV_1 and TLC, with no change or a possible increase in the FEV_1/FVC ratio (Romer 2009; Carlin et al 2009). Patients with interstitial fibrosis may show a low diffusing capacity, and neuromuscular diseases may reduce maximal inspiratory and expiratory pressures (Carlin et al 2009; Holland & Hill 2008).

A kyphosis is a skeletal abnormality that may result in physical lung restriction. Although primary kyphotic curves are normal for humans, an abnormal kyphosis, hyperkyphosis or problematic kyphosis may be referred to as kyphotic (Bloomfield et al 1994; Magee 2008) and several different descriptions are used for a kyphotic posture. To be classified with a thoracic kyphosis (increased flexion) a person must have an excessive curvature, typically in the thoracic spine (Kendall et al 2005). This abnormal (primary) curve of the thoracic spine is often referred to as a 'round back' or 'rounded shouldered posture' (Norris 2008). In other cases hunchbacks or humpbacks (also known as gibbus with an anterior wedging of vertebrae and normal pelvic inclination −30°) could be also the cause of kyphosis (Magee 2008). Dowager's hump is associated with height reduction, especially in postmenopausal women (Magee 2008). Kyphosis normally involves the thoracic spine, but can also occur in the lumbar spine or cervical spine (Kendall et al 2005). Normal kyphotic curves are between 20–50 degrees, bigger than 50 degrees are hyperkyphotic (Fon et al 1980; Stricker 2002).

For the treatment of kyphosis, it is important to distinguish between the different types of kyphosis. Postural kyphosis is abnormality due to poor postural behaviour like slouching, and appears usually between 9 and 12 years of age (Dommisse 1998; Stricker 2002). Postural kyphosis is usually within normal ranges (radiologically), but is accompanied with a flattened anterior chest. Because it does not involve the ossification of the vertebrae it can be corrected by physical activity, a conscious effort, or exercise (Dommisse 1998; Walker 2009). A 'round back' is the result of tight muscle groups for long periods of time (Magee 2002).

Congenital or primary kyphosis (not linked to any other cause) refers to a person born with hyperkyphotic curve, possibly accompanied with heart and kidney problems (Dommisse 1998). Another form of primary structural kyphosis is juvenile kyphosis, also referred to as Scheuermann's disease (Murray et al 1993). Because of faster growth in the posterior sections of the vertebrae, the vertebral bodies appeared to be more wedge-shape than normal. There is an anterior wedging of more than 5 degrees, within more than three contiguous vertebrae and at least 5 degrees per vertebrae with a curve of more than 50 degrees (Loder 2001). Scheuermann's disease normally appears in the mid-thoracic and thoracolumbar areas (Dommisse 1998), and is accompanied by Schmorl's nodes (small disc herniations). The onset of Scheuermann's disease appears during the adolescent growth spurt and increases with age up to 20 degrees in childhood, 25 degrees in adolescence, and 40 degrees in adulthood (Wenger & Frick 1999; Dommisse 1998; Hinman 2004). It is possible that genetic factors are responsible for the onset of the condition (Wenger & Frick 1999).

Hyperkyphosis is associated with ineffective pulmonary function and pulmonary death (Kado et al 2004, 2005) due to the inability of the chest wall to comply with the breathing demands (Kendall et al 2005). The normal function of other internal organs (Ehrman et al 2009) may also be restricted. Breathing patterns differ in children (abdominally), women (upper thoracic), men (upper and lower thoracic) and in older adults (lower thoracic and abdominal area) (Magee 2008). As the rounding of shoulders is taking place, the neck and head are moved in a forward position. Kyphosis does have a restrictive nature and the depressed chest will affect the intercostals spaces and action of accessory muscles. The upper and lateral fibres of internal oblique, the shoulder adductors and pectoralis minor are tightened. On the other hand, the thoracic spine extensors, middle trapezius and lower trapezius are lengthened. See Chapter 11, case study 2, for further consideration of thoracic hyperkyphosis.

EXERCISE AND RESPIRATORY CONDITIONS

Exercise testing for COPD (bronchitis, emphysema) and asthma

Patients with mild to moderate COPD may not present any symptoms of the disease until an increased demand is placed on the respiratory system. However, patients with severe disease may have such a reduced functional capacity that even simple ADL are difficult. Exercise testing can be used to detect the extent of COPD effects on heart rate, blood pressure, aerobic capacity, oxygen uptake, oxygen saturation, ventilation, lactate, muscle strength, flexibility and dyspnea (Rundell & Slee 2008). Clinical exercise testing guidelines from the ACSM and AACVPR should be followed (Thompson et al 2010). Lung function tests (FVC, FEV_1, FEV_1/FVC ratio, PEF_{25-75}, PEFR, TLC) should be performed prior to exercise testing. Patients who normally take bronchodilators should take their medication before starting an exercise test (Ong et al 2004). Patients with severe COPD who require supplemental oxygen during ADL and for exercise, should be tested using an elevated fraction of inspired oxygen that equates with the flow rate provided by their supplementary oxygen. Contraindications to exercise testing include unstable cardiac conditions (eg: unstable angina); severe hypoxemia; orthopaedic conditions that restrict exercise; neurological impairment and psychiatric disorders. Appropriate modes of exercise testing are shown in Table 4.4.

Exercise prescription for COPD

COPD patients suffer from varying degrees of exercise intolerance, and the airflow limitation greatly increases the work of breathing during exercise. Exercise-induced dyspnea, hypercapnea and hypoxemia will limit exercise capacity, and pulmonary function should be maximised with pharmacotherapy during exercise (Carlin et al 2009). Despite these limitations, a meta-analysis of 31 randomised controlled trials (RCTs)

Table 4.4 Exercise testing recommendations and guidelines for COPD

Clinical test	Mode	Protocols	Clinical measures
Cardiovascular	Treadmill Cycle 6MWT MST Step	8–12 min duration GXT using small increments (ramped cycle 10, 15 or 20 W/stage; TM 1–2 METs/stage) Incremental step test, 2 min step test or Queen's College step test	HR, 12 lead ECG BP RPE, RPD O_2 saturation Peak VO_2 Ventilation and gas exchange Blood lactate Distance or power
Strength	Isokinetic 3 or 5RM Sit to stand Wall or floor push-ups Modified sit-up test Hand grip strength	3, 5 or 10RM Reps per 30 sec or per min Kg per hand	Peak torque 3, 5 or 10RM Maximum number of reps or to fatigue Kg
Flexibility	Sit and reach Goniometer Apley's shoulder test Balance Gait analysis	Hip, hamstring and lower back flexibility Shoulder flexibility Stork stand or postural sway test	Range of motion, coordination, balance and motor control

Note: MST = Modified Shuttle Test; GXT = Graded Exercise Test; TM = Treadmill.
(Source: adapted from Swank et al 2009; ACSM 2010)

reviewed for the Cochrane Collaboration found that rehabilitation exercise training significantly improved QoL, functional capacity and maximal exercise capacity (Barnes & Wellington 2003; Lacasse et al 2008). While the effect of the exercise intervention depends on the severity of the COPD, there is overwhelming evidence that exercise is a vital part of pulmonary rehabilitation. Quality of life, dyspnea, anxiety and depression, mastery and self-efficacy, fatigue, aerobic exercise tolerance and strength are all significantly improved by exercise training (Lacasse et al 2008).

Lung function testing should be conducted before the prescription of exercise (Cooper 2001; Carlin et al 2009), as inspiratory capacity is a measure of hyperinflation and correlates with dyspnea and exercise capacity. An electrocardiogram (ECG) should also be conducted to determine if cardiac diseases are also present. A pulse oximeter is recommended during any exercise with COPD patients, as hypoxemia may occur. ACSM also suggest that haemoglobin be measured to determine the duration of hypoxemia. The ATS and ACSM state that stage 11 and 111 patients (see Tables 4.2 and 4.3) have significant impairment to airflow, QoL and exercise tolerance, and are thus at risk of early onset of hypoxemia and fatigue. Both ventilatory and peripheral muscles may fatigue during exercise, as skeletal muscle exercise endurance is limited by muscle wasting and peripheral oxygen delivery, and ventilatory muscles reduce in strength. Muscle biopsies have shown reduced type 1 oxidative fibres and increased type 2 glycolytic fibres in COPD patients (Casaburi 2001; Storer 2001), suggesting an earlier onset of anaerobic threshold and fatigue (Casaburi 2001; Kim et al 2008). Furthermore COPD patients show an increased inflammatory response with hypoxia, and therefore an increase in reactive oxygen species, combined with muscle atrophy, altered muscle substrate metabolism, reduced oxidative enzyme activity, and reduced capillary density, all suggestive of skeletal muscle dysfunction (Bernard et al 1998).

Exercise guidelines proposed by ACSM, AHA, AACVPR and similar groups suggest that a *minimum* of three exercise sessions per week is sufficient to improve functional capacity in COPD patients, and that five or more sessions per week may provide superior benefits. Ideally, an exercise regime should incorporate aerobic or endurance-type exercise, strength training and flexibility training. Cochrane reviews also suggest that home-based exercise programs, as well as fitness centre or clinically supervised exercise sessions, are capable of improving health and fitness in COPD patients (Lacasse et al 2007; Romer 2009).

The thresholds for determining exercise intensity with COPD include the extent of skeletal muscular deconditioning, onset of anaerobic threshold, dyspnea and ventilatory limitations (eg: hypoventilation, hypercapnia, hypoxemia), cardiovascular limitations (eg: tachycardia, ischaemia, hypertension, pulmonary oedema) and the extent of anxiety and fear of exercising. Evidence suggests that chronic responses to exercise in COPD patients depend upon the initial fitness status of the patient, the extent of COPD, and the use of bronchodilators and supplemental oxygen (Garrod et al 2008). Regular aerobic exercise will increase VO_{2peak}, maximal work rate, 6 minute walk test (6MWT) time, anaerobic and lactate thresholds, exercise efficiency, motor unit recruitment, whilst reducing resting and sub-maximal exercise heart rates, resting and sub-maximal exercise blood pressure, rate of perceived exertion, dyspnea, minute ventilation and anxiety (Bourjeily & Rochester 2000; Butcher & Jones 2006; Garrod et al 2008; Nakamura et al 2008). Interval training is recommended for severely de-conditioned COPD patients (Butcher & Jones 2006; Puhan et al 2006; Varga et al 2007) with a goal of increasing exercise tolerance to the point where steady state aerobic exercise can be maintained. In fact, high intensity, short intervals of training have resulted in significant improvements in aerobic capacity and exercise tolerance, with no oxygen desaturation in many patients with mild to moderate COPD (Butcher & Jones 2006; Puhan et al 2006; Arnardottir et al 2007).

Evidence-based guidelines advise the use of resistance training to increase or maintain lean muscle mass, including respiratory muscles such as the intercostals and diaphragm (Bernard et al 1998; Storer 2001; Nici et al 2006; Ries 2008), and flexibility training is also advised to maintain joint range of motion and coordination (Crowe et al 2005; Geddes et al 2008; Nelson et al 2007). There is recent evidence to support the use of inspirational muscle training (IMT) to reduce dyspnea and improve exercise capacity (Ambrosino & Strambi 2004; Gosselink 2004; Reid et al 2008; Decramer 2009) especially when used in conjunction with an exercise program, but Ries (2008) stated that there was not enough evidence to recommend that IMT be used as an essential part of pulmonary rehabilitation. There is no optimal protocol for exercise prescription for COPD (Butcher & Jones 2006) but current guidelines for healthy older adults (Nelson et al 2007) and reviews (Lacasse et al 2008; Puhan et al 2005a, 2008; O'Shea et al 2004; Storer 2001) provide a sound physiological base to prescribe exercise programs. This evidence suggests that strength training 2–3 times per week, with 1–3 sets of 8–10 repetitions is safe and will also produce significant improvements in patients with mild or moderate COPD (O'Shea et al 2004; Puhan et al 2005b). Guidelines suggest using intensities varying between 50–85% of 1RM (Storer 2001), but patients with severe COPD may be more limited. Other studies recommend the use of therabands, machine weights for patients with poor muscular control, body weight, free weights and aqua resistance.

Exercise prescription for asthma

A meta-analysis of physical training for asthmatics by the Cochrane Collaboration (Ram et al 2005; Robinson et al 2005) found that habitual physical activity increased cardiopulmonary fitness (VO_{2peak}, maximum work rate, maximum heart rate, maximum ventilation) but lung function was not improved. The authors noted that many patients reported that asthmatic symptoms were reduced when they were fitter, but the physiological basis for these claims has not been substantiated. However there is evidence that regular exercise lowers the minute ventilation of mild and moderate exercise, which may delay the onset of exercise-induced asthma (EIA), and exercise may also reduce the perception of breathlessness, possibly by strengthening the respiratory muscles (Ram et al 2005; Robinson et al 2005; Garrod et al 2008).

The consensus in the literature and from the ATS and ACSM is that asthma patients should avoid obvious environmental triggers when exercising (such as dust, cold dry air, and air pollutants) and should use their prescribed medications as directed by their physician (Thompson et al 2010). To reduce the risk of EIA, patients should use inhaled bronchodilator therapy (2 to 4 puffs) 15 minutes before starting to exercise, and should warm up gradually at a low to moderate intensity for at least 10 minutes (Anderson & Kippelen 2008; Rundell & Slee 2008). As sustained exertion tends to produce asthma symptoms, short intense intervals of exercise may not bring on EIA. Exercise testing is therefore very important to diagnose EIA, as the onset of symptoms may vary between chronic asthma due to purely environmental triggers, and actual EIA. EIA is usually diagnosed with pulmonary testing, a decrease in FEV_1 or PEF rate of $\geq 15\%$ following a steady state exercise challenge (McFadden & Gilbert 1994; Rundell & Slee 2008). The exercise protocols include both treadmill and cycle, with a work rate preferably 80–90% of the client's predicted VO_{2max} or maximum heart rate (McFadden & Gilbert 1994; Rundell & Slee 2008), and lasting 6–8 minutes. Ideally relative humidity should be < 50% with temperatures between 20–25 degrees Celsius.

There is overwhelming evidence that regular exercise, be it recreational activities or sports, improves functional capacity and QoL for asthmatics, and that people with mild to moderate asthma are not limited by the type of exercise they can do (Robinson et al 2005). Swimming or aqua exercise is recommended because the air is often warmer and moister, thus avoiding the asthma trigger of cold, dry air. Barnes and Wellington (2003), and Ambrosino and Strambi (2004), also reviewed inspiratory muscle training studies, and found that the subjects showed significant improvements in maximum inspiratory pressure, but for other outcomes (inspiratory muscle endurance, asthma symptoms, medication use, acute exacerbations) the findings were less clear. Oxygen supplementation during exercise was also recommended for severe asthmatics, because it reduced desaturation during exercise, allowing higher exercise intensity and increased exercise tolerance (Ambrosino & Strambi 2004; Nonoyama et al 2007)

Exercise testing for CF

Lung function has often been viewed as the 'golden standard' for measuring pulmonary disease and expected outcome (including in CF patients), however, it is not possible or accurate to predict exercise tolerance or functional ability of people with CF from lung function results (Balfour-Lynn et al 1998). The most accurate tests are VO_{2peak} measurements performed in appropriate laboratories with exhaled air analysis and treadmill or bicycle ergometry. Informal field tests like the modified shuttle test (MST) and the 6-minute walk test (6MWT) are inexpensive to implement and some evidence suggests that children with CF prefer the field tests above the clinical settings (Selvadurai et al 2003). The MST test has been validated in both children (Rodgers et al 2002) and adults (Bradley et al 1999) with CF. The MST test is indicated to be complementary to lung function testing and applicable when formal laboratory exercise testing is not possible (Cox et al 2006). Results obtained from formal and/or informal exercise testing will enable the clinical exercise therapist to prescribe an appropriate training program, however, these training programs may be erroneous due to exacerbation of inflammation in the lungs.

Exercise prescription for CF

Appropriate regular physical exercise enhances cardiovascular fitness, increases functional capacity and improves QoL (Yankaskas et al 2004). Regular physical activity has also been indicated to improve pulmonary gas exchange, exercise capacity and overall clinical condition. A study by Nixon et al (2001) who compared habitual physical activity and aerobic fitness in 30 children and adolescents with CF with healthy control subjects found CF subjects to be smaller and less fit than the controls. CF subjects participated in less vigorous exercise than the control subjects. Unstructured physical activity may also be applied to improve functional capacity in patients with CF: A study from Ireland indicated that children with CF use trampolining as an adjunct to regular physiotherapy (Curran & Mahony 2008).

Although considerable variation has been found in the results of exercise intervention on the variables determined in persons living with CF, exercise has increased the work capacity, cardiorespiratory fitness, ventilatory muscle endurance and immune function. Increased exercise has not improved pulmonary function, but has reduced the deterioration of lung function, thus improving QoL and activities for daily living (Orenstein et al 2004).

Results obtained from exercise interventions are dependent on compliance and intensities of training, with the best results obtained with supervised programs (Orenstein et al 2004; Bradley & Moran 2008). Cardiovascular training resulted in significantly better peak aerobic capacity, activity levels and QoL after a 1 month intervention of in-hospital patients (Selvadurai et al 2002). A 6-month aerobic and resistance training program indicated that pulmonary function improved with endurance training, but not with resistance training (Sahlberg et al 2008). A systematic review investigating oxygen therapy for cystic fibrosis reported that oxygen supplementation during exercise improved oxygenation, but mild hypercapnia resulted. Participants with oxygen therapy were also able to exercise for significant longer duration, but other exercise parameters were not altered (Elphick & Mallory 2009).

Additional to aerobic exercise, patients with CF should also perform resistance exercise. Patients with CF showed decreased muscle strength, abdominal strength, arm, shoulder and quadriceps muscle strength (Sahlberg et al 2005). Children with CF who received resistance training indicated an improved weight gain (total mass, as well as fat free mass), lung function and leg strength

compared to the aerobically trained children with CF (Selvadurai et al 2002) during in-hospital exercise and 1 month after discharge. Due to the effect of muscle wasting in CF and the consequent loss of muscle function, a pilot study investigated the effect of whole-body vibration on muscle function of adult patients with CF (Rietschel et al 2008). The results indicated that significant improvements were only observed in a chair-rising test and one and two leg jumps with no changes in the pulmonary function tests.

A systematic review on RCTs with the focus of improving pulmonary function and fitness in children (van Doorn 2009) reported a significant improvement in pulmonary function for short-term in-hospital aerobic and strength interventions. Significant strength gains were also found from strength training interventions. The findings are, however, limited due to only four RCTs meeting the inclusion criteria. A review of CF training studies for the Cochrane Collaboration by Bradley and Moran (2008) found that a mixed model approach to exercise prescription (aerobic plus strength training) produced improvements in exercise capacity and QoL, but that results were inconsistent across studies.

Although total body exercises are often prescribed for persons with CF, specific training of the respiratory muscles is also a recommended training approach. The production of thick tenacious secretions in the airways places an increased demand on the inspiratory muscles of CF patients. These secretions cause an increase in the airway resistance and higher minute ventilation due to ventilation-perfusion mismatch (Pinet et al 2003). A decrease in nutritional intake due to pancreatic insufficiency and an ongoing catabolic state because of chronic infection can lead to a loss of muscle mass (Pinet et al 2003). Similar to limb muscle, inspiratory muscle can be trained in people with COPD (Reid & Samrai 1995; Geddes et al 2008). Results from a systematic review (Reid et al 2008) found only two RCTs. One study found a significant increase in inspiratory muscle strength and endurance (de Jong et al 2001) while the other study did not measure inspiratory muscle endurance (Enright et al 2004). Lack of RCTs together with small sample sizes makes it impossible to draw a conclusion (Houston et al 2008). Differences in respiratory muscle strength in adolescents and adult patients with CF indicated that female CF patients showed more impaired lung function than male patients (Dunnink et al 2009).

Behavioural interventions for CF

Management and treatment of CF has improved in past decades, and physical training, airway clearance and conventional physiotherapy have been shown to increase QoL, exercise capacity and dyspnea (Bradley et al 2005; Houston et al 2008). More specifically, aerobic exercise and strength training can improve aerobic capacity, muscle strength and endurance, flexibility, coordination, onset of fatigue and body composition (Gruber et al 2008; Bradley et al 2005; Houston et al 2008). Some studies have shown improved pulmonary function (TLC, FEV_1), although much of the literature does not support these improvements (Houston et al 2008). Most research suggests that long-term training provides more substantial improvements in health, fitness and QoL (Bradley et al 2005; Bradley & Moran 2008; Gruber et al 2008).

Exercise testing for restrictive respiratory conditions

As with COPD, lung function tests should be performed on patients with restrictive pulmonary conditions, and exercise testing will determine the effects of restriction during exertions. Most restrictive lung diseases produce an abnormal exercise response. Interstitial lung conditions will primarily produce gas exchange abnormalities, but neuromuscular weaknesses may result in the inability to increase ventilation with exercise (Holland & Hill 2008; Carlin et al 2009). All restrictive lung diseases will show a reduced FVC and TLC (Carlin et al 2009). Decreased lung volumes result in a collapse of smaller airway units and a decrease in the functional alveolar-capillary interface, thus leading to reduced gas exchange, as well as reduced diffusion capacity. Chronic inflammation of the interstitium and alveoli leads to fibrosis, reduced lung compliance and increased lung stiffness (Carlin et al 2009).

During exercise testing (see Table 4.4), it is common to note dyspnea, reduced VO_{2peak}, reduced work rate, reduced V_T with increased respiratory rates at sub-maximal workloads, increased dead space ventilation, and arterial oxygen desaturation combined with unchanged $PaCO_2$ during exercise. Patients will breathe in rapid, shallow breaths during exercise. Hypoxemia may also occur as a result of vasoconstriction, pulmonary hypertension and destruction of pulmonary vascular beds (Holland & Hill 2008). Patients with neuromuscular conditions will be restricted due to muscular limitations, and their gas exchange will be normal. However their tidal volume will not increase with exercise although their ventilatory rate will increase until it reaches its limits at the end of exercise. Patients with pleural conditions or a kyphosis will have a similar response. The choice of a cardiorespiratory exercise test will depend on the extent of the patient's limitations. For example, the 6MWT may be a more functional and appropriate walking test than an incremental treadmill test for patients who are severely restricted. Strength tests will be affected by neuromuscular conditions, and patients with thoracic or kyphotic abnormalities may have difficulty with some flexibility tests.

Exercise prescription for restrictive respiratory conditions

Restrictive pulmonary conditions will limit exercise capacity because of the inability of the lung to expand normally. There is a mismatch between ventilation and perfusion, exercise-induced hypoxemia, an increase in ventilatory rate, and possibly there may be pulmonary hypertension (Cooper & Storer 2009). While airflow is usually not impeded, lung elasticity and recoil is affected. Thus, restrictive pulmonary patients will have a low exercise capacity, an increased breathing rate, dyspnea and hypoxemia. Patients with pulmonary hypertension may also have associated cardiac and hypertensive conditions (Holland & Hill 2008; Cooper & Storer 2009), with disturbances in ventilatory control. A meta-analysis of restrictive respiratory exercise rehabilitation by the Cochrane Collaboration (Holland & Hill 2008) found that exercise produced no adverse effects and improved 6MWT distance, dyspnea, maximal ventilation and QoL. However, there was insufficient data to establish: (a) whether maximal exercise capacity was significantly improved; (b) the effects of exercise training on patients with severe interstitial lung disease and desaturation; and (c) the long-term effects of exercise on restrictive disease patients. Furthermore, most of the reviewed studies examined only aerobic training, and there was little data on the effects of strength training for restrictive pulmonary patients. ACSM and AACVPR guidelines suggest that exercise should be combined with other components of rehabilitation such as education and self-management (Effing et al 2007); regular patient assessment (lung function testing, body composition, QoL surveys); nutritional intervention; pharmacological intervention (Cooper & Storer 2009); and medically prescribed supplemental oxygen (Thompson et al 2010). Self-management may include breathing techniques to improve respiratory muscle strength, inspiratory mouth pressure and work capacity (Budweiser et al 2006; Holland & Hill 2008). To date, the general exercise recommendations for restrictive pulmonary disease are similar to those for COPD, with the additional warning that higher intensity exercise is probably not suitable for patients who de-saturate heavily. Therefore, low to moderate intensity aerobic exercise, including interval training, low to moderate intensity resistance training, flexibility training and ventilatory muscle training may be included.

For kyphotic conditions, research suggests that deep breathing exercises will help stretch intercostals and upper parts of abdominal muscles (eg: pursed lips breathing) (Kendall et al 2005; Norris 2008). Strengthening of the thoracic spine extensors, middle and lower trapezius (Kendall et al 2005; Norris 2008) and stretch (if shortened) the pectoralis minor, shoulder adductors, and internal rotators (Kendall et al 2005; Norris 2008) may also assist in improved breathing.

Because of the fear of breathlessness during effective respiratory exercises, the practitioner must ensure confidence and cooperation from the patient whilst training respiratory muscles for strength and endurance. Relaxation therapy has several advantages such as a decrease in oxygen consumption, deeper breathing to prevent dyspnea and a decrease in the overuse of accessory muscles (Kendall et al 2005). Lung volumes could be influenced negatively by the imbalance of muscle structures because of a poor posture. The exercise practitioner must also give attention to the improvement of general health, coordination and optimal body composition (Kendall et al 2005) to assist in patient rehabilitation. In a summary of recommendations for pulmonary rehabilitation, Ries (2008) advised a 12-week rehabilitation program (more effective than 6 weeks) and strongly recommended strength training for the upper body, as well as endurance training, as part of the program.

Contraindications and precautions

Contraindications for exercise in clients with obstructive and restrictive respiratory conditions are:

- diagnosed cardiovascular symptoms such as severe angina, recent myocardial infarction, uncontrolled hypertension, atrial or ventricular fibrillation, right heart failure, congestive heart failure, severe aortic stenosis, uncontrolled arrhythmias, presence of thrombi, active or suspected myocarditis or pericarditis
- uncontrolled metabolic disease
- pulmonary symptoms at rest.

Precautions: clients with these conditions concurrent with obstructive or restrictive respiratory disease may exercise with caution:

- intermittent claudication
- two or more of the ACSM risk factors for cardiovascular disease (ACSM 2010), such as diagnosed cardiovascular disease, smoking, obesity, hyperlipidemia, hypertension, a family history of heart disease, a sedentary lifestyle
- pulmonary symptoms at rest, such as oxygen desaturation below 88%, dyspnea, hyperventilation, hypoventilation
- asthmatic symptoms, such as breathlessness, chest constriction and wheezing, and severe environmental triggers for asthma
- neuromuscular, neurological or musculoskeletal conditions that are exacerbated by exercise
- significant or severe emotional or mental conditions, such as psychosis or acute anxiety.

Summary of key lessons

- Respiratory diseases include obstructive and restrictive pulmonary diseases and conditions.

- Chronic obstructive pulmonary diseases (COPD) include chronic bronchitis, emphysema, cystic fibrosis and obstructive bronchiolitis. Asthma is a reversible obstructive and inflammatory condition.

- Restrictive pulmonary conditions include interstitial lung diseases (eg: asbestosis, silicosis), chronic infections, sarcoidosis, neoplastic disorders, vascular disorders, drug injury, fibrotic disorders and kyphosis.

- Pulmonary rehabilitation is multidisciplinary and includes patient assessment, disease and self-management, exercise training, pharmacological interventions, breathing techniques and nutritional education.

- Lung function testing (spirometry) should be conducted before the prescription of exercise, in conjunction with assessment of functional capacity (aerobic, strength, flexibility), to determine exercise tolerance.

- Evidence suggests that mixed-model exercise programs (aerobic, strength and flexibility) will improve functional capacity, dyspnea, QoL and exercise tolerance.

REFERENCES

Ambrosino N, Strambi S (2004) New strategies to improve exercise tolerance in chronic obstructive pulmonary disease. *European Respiratory Journal*, 24:313–22

American College of Sports Medicine (ACSM) (2010) *ACSM's Resource Manual for Guidelines for Exercise Testing and Prescription* (6th ed). Philadelphia: Wolters Kluwer: Lippincott Williams & Wilkins

Anderson G (2006) Current issues with beta2-adrenoceptor agonists: pharmacology and molecular and cellular mechanisms. *Clinical Review of Allergy and Immunology*, 31(2,3):119–30

Anderson S, Holzer K (2000) Exercise-induced asthma: is it the right diagnosis in elite athletes? *Journal of Allergy and Clinical Immunology*, 106(3):419–28

Anderson S, Kippelen P (2008) Airway injury as a mechanism for exercise-induced bronchocosntriction in elite athletes. *Journal of Allergy and Clinical Immunology*, 122(2):225–35

Arnardottir R, Boman G, Larsson K, et al (2007) Interval training compared with continuous training in patients with COPD. *Respiratory Medicine*, 101:1196–204

Australian Centre for Asthma Monitoring (2006) *Asthma and chronic obstructive pulmonary disease among older people in Australia* (Report No. ACM 7). Canberra: Australian Institute of Health and Welfare. Cat. No. ACM 7 ISBN-13 9781 74024 6064

—— (2008) *Asthma in Australia 2008*. Australian Institute for Health and Welfare (AIHW) Asthma Series no. 3. Cat. no. ACM 14. Canberra: AIHW

Barnes N, Wellington S (2003) Inspiratory training for asthma. *Cochrane Database of Systematic Reviews*, (1):1–23

Baroffio M, Barisione G, Crimi E, et al (2009) Noninflammatory mechanisms of airway hyper-responsiveness in bronchial asthma: an overview. *Therapeutic Advances in Respiratory Disease*, 3:163–74

Bernard S, LeBlanc P, Whittom F, et al (1998) Peripheral muscle weakness in patients with chronic obstructive pulmonary disease. *American Journal of Respiratory and Critical Care Medicine*, 158(2):896–901

Bloomfield J, Ackland T, Elliot B (1994) *Applied Anatomy and Biomechanics in Sport*. Melbourne: Blackwell Scientific Publications, p 374

Bourjeily G, Rochester C (2000) Exercise training in chronic obstructive pulmonary disease. *Clinical Chest Medicine*, 21(4):763–81

Bradley J, Howard J, Wallace E, et al (1999) Validity of a modified shuttle test in adult cystic fibrosis. *Thorax*, 54: 437–9

Bradley J, Moran F (2008) Physical training for cystic fibrosis. *Cochrane Database of Systematic Reviews*, (1):1–52

Bradley J, Moran F, Elborn J (2005) Evidence for physical therapies (airway clearance and physical training) in cystic fibrosis: an overview of five Cochrane systematic reviews. *Respiratory Medicine*, 100:191–201

Budweiser S, Moertl M, Jorres R, et al (2006) Respiratory muscle training in restrictive thoracic disease: a randomized controlled trial. *Archives of Physical Medicine and Rehabilitation*, 87:1559–1565

Butcher S, Jones R (2006) The impact of exercise training intensity on changes in physiological function in patients with chronic obstructive pulmonary disease. *Sports Medicine*, 36(4):307–25

Carlin B, Bigdeli G, Kaplan, P (2009) Diagnostic procedures in patients with pulmonary diseases. In: DeJong A, J Ehrman (eds), *ACSM's Resource Manual for Guidelines for Exercise Testing and Prescription* (6th ed). Baltimore, ML: Wolters Kluwer: Lippincott Williams & Wilkins, pp 375–90

Carlsen K, Engh G, & Mork, M (2000) Exercise-induced bronchoconstriction depends on exercise load. *Respiratory Medicine*, 94:750–5

Casaburi R (2001) Skeletal muscle dysfunction in chronic obstructive pulmonary disease. *Medicine and Science in Sports and Exercise*, 33 (7, Suppl):S662–70

Cooper C, Storer T (2009) Exercise prescription in patients with pulmonary disease. In: Swain D, Ehrman J (eds), *ACSM's resource Manual for Guidelines for Exercise Testing and Prescription* (6th ed). Baltimore, ML: Wolters Kluwer: Lippincott Williams and Wilkins, pp 575–99

Cooper P (2001) Exercise in chronic pulmonary disease: aerobic exercise prescription. *Medicine and Science in Sports and Exercise*, 33(7, Suppl):S671–9

—— (2001) Exercise in chronic pulmonary disease: limitations and rehabilitation. *Medicine and Science in Sports and Exercise*, 33(7, Suppl):S643–6

Cox N, Follett J, McKay, K (2006) Modified shuttle test performance in hospitalized children and adolescents with cystic fibrosis. *Journal of Cystic Fibrosis*, 5:165–70

Crowe J, Reid W, Geddes E, et al (2005) Inspiratory muscle training compared with other rehabilitation interventions in adults with chronic obstructive pulmonary disease: a systematic literature review and meta-analysis. *COPD*, 2(3), 319–29

Curran J, Mahony, MJ (2008) Trampolining as an adjunct to regular physiotherapy in children with cystic fibrosis. *Irish Medical Journal*, 101(1):188

Cystic Fibrosis Foundation (2008) *Patient Registry 2000 Annual Data Report*: Cystic Fibrosis Foundation. Bethesda, Maryland: Patient Registry

Davis P, Drumm M, Konstan M (1996) Cystic Fibrosis. *American Journal of Respiratory and Critical Care Medicine*, 154:1229–56

de Jong W, van Aalderen W, Kraan J, et al (2001) Inspiratory muscle training in patients with cystic fibrosis. *Respiratory Medicine*, 9:531–6

Decramer, M (2009) Response of the respiratory muscles to rehabilitation in COPD. *Journal of Applied Physiology*, 107(3):971–6

Dommisse G (1998) Scheuermann's disease and postural kyphosis. *South African Journal of Bone and Joint Surgery*, 8(3):48–51

Dunnink M, Doeleman W, Trappenburg J, et al (2009) Respiratory muscle strength in stable adolescents and adult patients with cystic fibrosis. *Journal of Cystic Fibrosis*, 8:31–6

Effing T, Monninkhof E, van der Valk P, et al (2007) Self-management education for patients with chronic obstructive pulmonary disease. *Cochrane Database of Systematic Reviews*, (1):72

Ehrman J, Gordon P, Visich P, et al (2009) *Clinical Exercise Physiology* (2nd ed). Champaign, IL: Human Kinetics, p 691

Ellphick H, Mallory G (2009) Oxygen therapy for cystic fibrosis. *Cochrane Database of Systematic Reviews*, (1)

Enright S, Chatman K, Ionescu A, et al (2004) Inspiratory muscle training improves lung function and exercise capacity in adults with cystic fibrosis. *Chest*, 126:405–11

Fon G, Pitt M, Thies A (1980) Thoracic kyphosis: range in normal subjects. *American Journal of Roentgenology*, 134:979–83

Garrod R, Brooks D, Lasseron T, et al (2008) Supervised physical exercise training for chronic obstructive pulmonary disease: long-term efficacy and safety. *Cochrane Database of Systematic Reviews*, (1):5

Geddes E, O'Brien K, Reid W, et al (2008) Inspiratory muscle training in adults with chronic obstructive pulmonary disease: an update of a systematic review. *Respiratory Medicine*, 102(12):1715–29

Gosselink R (2004) Breathing techniques in patients with chronic obstructive pulmonary disease. *Chronic Respiratory Disorders*, 1:163–72

Gruber W, Orenstein D, Braumann K, et al (2008) Health-related fitness and trainability in children with cystic fibrosis. *Pediatric Pulmonology*, 43:953–64

Harris-Eze A, Sridar G, Zintel T, et al (1996) Role of hypoxemia and pulmonary mechanics in exercise limitation in interstitial lung disease. *American Journal of Respiratory and Critical Care Medicine*, 154:994–1001

Hinman M (2004) Comparison of thoracic kyphosis and postural stiffness in younger and older women. *The Spine Journal*, 4(4):413–17

Holland A, Hill C (2008) Physical training for interstitial lung disease. *Cochrane Database of Systematic Reviews*, (1):1–62

Houglum P (2005) *Therapeutic Exercise for Musculoskeletal Injuries* (2nd ed). Champaign, IL: Human Kinetics

Houston B, Mills N, Solis-Moyer A (2008) Inspiratory muscle training for cystic fibrosis. *Cochrane Database of Systematic Reviews*, (1):1–38

Kado DM, Huang MH, Barrett-Connor E, et al (2005) Hyperkyphotic Posture and Poor Physical Functional Ability in Older Community-Dwelling Men and Women: The Rancho Bernardo Study. *Journal of Gerontology*, Series A: Biological Sciences and Medical Sciences, 60:633–37

Kado DM, Huang MH, Karlamangla AS, et al (2004) Hyperkyphotic posture predicts mortality in older community-dwelling men and women: a prospective study. *Journal of the American Geriatrics Society*, 52(10):1662–7

Kendall F, McCreary E, Provance P, et al (2005) *Muscle Testing and Function; with Posture and Pain* (5th ed). Baltimore: Williams and Wilkins

Kim H, Mofarrahi M, Hussain S (2008) Skeletal muscle dysfunction in patients with chronic obstructive pulmonary disease. *International Journal of Chronic Obstructive Pulmonary Diseases*, 3(4):637–58

Koh M, Tee A, Lasserson T, et al (2007) Inhaled corticosteroids compared to placebo for prevention of exercise induced bronchoconstriction. *Cochrane Database of Systematic Reviews*, (1):1–31

Kolber H (1998) Cystic fibroses and physical activity: an introduction. *International Journal of Sports Medicine*, 92–5

Lacasse Y, Goldstein R, Lasseron T, et al (2006) Pulmonary rehabilitation for chronic obstructive pulmonary disease. *Cochrane Database of Systematic Reviews*, (1):47

Loder R (2001) The sagittal profile of the cervical and lumbosacral spine in Scheuermann thoracic kyphosis. *Journal of Spinal Disorders*, 14(3):226–31

Magee D (2008) Thoracic (Dorsal) Spine. In: Magee D (ed.), *Orthopedic Physical Assessment* (5th ed). St Louis, Missouri: Saunders Elsevier, pp 476–8

Marshall B, Samuelson M (1998) Basic therapies in cystic fibrosis: does standard therapy work? *Clinical Chest Medicine*, 19:487–504

Mason R, Broaddus C, Murray J, et al (2005) Part lll: Clinical respiratory medicine. In: Murray J, Nadel J (eds), *Murray and Nadel's Textbook of Respiratory Medicine* (4th ed). New York: Elsevier

McFadden E, Gilbert I (1994) Exercise-induced asthma. *New England journal of Medicine*, 330(19):1362–7

McGill S (2002) *Low Back Disorders: Evidence-based Prevention and Rehabilitation*. Champaign, IL: Human Kinetics

Mehrsheed S, Robert H, Christine A, et al (2005) Balance disorder and increased risk of falls in osteoporosis and kyphosis: signifiance of kyphotic posture and muscle strength. *Osteoporosis International*, 16(8):1004–10

Murray P, Weinstein S, Spratt K (1993) The natural history of long-term follow-up of Scheuermann Kyphosis. *Journal of Bone and Joint Surgery*, 75:236–47

Nakamura Y, Tanaka K, Shigematsu R, et al (2008) Effects of aerobic training and recreational activities in patients with chronic obstructive pulmonary disease. *International Journal of Rehabilitation Research*, 31(4):275–83

Nelson M, Rejeski W, Blair S, et al (2007) Physical activity and public health in older adults: recommendations from the American College of Sports Medicine and the American Heart Association. *Medicine and Science in Sports and Exercise*, 39(8):1435–45

Newall C, Stockley R, Hill S (2005) Exercise training and inspiratory muscle training in patients with bronchiectasis. *Thorax*, 60:943–8

Nici L, Donner C, Wouters E (2006) American Thoracic Society/European Respiratory Society statement on pulmonary rehabilitation. *American Journal of Respiratory and Critical Care Medicine*, 173:1390–413

Nixon P, Orenstein D, Kelsey S (2001) Habitual physical activity in children and adolescents with cystic fibrosis. *Medicine and Science in Sports and Exercise*, 33(1):30–5

Nonoyama M, Brooks D, Lacasse Y, et al (2007) Oxygen therapy during exercise training in chronic obstructive pulmonary disease. *Cochrane Database of Systematic Reviews*, (1):67

Norris C (2008) *Back Stability: Integrating Science and Therapy* (2nd ed). Champaigne, IL: Human Kinetics

O'Donnell D (2001) Ventilatory limitations in chronic obstructive pulmonary disease. *Medicine and Science in Sports and Exercise*, 33(7):S647–55

O'Shea S, Taylor N, Paratz J (2004) Peripheral muscle strength training in COPD: a systematic review. *Chest*, 126:903–14

Ong K, Chong W, Soh C, et al (2004) Comparison of different exercise tests in assessing outcomes of pulmonary rehabilitation. *Respiratory Care*, 49(12):1498–503

Orenstein D, Hovell M, Mulvihill M, et al (2004) Strength vs aerobic training in children with cystic fibrosis: a randomized controlled trial. *Chest*, 126(4):1204–14

Pauwels R, Buist A, Ma P, Jenkins C, aHurd S (2001) Global strategy for the diagnosis, management, and prevention of chronic obstructive pulmonary disease: National Heart, Lung, and Blood Institute and World Health Organisation Global Initiative for Chronic Obstructive Pulmonary Disease (GOLD): executive summary. *Respiratory Care*, 46:798–825

Pinet C, Cassart M, Scillia P (2003) Function and bulk of respiratory and limb muscles in patients with cystic fibrosis. *American Journal of Respiratory and Critical Care Medicine*, 335179–88

Puhan M, Busching G, Schunemann H, Vanoort E, Zaugg C, Frey M (2006) Interval versus continuos high-intensity exercise in chronic obstructive pulmonary disease: a randomized trial. *Annals of Internal Medicine*, 145(11):816–25

Puhan M, Scharplatz M, Troosters T, et al (2005a) Respiratory rehabilitation after acute exacerbation of COPD may reduce risk for readmission and mortality — a systematic review. *Respiratory Research*, 6:54–66

Puhan M, Scharplatz M, Troosters T, Walters E, Steurer J (2008) Pulmonary rehabilitation following exacerbations of chronic obstructive pulmonary disease. *Cochrane Database of Systematic Reviews*, (1):32

Puhan M, Schunemann H, Frey M, et al (2005b) How should COPD patients exercise during respiratory rehabilitation? Comparison of exercise modalities and intensities to treat skeletal muscle dysfunction. *Thorax*, 60(5):367–75

Rabe K, Hurd S, Anzueto A (2007) Global strategy for the diagnosis, management and prevention of chronic obstructive pulmonary disease: GOLD executive summary. *American Journal of Respiratory and Critical Care Medicine*, 176:532–55

Ram F, Robinson S, Black P, et al (2005) Physical training for asthma. *Cochrane Database of Systematic Reviews*, 1(4): CD001116 DOI:10.1002/14651858

Reid W, Geddes E, O'Brien K, et al (2008) Effects of inspiratory muscle training in cystic fibrosis: a systematic review. *Clinical Rehabilitation*, 22:1003–13

Reid W, Samrai B (1995) Respiratory muscle training for patients with chronic obstructive pulmonary disease. *Physical Therapy*, 75(11):996–1005

Ries A (2008) Pulmonary Rehabilitation: Summary of an evidence-based guideline. *Respiratory Care*, 53(9): 1203–207

Rietschel E, Van Koningsbruggen S, Fricke O, et al (2008) Whole-body vibration: a new therapeutic approach to improve muscle function in cystic fibrosis. *International Journal of Rehabilitation Research*, 31(3):253–6

Robinson S, Black P, Picot J (2005) Physical training for asthma. *Cochrane Database of Systematic Reviews*, (4):1–24

Rodgers D, Smith P, John N, et al (2002) Validity of a modified shuttle walk test as measure of exercise tolerance in paediatric CF patients. *Journal of Cystic Fibrosis*, 1 (Suppl):22

Romer L (2009) Pathophysiology and Treatment of Pulmonary Disease. In: Womack C, Ehrman J (eds), *ACSM's Resource Manual for Guidelines for Exercise Testing and prescription* (6th ed). Baltimore, ML: Wolters Kluwer: Lippincott Williams & Wilkins, pp 119–38

Rundell K, Slee J (2008) Exercise and other indirect challenges to demonstrate asthma or exercise-induced bronchoconstriction in athletes. *Journal of Allergyand Clinical Immunology*, 122:238–46

Sahlberg M, Erikssons B, Strandvik B (2008) Cardiopulmonary data in response to 6 months of training in physically active adult patients with classic cystic fibrosis. *Respiration*, 76(4):413–20

Sahlberg M, Svantesson U, Thomas E, et al (2005) Muscle strength and function in patients with cystic fibrosis. *Chest*, 127(5):1587–92

Schneiderman-Walker J, Pollock S, Corey M (2000) A randomized controlled trial of a 3-year home exercise program in cystic fibrosis. *Journal of Paediatrics*, 136:304–10

Selvadurai H, Blimkie C, Meyers N, et al (2002) Randomized controlled study of in-hospital exercise training programs in children with cystic fibrosis. *Pediatric Pulmonology*, 33(3):194–200

Selvadurai H, Cooper P, Meyers N (2003) Vaildation of shuttle test in children with cystic fibrosis. *Pediatric Pulmonology*, 35:133–8

Shahin B, Germain M, Kazem A, Annat G (2008) Benefits of short inspiratory muscle training on exercise capacity, dyspnea and inspiratory fraction in COPD patients. *International Journal of Chronic Obstructive Pulmonary Diseases*, 3(3):423–7

Sietsema K (2001) Cardiovascular limitations in chronic pulmonary disease. *Medicine and Science in Sports and Exercise*, 33(7, Suppl):S656–61

Steinsbekk A, Lomundal B (2009) Three-year follow-up after a two-year comprehensive pulmonary rehabilitation program. *Chronic Respiratory Disease*, 6:5–11

Storer T (2001) Exercise in chronic pulmonary disease: resistance exercise prescription. *Medicine and Science in Sports and Exercise*, 33(7):S680–92

Stricker S (2002) The maligned adolescent spine — part 2: Scheuermann's kyphosis and spondylolisthesis. *International Pediatrics*, 17(3):135–417

Swank A, Berry M, Woodard M (2009) Chronic Obstructive Pulmonary Disease. In: Ehrman J, Gordon P, Visich P, Keteyian S (eds). *Clinical Exercise Physiology* (2nd ed). Champaign, IL: Human Kinetics

Tan R, Spector S (1998) Exercise-induced asthma. *Sports Medicine*, 25(1):1–6

Thomas J, Cook D, Brooks D (1995) Chest physical therapy management of patients with cystic fibrosis: a meta-analysis. *American Journal of Respiratory and Critical Care Medicine*, 151:846–50

Thompson WR, Gordon NF, Pescatello LS (eds) (2010) *ACSM's guidelines for exercise testing and prescription* (8th ed). Baltimore, MD: Lippincott Williams & Wilkins

van Doorn N (2009) Exercise programs for children with cystic fibrosis: A systematic review of randomised controlled trials. *Disability and Rehabilitation*, 26:1–9

Varga J, Porszasz J, Boda K, et al (2007) Supervised high intensity continuous and interval training vs. self-paced training in COPD. *Respiratory Medicine*, 101:2297–304

Wenger D, Frick S (1999) Scheuermann kyphosis. *Spine*, 24(24):2630–9

Yankaskas J, Marshall B, Sufian B, et al (2004) Cystic fibrosis adult care: Consensus Conference report. *Chest*, 125(1)1–39

Zach M, Purrer B, Oberwaldner B (1981) Effect of swimming on forced expiration and sputum clearance in cystic fibrosis. *Lancet*, 2(8257), 1201–3

Chapter 5

Exercise as therapy in neurological conditions

Alan Pearce and Meg Morris

Assumed concepts

This chapter is based on the assumption that readers already understand key concepts and have some fundamental knowledge of:

- the human nervous system
- principles of resistance training, particularly between concentric, eccentric, isotonic, isometric, and isokinetic training
- the differences between brain injury, neurological and neurodegenerative conditions, and neuromuscular conditions.

INTRODUCTION

Neurological conditions are those that affect the central nervous system (CNS), peripheral nervous system (PNS), or the autonomic nervous system (ANS). These conditions can include acquired brain injury (ABI), neurodegenerative conditions, neuromuscular conditions, tumours and other conditions. ABI can result from traumatic brain injury (TBI) following serious trauma to the head, or non-TBI such as stroke, brain tumours or infections. Neurodegenerative conditions result from progressive deteriorations of neurons leading to cognitive, sensory or motor dysfunction. Common examples include Parkinson's disease, motor neurone disease, Huntington's disease and multiple sclerosis. Neuromuscular conditions include such conditions as muscular dystrophy, polio, myasthenia gravis and myopathies.

Relatively little is known about the pathophysiology and aetiology of some neurological conditions (Thickbroom & Mastaglia 2009), which can make rehabilitation challenging. In many neurological conditions, therapy aims to reduce the impact of the impairments and disabilities or degeneration on the person and their families. The effectiveness of exercise as a mode of therapy varies across conditions and will be discussed during the course of this chapter. Other factors such as the person's age, medications, lifestyle habits and comorbid conditions can affect the outcomes of prescribed exercise therapy, however these lie outside of the scope of this chapter. Although exercise needs to be tailored to the type of condition and individual differences, there is growing evidence to suggest that some forms of exercise, whether motor skill training, balance training or resistance training, have the potential to influence neural networks. The historical view that the adult brain is structurally stable and incapable of change or recovery has now been challenged by motor control models that assume neuroplasticity and the ability to improve with practice (Pascual-Leone et al 1995; Pearce et al 2000; Thickbroom & Mastaglia 2009).

The evidence for neuroplasticity is rapidly accumulating and is now well regarded (see Doidge 2008; Thickbroom & Mastaglia 2009). It is not so much a case of how change occurs but, rather, what methods of training are available to facilitate this process (Thickbroom & Mastaglia 2009). In discussing the benefits of exercise in adults, Fox et al (2006) have suggested five principles to promote neuroplasticity: (1) intensive exercise maximises synaptic changes augmenting plasticity; (2) performance of complex tasks promotes neural adaptation; (3) tasks that are rewarding increase dopamine levels, promoting learning/relearning; (4) neurons responsive to dopamine are highly receptive to exercise, but also to inactivity; and (5) where exercise is introduced at an earlier stage of a progressive disease, progression hypothetically may be slowed.

This chapter will explore the concept of neuroplasticity. The techniques to measure plasticity non-invasively will be outlined, with examples from published research in skill and strength training. The discussion will then lead to current research on the effectiveness of exercise training on traumatic and non-traumatic ABI (particularly in relation to stroke) and neurodegenerative conditions (Parkinson's disease, motor neurone disease, and multiple sclerosis).

METHODS TO MEASURE THE HUMAN CORTICOSPINAL SYSTEM

Several methods are now available to measure activity in the nervous system. These include imaging technologies as well as electrical and magnetic stimulation techniques. Many investigations have combined several of these techniques concurrently in studies measuring neuroplasticity. A number of these techniques will be discussed in this section, that particularly relate to the neural adaptations following training. For further information regarding other types of non-invasive neurological measurement methods,

such as nerve conduction studies, including the Hoffman Reflex (H-Reflex), M-wave (or M-response) and twitch interpolation technique, the reader is directed to Latash (2008).

Functional neuroimaging techniques

Functional imaging techniques include technologies such as positron emission tomography (PET) and functional magnetic resonance imaging (fMRI). Both PET and fMRI techniques are non-invasive, in that they do not involve procedures that enter the body, such as cutting or inserting any measurement devices under the skin or through the skull. PET indirectly measures in an individual the flow of blood to various parts of the brain that are marked with a radioactive tracer marker, taken by the participant prior to scanning, to measure the haemodynamic changes associated with neuronal activity that can be associated with task related or goal related movement. Major advantages of PET include rapid and reliable assessment of neurological conditions such as epilepsy and various dementias as well as quantifying neurophysiological processes of neural networks during sensorimotor task performance. PET imaging also has some limitations and disadvantages. PET images can not assess the function of an area of the brain being assessed. Despite revealing high resolution neuroanatomical images, these images cannot alone prove physiologically an area is essential for a motor function (Hallett 2000); and although the radioactive components used in PET imaging do not last for any extended period, participants cannot undergo an infinite number of scans, limiting the use of PET as a research tool. The technology required to perform PET scans limits the number of PET scanners available in institutions to conduct research.

fMRI is a recently developed form of neuroimaging focused on measuring haemodynamic responses (known as blood-oxygen-level dependant or BOLD) in the brain. The advantage of fMRI over PET is the relatively lower radiation exposure during scanning as well as the greater availability of the technology. Similar to PET scanning, spatial resolution of fMRI is high, however temporal resolution is relatively poor due to measurement of BOLD activity in the brain, rather than neuroelectrical activity. Also, similar to PET scanning, fMRI is unable to provide direct evidence of areas directly involved with motor function (Hallet 2000).

Creating neuroimages via magnetic fields produced by brain electrical activity, magnetoencephalography (MEG) allows for temporal measurements of multiple sites over the cerebral cortex. In terms of temporal resolution EEG and MEG are similar as both are generated by the same neurophysiological processes. MEG differs from EEG in that it allows for superior spatial resolution as the boney tissue of the skull provides less distortion to the magnetic fields generated (Cohen & Cuffin 1983). Conversely, a major disadvantage of MEG is that activity signals are extremely small, and the technology requires specialised shielding to eliminate artefact found in typical laboratory environments. MEG has been used to show cortical reorganisation (plasticity) in a landmark study by Elbert and colleagues (1995) who demonstrated changes in the cortical representation

of the fingering hand of expert violin players. Reorganisation, demonstrating neuroplasticity, not only correlated to the amount of control required by the fingering digits, for example, the thumb used for stabilising the neck of the violin showing little change, but also to the length of experience in playing the violin; the longer the overall time, the greater the reorganisation.

Brain stimulation

Alternative to neuroimaging methods, it is also possible to study the brain using electromagnetic stimulation. Non-invasive brain stimulation, most notably, transcranial magnetic stimulation (TMS), was first developed in 1982. Commercially available stimulators (see Figure 5.1) suitable for human study have been available since 1985 (Barker et al 1985) with minimal risk to healthy individuals (Wasserman 2002). Although quite rare, individuals may experience mild discomfort

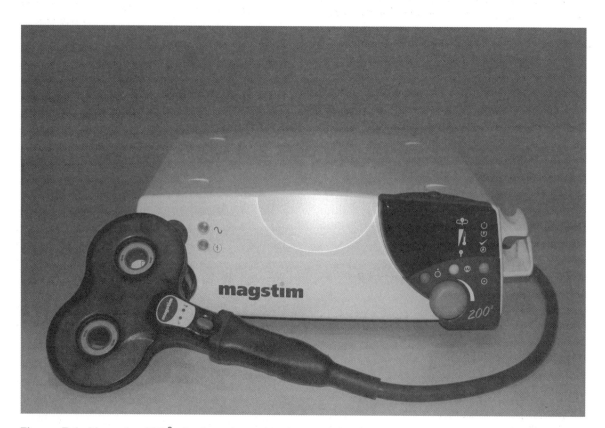

Figure 5.1 Magstim 200^2 single pulse stimulator with a 'figure of eight' magnetic coil. The figure of eight coil contains two small magnets in reverse polarity enabling a more focused electromagnetic impulse than the standard circular coil

(Source: from authors' own image collection)

such as local pain on the scalp musculature or a headache. However, since the introduction of commercially available single pulse stimulators, only three cases of seizure have been reported in adult patients with large cerebral infarcts or other lesions, with no adverse reports in healthy individuals (Wasserman 2002).

TMS employs time varying magnetic fields that induce electrical currents in conductive tissues such as neural tissue, with the induced electric field being proportional to the rate of the magnetic field. If the current induced by the electric field is of sufficient amplitude and duration, it will depolarise neural tissue, recorded and measured as a motor evoked potential (MEP) in the electromyogram (EMG) of the target muscle. Figure 5.2 illustrates the measurable components of an MEP. For more information on the physics and mechanism underpinning TMS, the reader is directed to Hallet (2000).

The MEP is a relatively synchronous muscle response that can be measured on the EMG (Hallet 2000). The amplitude of a MEP is influenced by inhibitory and excitatory interconnections descending on the motor neurone pool at the time of stimulation (Hallett 2000), with the amplitude of MEPs differing between individuals (Wasserman 2005). When controlled for torque and type of motor task, the MEP is a reliable measure (Kamen 2004; van Hedal et al 2007), allowing for confident interpretation of changes following acute or chronic interventions. Moreover, investigators will use a MEP/M-wave ratio to further normalise individual MEP variations between participants (Pearce et al 2000; Kidgell & Pearce 2010).

TMS also has the ability to be used as an imaging technique, illustrating topographical representation of muscles on the motor cortex in healthy (Wilson et al 1993; Pearce et al 2000) and diseased groups (Byrnes et al 1999; Thickbroom et al 2006). Using a methodology based on a latitude and longitude system, TMS can be employed to stimulate a number of areas overlying the motor cortex systematically. Averaging the MEP waveforms over each site, topographical maps can be generated to provide a representation of the muscle targeted during stimulation. Examples of these maps are presented in Figure 5.3. A number of these studies, using this technique,

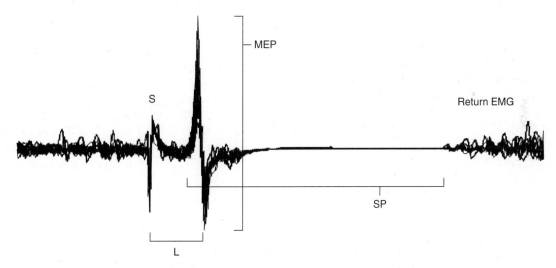

Figure 5.2 The components of a MEP as recorded on EMG. Overlayed image of 20 sweeps, obtained from the first dorsal interosseous (FDI) muscle following TMS over the contralateral motor cortex, illustrating the reliability of the MEP when the muscle is controlled for contraction level. The MEP is visible approximately 20–25ms following cortical stimulation (S). This is termed latency (L). MEP amplitude is calculated by cursoring the peak to peak value of the MEP. Silent period (SP) is measured by cursoring onset of MEP to return of EMG activity

(Source: image from Pearce 2000)

will be discussed later in this chapter to illustrate neuroplasticity.

A major difference between neuroimaging techniques and TMS is that TMS has the ability to not only show excitation but inhibition of the CNS, thereby demonstrating an area's direct influence on a motor performance. There are a number of studies that have directly shown increased excitability (Pascual-Leone et al 1995) in a cortical motor area during task activation or, conversely, use TMS to transiently suppress or interfere with motor regions of the cerebral cortex, providing stronger evidence of regions directly involved in a task (Rothwell 1994). It is for this reason that TMS has been pivotal in a variety of research in neurophysiology and motor control, which will be discussed further in this chapter. Many studies now combine both spatial imaging of fMRI with time resolution techniques such as TMS to investigate areas of the brain directly involved with motor function (Bohning et al 1999; Foylts et al 2000; Kuhtz-Buschbeck et al 2003).

NEUROPLASTICITY

The term 'plasticity', referring to adaptability and reorganisation of the brain (Thickbroom & Mastaglia 2009), is now regularly used. However, arguments that the brain is adaptable and has the ability to change based on experience, regardless of age (Disterhoft & Oh 2006) have been apparent for approximately 350 years (Doidge 2008). Early cytoarchitectural work by Ramón y Cajal, Ioan Minea and Gheorghe Marinesco in the late 19th and early 20th centuries (Jones 2000) questioned but did not refute outright 'localisation'. Described colloquially (Doidge 2008) as 'one function, one location' (p 17), localisation was interpreted as one part of the brain has one dedicated hardwired location or more globally as structural stability of the neocortex (Rioult-Pedotti & Donoghue 2003). Attempts to refute localisation, in the 1960s and 1970s, where not initially accepted in the neuroscience field, despite persuasive evidence from micro-stimulation studies in monkeys (Paul et al 1972; Merzenich et al 1983). It was not until the late 20th century that the technology would allow for unequivocal evidence for neuroplasticity. It is now not a case of investigating if plasticity occurs, but rather the degree and variations in

the form of plasticity (Disterhoft & Oh 2006; Thickbroom & Mastaglia 2009).

Mechanisms underpinning neuroplasticity

Several mechanisms underpin the phenomena of neuroplasticity in humans (Rioult-Pedotti & Donoguhue 2003), providing evidence against the traditional view of a structurally fixed cerebral cortex. Rapid neuroplastic changes, reflected as increased excitability of the neuromuscular pathway projecting from the M1 to the muscles, have been shown to occur following acute sensory and peripheral manipulation interventions, such as electrical stimulation (Fuhr et al 1992), limb amputation or immobilisation (Cohen et al 1991), nerve deafferentation or anaesthesia (Brasil-Neto et al 1992); or motor control tasks such as motor learning (Pascual-Leone et al 1995), and precision fine control of motor tasks (Lemon et al 1995; Pearce & Kidgell 2009, 2010). Suggestions for these rapid changes include 'unmasking' of pre-existing connections in the M1 (Huntley 1997) where older neural pathways, potentially made redundant due to newer pathways taking over, reactivate. There have also been suggestions of changes in balance between excitatory or inhibitory inputs between neurons thereby increasing the excitability or inhibiting existing neural connections (Jacobs & Donoghue 1991). A suggestion still open to conjecture (Rioult-Pedotti & Donoghue 2003) is the activation of existing or 'silent synapses', defined as an existing anatomical connection between synapses but neurotransmitter release does not result in excitation between neurons (Liao et al 1995). The activation of silent synapses has been shown experimentally (Liao et al 1999) and in animal models (Atwood & Wojtowicz 1999), however, there is little evidence of the existence of silent synapses in the mature human nervous system. Although, as proposed by Rioult-Pedotti and Donoghue (2003), the activation of silent synapses is a theoretically plausible component underpinning neuroplasticity.

Alternatively, longer-term neuroplastic changes can be attributed to the mechanisms of long-term potentiation (LTP) or long-term depression or inhibition (LTD or LTI; Martin et al 2000). LTP refers to a persistent increase in synaptic efficacy between neurons and has been suggested as a mechanism to consolidate learning. Alternatively,

LTD increases the inhibition between neurones actively weakening the synapse. LTP has been demonstrated to be involved in the learning as well as the retention of motor skills (Rioult-Pedotti et al 2000) as well as long-term expert motor performance (Pearce et al 2000).

Motor learning and memory of skills has also been attributed to new synapses (synaptogenesis) or remodelling of existing synapses (synaptic remodelling) underpinning LTP (Martin et al 2000). Evidence of increased synapses per neuron following a period of motor skill learning have been shown in M1 (Kleim et al 1996) and the cerebellum (Kleim et al 1998). However, contradictory evidence has been presented with a number of studies showing evidence for increased synapse numbers (Engert & Bonhoeffer 1999; Toni et al 1999) or no change (Sorra & Harris 1998; Bourgeois et al 1999) following learning or LTP induction. For further reading on LTP and the generation of new synapses the reader is directed to review by Geinisman (2000), and Benowitz and Carmichael (2010).

Evidence for neuroplasticity

Non-invasive imaging and stimulation techniques have shown the human CNS to be able to change based on the repeated performance functional motor control tasks (Rao et al 1993; Pearce & Kidgell 2009, 2010). For example, fMRI studies have shown changes in cortical activation associated with simple and complex finger movements (Rao et al 1993). Similarly TMS studies have shown increased corticospinal excitability, in hand muscles, during movements requiring greater precision control (Lemon et al 1995; Pearce & Kidgell 2009, 2010). This illustrates the ability of the CNS to rapidly modify its output based on the motor task performance required.

Some of the first evidence to support neuroplasticity in the human corticospinal system was provided by Pascual-Leone et al (1995). Using TMS mapping, they demonstrated changes in the cortical representation of an intrinsic hand muscle following a period of short-term motor practice of 5 days, as well as changes during the acquisition phase of a simple motor task. Long-term motor practice has also shown neuroplastic changes in sensorimotor representation in expert musicians (Elbert et al 1995) and elite racket sport athletes (Pearce et al 2000).

Evidence is accumulating showing that brain plasticity and adaptation can occur post-ABI or during the course of a progressive neurodegenerative condition (Thickbroom et al 2006; Lee et al 2000; Benowitz & Carmichael 2010). Evidence from fMRI, MEG and TMS studies has illustrated the occurrence of functional reorganisation of the motor cortex following stroke (Traversa et al 1997; Rossini et al 1998; Byrnes et al 1999), dystonia (Byrnes et al 1998), Parkinson's disease (PD; Thickbroom et al 2006) and multiple sclerosis (MS; Lee et al 2000).

Byrnes and colleagues (1999), demonstrated corticomotor reorganisation in 16 individuals (17–72 years of age) who had recovered varying degrees of motor function following a sub-cortical stroke, sparing M1. Using the TMS mapping (Wilson et al 1993), these investigators illustrated significant alterations in the representation of the affected to unaffected abductor pollicis brevis (APB) muscles in 12 of a sample of 16 patients as early as 4 weeks. Using the same TMS mapping technique, Thickbroom et al (2006) investigated the motor cortex representation projecting to the APB muscle in patients with idiopathic PD correlating the differences between the inter hemispheric map representations to the severity of PD symptoms, via the use of the Unified Parkinson's Disease Rating Scale (UPDRS). The greater the difference in the maps (Figure 5.3) the greater the UPDRS scale between hands (r = 0.60; p = 0.018). Cortical reorganisation has also been shown in patients with multiple sclerosis. Using fMRI, Lee et al (2000) compared 12 MS patients with 12 healthy age matched controls during simple flexion-extension 'tapping' movements of the fingers. MS patients showed greater relative supplementary motor area activation in comparison to the control group. Moreover, all patients showed alterations (posterior shifts) in the centre of activation in the sensorimotor cortex relative to unimpaired people.

The examples provided illustrate neuroplasticity in the human sensorimotor cortex in response to acute, short-term and long-term practice in unimpaired individuals as well as in some people with neurodegenerative or neuromuscular conditions. Apart from the short-term studies of Pascual-Leone et al (1995), these studies have been 'snap shot' investigations demonstrating experience dependant plastic changes, rather than

Left hemisphere   Right hemisphere

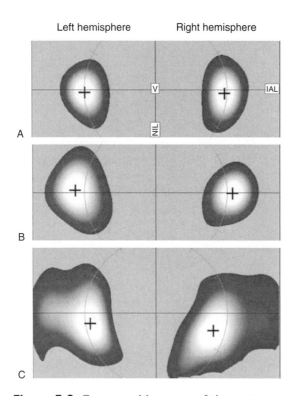

Figure 5.3 Topographic maps of the motor representation of left and right abductor pollicis brevis muscle. Map of a control participant (A), illustrating interhemispheric symmetry in map position (as shown by the black cross). (B-C) Maps from Parkinson's disease patients showing a laterally displaced map (B) and medially displaced map (C) with enlarged map area (C).
V: vertex; NIL: nasion-inion line; IAL: inter-aural line; arcs indicate 6cm from vertex

[Source: reproduced with permission from Thickbroom et al. Motor cortex reorganisation in Parkinson's disease; published by Elsevier, 2006]

intervention studies. The next section will discuss exercise therapy in health and disease. It should be noted that contraindications exists with any exercise rehabilitation program. Prior to starting any exercise program, the patient should seek advice from their medical practitioner to ensure that they are ready and able to exercise.

Neuroplasticity and exercise in unimpaired people

The premise that exercise has the potential to benefit people with neurological conditions is strengthened by recent data illustrating neural adaptations following exercise interventions in healthy models. Short-term (4 weeks or less) strength training studies have shown increases in strength in the absence of muscle hypertrophy with increased associated corticospinal excitability (Beck 2007; Griffen & Cafferelli 2007; Kidgell & Pearce 2009), or reduced silent period (SP) duration (Kidgell & Pearce 2010). Resistance training of one limb has also been shown to be associated with an increase in strength in the opposite, non-trained arm in absence of muscle hypertrophy (Farthing & Chilibeck 2005).

Studies directly investigating cortical mechanisms underpinning cross education support the concept of neuroplasticity. Farthing et al (2007) investigated cortical activation, using fMRI, following a 6-week period of unilateral right limb training of a novel exercise task (maximal isometric ulnar deviation). After the training period, scans demonstrated enlarged cortical activation in the contralateral sensorimotor cortex (left hemisphere) and left temporal lobe suggesting adaptations within memory areas associated with motor learning and training which may have implications for rehabilitation. Unilateral strength training has also shown corticospinal changes with several recent TMS investigations showing increased MEP amplitude following 4 weeks moderate to high intensity strength training (Lee et al 2009; Kidgell & Pearce 2009).

The effect of limb immobilisation with resistance training of the non-immobilised limb has also been investigated. Farthing et al (2009) immobilised by casting one limb and exercised the non-immobilised limb of one group (trained group), three times per week for 3 weeks, and compared strength and muscle cross sectional area to an untrained group, who had one limb immobilised but with no training, and a control (no immobilisation or exercise). Participants in the trained group with immobilisation showed increased strength in the trained arm, but also showed no change in strength or muscle thickness in the immobilised arm. The untrained group with immobilisation showed significant declines in strength and muscle thickness. Although neurophysiological measures where not taken, Farthing et al (2009) suggested that cross-education strength training attenuated the loss of strength and muscle morphology which may have implications for exercise rehabilitation strategies.

EXERCISE THERAPY FOR ACQUIRED BRAIN INJURY

Stroke

Rehabilitation is now well established as a standard intervention for people who have experienced a stroke. Rehabilitation can incorporate a range of interventions, such as task oriented training, progressive resistance strength training exercises (Ada et al 2007; Pak et al 2008; Wevers et al 2009), robot and treadmill based facilitation techniques (Hesse et al 2008; Brewer et al 2007), constraint-induced therapy (Bonaiuti et al 2007), hydrotherapy (Mehrholz et al 2010), motor skill training (eg: mirroring or external feedback) (French et al 2010; Subramanian et al 2009; Ezendam et al 2009) and falls prevention education. Physiotherapists and other rehabilitation clinicians select the most appropriate interventions for each individual based on the type and severity of stroke, capacity for motor skill learning, age, physical capacity and prevalence of co-existing conditions. Given that many patients have weakness as a result of the stroke, reduced physical activity or co-existing conditions, strength training exercises are frequently incorporated into the person's rehabilitation program (Morris et al 2004).

In terms of the overall effectiveness of exercise therapy post-stroke, several studies have focused on strength, flexibility or aerobic training regimes. Strength training as a mode of neurological rehabilitation has been a controversial topic with some authors suggesting that resistance training might provide an overload that can sometimes increase spasticity (Bobath 1990; Davies 1990). Other studies using progressive resistance training have provided evidence that spasticity does not always occur with resistance training (Sharpe & Bower 1997; Smith et al 1999; Teixeira-Salmela et al 1999). For a review of these studies the reader is referred to Brownlee and Durward (2005).

An early Cochrane review by Saunders et al (2004) was unable to ascertain whether muscle strength training had exercise therapy benefits in neurological conditions. This was despite a review by Morris et al (2004) showing that progressive strength training was increasingly being used in clinical practice. The studies reviewed indicated positive outcomes, including increased muscular strength without increased occurrence of spasticity

or reduced range of movement. More recently, Yang et al (2006) demonstrated benefits of a 4-week task-orientated resistance training program for stroke patients with lower limb paresis. Exercises included functional tasks such as moving from sitting to standing and stepping up and down a series of steps. Resistance was limited to own body weight, and overload comprised of increased repetition or complexity of the task. The results showed significant improvements in strength and all functional tests (except in the step test of the unaffected limb) with participants who undertook the training. There were also significant between group increases in muscle strength and functional outcomes. Although the results were positive, the comparison was with a no-treatment control group. Further studies could compare training that incorporates the performance of daily activities and functional tasks with generic strength training.

Although treadmill training is frequently used in stroke rehabilitation, the use of treadmills as a rehabilitation method post-stroke is only just beginning to be a major emphasis of therapy (Ada et al 2010; Mosley et al 2005; Hesse et al 2008). da Cunha (2002) reported improvements in walking economy with treadmill training, but cautioned against the interpretation and generalisation of results due to the small sample size. A meta-analysis by Mosley et al (2009) yielded no differences between treadmill walking and other physiotherapy interventions. It was suggested participant diversity contributed to limited statistical power of the meta-analysis. More recently, a randomised trial in 126 sub-acute stroke patients reported that weight supported treadmill training resulted in more people walking independently and earlier than those who walk overground without weight-bearing assistance (Ada et al 2010). Weight-bearing treadmill training may also result in better walking capacity and perception of walking compared to overground walking (Dean et al 2010). Refer to Chapter 15, case study 1, for a detailed case study of the use of exercise post-stroke.

There are numerous other exercise interventions that can be considered post-stroke; such as hydrotherapy (Mehrholz et al 2010), tai chi (Au-Yeung et al 2009), yoga (Lynton et al 2007), electrical or vibration stimulation (Meilink et al 2008; Paoloni et al 2009), robot assisted therapy (Prange et al 2006) and constraint induced therapy (Bonaiuti et al 2007). These are awaiting verification with large randomised controlled trials. Currently the evidence for the beneficial effects of aquatic exercise for people with stroke remains equivocal. A Cochrane review is currently being undertaken (Mehrholz et al 2010) to evaluate the effectiveness of aquatic exercise. Clinically, it is suggested that water-based exercises may have the potential to improve activities of daily living and other physiological aspects, such as cardiovascular fitness, following a stroke. Robot assisted therapy is also emerging as a potential rehabilitation strategy for upper limb hemi-paresis post-stroke. A systematic review concluded that robot assisted rehabilitation post-stroke led to both short and long-term improvements in upper limb motor control, and that robot assisted therapy may result in greater improvements in motor control than conventional therapy (Prange et al 2006).

Cerebral palsy

Cerebral palsy (CP) is a chronic neurological condition caused by a lesion to the developing brain, affecting motor function in adulthood, characterised by deficits in movement and postural control. Exercise, particularly strength training, has been purported as an approach to improving and maximising function in people with CP. Refer to Chapter 7 for more information regarding CP in children, and Chapter 15 case study 2 for a detailed account of the use of exercise therapy by an adult with CP.

EXERCISE THERAPY FOLLOWING TRAUMATIC BRAIN INJURY

According to Gormley and Hussey (2005), traumatic brain injury (TBI) is classified as primary when the damage is at time of impact; and secondary in response to the primary injury. Gormley and Hussey (2005) proposed that exercise may have similar outcomes as for stroke patients, although this awaits empirical verification. Two recent reviews provided some evidence for exercise therapy post-TBI (Hassett et al 2008; Hellweg & Johannes 2008). These agreed with Gordon et al (1998) and Jackson et al (2001) that cardiovascular exercise appears to be a safe intervention for many individuals. Hassett et al (2008) suggested that studies to date are insufficiently powered to

determine the effects of cardiovascular exercise in TBI. Nevertheless, Hellweg and Johannes (2008) found no evidence supporting the use of cardiovascular exercise therapy transferring to the functional level. Recent research by Williams and Morris (2009) has demonstrated the value of high level activities in TBI, such as stair descent, mini trampoline, jogging, running drills and lower limb strength exercises. For higher level participants, agility and plyometric exercises were beneficial for people with ABI, more than half of whom had a TBI. Following a 3-month exercise program, significant motor recovery in high level mobility was shown. Further research is required to determine whether gains positively impact on emotional, societal and quality of life (QoL) measures.

Strength training as a mode of therapy post-TBI has also been given relatively little attention. Morris et al (2009) recently completed a multiple case-study on the effectiveness of strength training in seven adults following TBI. A twice weekly program for 8 weeks led to increases in leg press strength in four participants and arm press strength in two participants. Two improved on the sit to stand test. Maximal gait speed and the Brain Injury Community Rehabilitation Outcome-39 (BICRO-39) scale scores did not change. Collectively, these studies show that more research (and specifically with regards to various exercise regimes) is warranted on the effectiveness of exercise therapy and TBI.

Only one experimental study has used TMS to investigate the cortical influences on the M1 following mild to moderate TBI (Christyakov et al 2001) which has been described earlier in this chapter. Future research should also incorporate neurophysiological measures (fMRI and/or TMS) to measure corticospinal changes associated with recovery.

EXERCISE THERAPY FOR NEURODEGENERATIVE CONDITIONS

Parkinson's disease

The benefits of exercise appear to have received greater attention in neurodegenerative conditions, such as Parkinson's disease (PD; see review by Goodwin et al 2008). It is now acceptable to suggest that exercise, particularly progressive resistance strength training, has the potential for neuroplastic changes, with animal models showing exercise may delay the onset of some symptoms (Faherty et al 2005). Locomotion training has also been suggested to be a suitable form of therapy, with suggestions for tailoring gait training over the progression of the condition provided by Morris et al (2010). A recent systematic review on exercise and physical functioning provided evidence of improvement in physical functioning in people with PD following a period of exercise. The interventions for the different studies reviewed varied in the type of exercises, number of exercise sessions per week and intervention durations.

The efficacy of specific types of exercise may vary across individuals (Dibble et al 2009). Morris and colleagues (2009), using a two-group randomised controlled trial (RCT), aimed to compare movement rehabilitation strategies, using cognitive strategies such as focusing attention on and responding to external cues to enhance functional movements (such as walking, turning, standing up from sitting and negotiating obstacles) to conventional musculoskeletal exercise therapy consisting of lower limb and trunk strengthening and stretching and postural alignment feedback during 2 weeks of inpatient hospital care. The movement strategy group showed improvements on the Unified Parkinson's Disease Rating Scale (UPDRS), 10m and 2 minute walk trials, balance and QoL assessment at discharge but at 3 months follow up showed some regression in the 2 minute walk and QoL assessment. The exercise group similarly demonstrated gains and that at 3 months only the 2 minute walk trial had shown regression. The authors conclude follow-up movement or exercise therapy continued at home or provided in outpatient clinics would benefit the individual and reinforce the need for sustained physical activity following discharge.

Dibble et al (2006, 2009) advocated high-intensity resistance training as a mode of exercise therapy for people with PD. They used high-intensity eccentric exercise protocol for 45–60 minutes per day, 3 days per week for 12 weeks; with results demonstrating improved muscular force, physical tests such as the 6 minute walk, gait speed, and timed up-and-go tests, and with PD symptoms measured using the UPDRS. These findings concur with previous reports investigating high-intensity resistance training in older and PD individuals (Churma 2007;

Hirsch et al 2003; Scandalis et al 2001; Toole et al 2000).

A growing body of evidence supports use of progressive resistance exercise for clinical and functional outcomes in people with PD (Falvo et al 2008; Hirsch et al 2003; Dibble et al 2006, 2009; Morris et al 2010). Whether therapeutic exercises slow disease progression or lead to improvements in motor performance remains open to question. Questions also remain on intensities and duration of training, as well as the minimal duration before benefits are noticeable. The mechanisms that underpin neuroplastic changes in those with PD who undertake exercise training are yet to be investigated. It has been shown that cortical reorganisation of the M1 occurs in those with PD, with changes in M1 representation of muscles correlating to the severity of the UPDRS (Thickbroom et al 2006; Figure 3). More research is required to measure neuroplastic changes underpinning the functional outcomes following exercise interventions.

Motor neuron disease

Suggestions regarding the potential beneficial effects of exercise have also been reported for people with motor neuron disease (MND). MND has several variants. The most common is amyotrophic lateral sclerosis (ALS), or sporadic MND, which is typically idiopathic. However, 10% of cases are familial where two or more family members are affected (Morris 2006). Kiernan (2009) argued that a largely unresolved area is the effect exercise has in attenuating the progression of ALS, possibly due to the mechanisms underlying degeneration in both idiopathic and familial ALS remaining undefined. A Cochrane review (Dal Bello-Haas et al 2008) cited two studies (one implementing moderate aerobic exercise, the other moderate intensity resistance training) meeting the criteria. Therefore meaningful interpretation on benefits of exercise for people with MND is not possible at this time. Kiernan (2009) noted that human studies are currently being conducted to address this question; however, animal studies have recently shown improved motor functioning following an exercise program of swimming compared to running in mice with ALS (Desforges et al 2009). ALS mice subjected to swimming showed significantly longer maintained grip strength of own body weight as well as significantly longer maintenance of normal locomotive activity than control ALS mice groups. Although encouraging, results from animal models need to be interpreted with caution as similar trials yet to be conducted in human populations with sporadic MND.

Multiple sclerosis

Growing evidence supports the use of exercise for some people with multiple sclerosis (MS). Twenty years ago patients with MS were sometimes advised against exercise, due to the reporting of fatigue with high intensity physical activity (Freal et al 1984; Krupp et al 1989). These symptoms have been shown to be due to increased corticospinal excitability from the motor cortex during exercise and have been associated with an increased rate of perceived exertion (Thickbroom et al 2006). However, symptoms of fatigue have been shown to be often transient (Brownlee & Durwood 2005), and the benefits of low to moderate exercise have been shown to increase aerobic threshold, perceptions of health and activity levels (Petajan et al 1996; Mostert & Kesselring 2002). A Cochrane review (Rietberg et al 2004) exploring exercise therapy with individuals with MS reported qualitative evidence in favour of exercise therapy compared to no exercise for measures in muscular power, exercise tolerance and mobility (balance and walking cadence). No evidence was observed for exercise training on muscular fatigue. Nevertheless, no deleterious effects were found in any studies presented in the review (Rietberg et al 2009). No data at present is available on the mechanisms underpinning these findings, although experimental studies on neurophysiological measures and cortical responses in MS (Jørgensen et al 2005; Thickbroom et al 2006) require further research to combine physiological measures underpinning functional outcomes being reported.

Other neurodegenerative conditions

In general terms, and using data mainly from mouse models (eg: Pang et al 2006; Biondi et al 2008), exercise has been postulated to have some neuroprotective effects for a range of neurodegenerative conditions such as Huntington's disease, Alzheimer's disease (see review by Cotman

et al 2006), Kennedy's disease and spinal muscular atrophy. Animal studies by Pang et al (2006) and Biondi et al (2008) demonstrated maze performance and wheel running, were associated with reduced progression of cognitive decline (Pang et al 2006) and a reduced rate of motor neuron death. Although positive data can be gleaned from these studies on the benefits of exercise for these conditions, human clinical trials have not yet been completed and therefore interpretation of the data should be viewed with caution. Moreover, similar issues remain, on the specifics and type of exercise that will most benefit the individual with a given condition.

Alternative exercise modalities, such as yoga and tai chi might be considered as options to address flexibility and are sometimes used in daily rehabilitation practice. Yoga and tai chi, as two of a number of modalities of therapy for epilepsy and dementia respectively, have been systematically evaluated via two Cochrane reviews (Ramaratnam & Sridharan 2002; Forbes et al 2008). Both reviews have proposed that further comparative trials are required to ascertain the benefits to people with neurological conditions.

CONCLUSION

The ability of the human brain to reorganise itself is no longer subject to conjecture. There is a growing body of evidence demonstrating changes in the brain, either as adaptations to facilitate improvement in function (skill or strength) or in response to alterations in the central or peripheral nervous systems through non-traumatic brain injury or neurodegeneration. There is also emerging evidence that exercise can have some beneficial effects when the dosage, content, and intensity are appropriate to individual needs. Further studies incorporating more robust methodological designs and measuring functional outcomes are required. Attention is also required to investigate the physiological mechanisms underpinning neuroplasticity with ABI and neurodegenerative conditions in order to fully ascertain the effectiveness of the exercises prescribed, and to determine appropriate training for individuals with these debilitating neurological conditions.

Summary of key lessons

- Neuroplasticity is a physiological process that can occur at all ages.

- Neural adaptations occur in the short term when the individual is challenged sufficiently in a movement task.

- Neuroplasticity is a long-term process requiring constant repetition balanced with variety of exercises. In strength training, altering the speed of movement, or changing the exercise, can stimulate the nervous system.

- Neural adaptation and plasticity have been shown to occur in those with neurological conditions, particularly with strength training.

- Some modalities of training, such as water-based exercises, tai chi and yoga, require further rigorous investigation on their effectiveness but might benefit some individuals with neurological conditions.

REFERENCES

Ada L, Dean CM, Morris ME (2007) Supported treadmill training to establish walking in non-ambulatory patients early after stroke. *BMC Neurology*, 7:29–35

Ada L, Dean CM, Morris ME, et al (2010) Randomised trial of treadmill walking with body weight support to establish walking in subacute stroke: the MOBILISE trial. *Stroke*, 4:1237–42

Atwood HL, Wojitowicz JM (1999) Silent synapses in neural plasticity: current evidence. *Learning and Memory*, 6:542–71

Au-Yeung SSY, Hui-Chan CWY, Tang JCS (2009) Short-form tai chi improves standing balance of people with chronic stroke. *Neurorehabilitation and Neural Repair*, 23:515–22

Barker AT, Jalinous R, Freeston IL (1985) Non-invasive magnetic stimulation of human motor cortex. *Lancet*, 2:1106–7

Beck S, Taube W, Gruber M et al (2007) Task-specific changes in motor evoked potentials of lower limb muscles after different training interventions. *Brain Research*, 1179:51–60

Benowitz LI, Carmichael ST (2010) Promoting axonal rewiring to improve outcome after stroke. *Neurobiology of Disease*, 37: 259–66

Biondi O, Grondard C, Lécolle S et al (2008) Exercise-induced activation of NMDA receptor promotes motor unit development and survival in a type 2 spinal muscular atrophy model mouse. *The Journal of Neuroscience*, 28: 953–62

Bliss TVP, Lomo T (1973) Long-lasting potentiation of synaptic transmission in the dentate area of the anesthetised rabbit following stimulation of the perforant path. *Journal of Physiology*, 232:331–56

Bobath B (1990) *Adult Hemiplegia: Evaluation and Treatment* (3rd edn). Oxford: Heinemann

Bohning DE, Shasri A, McConnell KA et al (1999) A combined TMS/fMRI study of intensity-dependent TMS over motor cortex. *Biological Psychiatry*, 45:385–94

Bonaiuti D, Rebasti L, Sioli P (2007) The constraint induced movement therapy: a systematic review of randomised controlled trials on the adult stroke patients. *Europa Medicophysica*, 43:139–46

Bourgeois J-P, Goldman-Rakic P, Rakic P (1999) Formation, elimination and stabilisation of synapses in the primate cerebral cortex. In: Gazzaniga M S (ed.) *Cognitive Neuroscience. A Handbook for the Field* (2nd edn). Cambridge: MIT Press, pp 23–32

Brasil-Neto JP, Cohen LG, Pasual-Leone A et al (1992) Rapid reversible modulation of human motor outputs after transient deafferentation of the forearm: a study with transcranial magnetic stimulation. *Neurology*, 42:1302–6

Brewer BR, McDowell SK, Worthen-Chaudhari LC (2007) Poststroke upper extremity rehabilitation: a review of robotic systems and clinical results. *Topics in Stroke Rehabilitation*, 14:22–44

Brownlee M, Durward B (2005) Exercise in treatment of stroke and otter neurological conditions. In: Gormley J, Hussey J (eds) *Exercise Therapy: Prevention and Treatment of Disease*. Oxford: Blackwell Publishing

Byrnes ML, Thickbroom GW, Phillips BA et al (1999) Physiological studies of the corticomotor projection to the hand after subcortical stroke. *Clinical Neurophysiology*, 110:487–98

Byrnes ML, Thickbroom GW, Wilson SA et al (1998) The corticomotor representation of upper limb muscles in writer's cramp and changes following botulinum toxin injection. *Brain*, 121:977–88

Chistyakov AV, Soustiel JF, Hafner H et al (2001) Excitatory and inhibitory corticospinal responses to transcranial magnetic stimulation in patients with minor to moderate head injury. *Journal of Neurology, Neurosurgery and Psychiatry*, 70:580–7

Churma T (2007) Rehabilitation for patients with Parkinson's disease. *Journal of Neurology*, 254(Suppl 4):IV/58–IV/61

Cohen D, Cuffin BN (1983) Demonstration of useful differences between the magnetoencephalogram and electroencephalogram. *Electroencephalography and Clinical Neurophysiology*, 56:38–51

Cohen LG, Bandinelli S, Findley TW, et al (1991) Motor reorganisation after upper limb amputation in man. *Brain*, 114:615–27

Cotman CW, Berchtold NC, Christie L-A (2006) Exercise builds brain health: key roles of growth factor cascades and inflammation. *Trends in Neurosciences*, 30:464–72

da Cunha IT, Lim PA, Qureshy H, et al (2002) Gait outcomes after acute stroke rehabilitation with supported treadmill training: a randomised controlled pilot study. *Archives of Physical Medicine and Rehabilitation*, 83:1258–65

Dal Bello-Haas V, Florence JM, Krivickas LS (2008) Therapeutic exercise for people with amyotrophic lateral sclerosis or motor neuron disease. *Cochrane Database of Systematic Reviews*, Issue 2, Art No: CD005229. DOI: 10.1002/14651858.CD005229.pub2

Davies PM (1990) *Right in the Middle*. Berlin: Springer-Verlag

Dean C, Ada L, Bampton J, et al (2010) Treadmill walking with body weight support in sub-acute non-ambulatory stroke improves walking capacity more than over-ground walking: a randomised trial. *Journal of Physiotherapy*, 56:97–103

Desforges S, Branchu J, Biondi O, et al (2009) Motoneuron survival is promoted by specific exercise in a mouse model of amyotrophic lateral sclerosis. *Journal of Physiology*, 587:3561–71

Dibble LE, Hale TF, Marcus RL, et al (2006) High-intensity resistance training amplifies muscle hypertrophy and functional gains in persons with Parkinson's disease. *Movement Disorders*, 21:1444–52

Dibble LE, Hale TF, Marcus RL, et al (2009) High intensity eccentric resistance training decreases bradykinesia and improves quality of life in persons with Parkinson's disease: a preliminary study. *Parkinsonism and Related Disorders*, 15:752–7

Disterhoft JF, Oh MM (2006) Learning, aging and intrinsic neuronal plasticity. *Trends in Neuroscience*, 29:587–99

Doidge N (2008) *The Brain That Changes Itself*. Melbourne: Scribe

Elbert T, Pantev C, Wienbruch C, et al (1995) Increased cortical representation of the fingers of the left hand in string players. *Science*, 270:305–7

Engert F, Bonhoeffer T (1999) Dendritic spine changes associated with hippocampal long-term synaptic plasticity. *Nature*, 399:66–70

Ezendam D, Bongers RM, Jannink MJA (2009) Systematic review of the effectiveness of mirror therapy in upper extremity function. *Disability Rehabilitation*, 31:2135–49

Faherty CJ, Shepherd KR, Herasimtschuk A, et al (2005) Environmental enrichment in adulthood eliminates neuronal death in experimental Parkinsonism. *Molecular Brain Research*, 134:170–9

Falvo MJ, Schilling BK, Earhart GM (2008) Parkinson's disease and resistive exercise: rationale, review, and recommendations. *Movement Disorders*, 23:1–11

Farthing JP, Borowsky R, Chilibeck P, et al (2007) Neuro-physiological adaptations associated with cross-education of strength. *Brain Topography*, 20:77–88

Farthing JP, Chilibeck PD, Binsted G (2005) Cross-education of arm muscular strength is unidirectional in right-handed individuals. *Medicine and Science in Sports and Exercise*, 37:1594–1600

Farthing JP, Krentz JR, Magnus CRA (2009) Strength training the free limb attenuates strength loss during unilateral immobilization. *Journal of Applied Physiology*, 106:830–6

Forbes D, Forbes S, Morgan DG, Markle-Reid M, Wood J, Culum I (2008) Physical activity programs for persons with dementia. *Cochrane Database of Systematic Reviews*, Issue 3. Art No: CD006489. DOI: 10.1002/14651858.CD006489.pub2

Fox CM, Ramig LO, Ciucci MR, et al (2006) The science and practice of LSVT/LOUD: neural plasticity principled approach to treating individuals with Parkinson's disease and other neurological disorders. *Seminars in Speech and Language*, 27:283–99

Foylts H, Kemeny S, Krings T, et al (2000) The representation of the plegic hand in the motor cortex: a combined fMRI and TMS study. *Neuroreport*, 11:147–50

Freal JE, Kraft GH, Coryell JK (1984) Symptomatic fatigue in multiple sclerosis. *Archives of Physical Medicine and Rehabilitation*, 65:135–8

French B, Thomas L, Leathley M, et al (2010) Does repetitive task training improve functional activity after stroke? A Cochrane systematic review and meta-analysis. *Journal of Rehabilitation Medicine*, 42:9–14

Fuhr P, Cohen LG, Dang N, et al (1992) Physiological analysis of motor reorganisation following lower limb amputation. *Electroencephalography and Clinical Neurophysiology*, 85:53–60

Geinisman Y (2000) Structural synaptic modifications associated wit hippocampal LTP and behavioural learning. *Cerebral Cortex*, 10:952–62

Goodwin VA, Richards, SH, Taylor RS, et al (2008) The effectiveness of exercise interventions for people with Parkinson's disease: a systematic review and meta-analysis. Movement Disorders 23:631–40

Gordon WA, Sliwinski M, Echo J, et al (1998) The benefits of exercise in individuals with traumatic brain injury: a retropsctive study. *Journal of Head Trauma and Rehabilitation*, 13:58–67

Gormley J, Hussey J (2005) (eds) *Exercise Therapy: Prevention and Treatment of Disease*. Oxford: Blackwell Publishing

Griffin L, Cafarelli E (2007) Transcranial magnetic stimulation during resistance training of the tibialis anterior muscle. *Journal of Electromyography and Kinesiology*, 17:446–52

Hallett M (2000) Transcranial magnetic stimulation and the human brain. *Nature*, 406:147–50

Hassett LM, Moseley AM, Tate R, et al (2008) Fitness training for cardiorespiratory conditioning after traumatic brain injury. *Cochrane Database of Systematic Reviews*, Issue 2, Art No: CD006123. DOI: 10.1002/14651858.CD006123.pub2

Hellweg S, Johannes S (2008) Physiotherapy after traumatic brain injury: a systematic review of the literature. *Brain Injury*, 22:365–73

Hesse S (2008) Treadmill training with partial body weight support after stroke: a review. *NeuroRehabilitation*, 23:55–65

Hirsch MA, Toole T, Maitland CG, et al (2003) The effects of balance training and high-intensity resistance training on persons with idiopathic Parkinson's disease. *Archives of Physical Medicine and Rehabilitation*, 84:1109–117

Huntley G W (1997) Correlations between patterns of horizontal connectivity and the extent of short-term representational plasticity in rat motor cortex. *Cerebral Cortex*, 7:143–56

Jackson D, Turner-Stokes L, Culpan J, et al (2001) Can brain injured patients participate in an aerobic exercise programme during early inpatient rehabilitation? *Clinical Rehabilitation*, 15:535–44

Jacobs KM, Donoghue JP (1991) Reshaping the cortical motor map by unmasking latent intracortical connection. *Science*, 251:944–7

Jones E G (2000) Plasticity and neuroplasticity. *Journal of the History of Neuroscience*, 9:37–9

Jørgensen LM, Nielsen JE, Ravnborg M (2005) MEP recruitment curves in multiple sclerosis and hereditary spastic paraplegia. *Journal of the Neurological Sciences*, 237:25–9

Kamen G (2004) Reliability of motor-evoked potentials during resting and active contraction conditions. *Medicine and Science in Sports and Exercise*, 36:1574–9

Kidgell DJ, Pearce AJ (2009) Neural adaptations following cross education strength training. *Journal of Science and Medicine in Sport*, (Suppl) 12:52–3

Kidgell DJ, Pearce AJ (2010) Corticospinal properties following short-term strength training of an intrinsic hand muscle. *Human Movement Science*, 29:631–41

Kiernan MC (2009) Amyotrophic lateral sclerosis and the neuroprotective potential of exercise. *The Journal of Physiology*, 587:3759–60

Kleim JA, Barbay S, Nudo RJ (1998) Functional reorganisation of the rat motor cortex following motor skill learning. *Journal of Neurophysiology*, 80:3321–5

Kleim JA, Lussing E, Schwarz ER, et al (1996) Synaptogenesis and FOS expression in the motor cortex of adult rat after motor skill learning. *Journal of Neuroscience*, 16:4529–35

Krupp LB, LaRocca NG, Muir-Nash J, et al (1989) The fatigue severity scale. Application to patients with multiple sclerosis and systemic lupus erythematosus. *Archives of Neurology*, 46:1121–3

Kuhtz-Buschbeck JP, Mahnkopf C, Holzknecht C, et al (2003) Effector-independent representation of simple and complex imagined finger movements: a combined fMRI and TMS study. *European Journal of Neuroscience*, 18:3375–87

Latash ML (2008) *Neurophysiological basis of movement* (2nd edn). Champaign: Human Kinetics

Lee M, Gandevia SC, Carroll T J, et al (2009) Short-term strength training does not change cortical voluntary activation. *Medicine and Science in Sports and Exercise*, 41:1452–60

Lee M, Reddy H, Johansen-Berg H, et al (2000) The motor cortex shows adaptive functional changes to brain injury from multiple sclerosis. *Annals of Neurology*, 47:606–13

Lemon RN, Johansson RS, Westling G (1995) Corticospinal control during reach, grasp and precision lift in man. *The Journal of Neuroscience*, 15:6145–56

Liao D, Zhang X, O'Brien R, et al (1999) Regulation of morphological postsynaptic silent synapses in developing hippocampal neurons. *Nature Neuroscience*, 2:37–43

Liao DN, Hessler A, Malinow R (1995) Activation of postsynaptically silent synapses during pairing-induced LTP in CA1 region of hippocampal slice. *Nature*, 375:400–4

Lynton H, Kligler B, & Shiflett S (2007) Yoga in stroke rehabilitation: a systematic review and results of a pilot study. *Topics in Stroke Rehabilitation*, 14:1–8

Martin SJ, Grimwood PD, Morris RGM (2000) Synaptic plasticity and memory: an evaluation of the hypothesis. *Annual Review of Neuroscience*, 23:649–711

Mehrholz J, Kugler J, Pohl M (2010) Water-based exercise for reducing disability after stroke (Protocol). *Cochrane Database of Systematic Reviews*, Issue 1. Art No: CD008186. DOI: 10.1002/14651858.CD008186

Meilink A, Hemmen B, Seelen HAM, et al (2008) Impact of EMG-triggered neuromuscular stimulation of the wrist and finger extensors of the paretic hand after stroke: a systematic review of the literature. *Clinical Rehabilitation*, 22:291–305

Merzenich MM, Kaas JH, Wall J, et al (1983) Topographic reorganisation of somatosensory cortical areas 3b and 1 in adult monkeys following restricted deafferentation. *Neuroscience*, 8:33–55

Morris ME (2006) Locomotor training in people with Parkinson's disease. *Physical Therapy*, 86:1426–35

Morris ME, Lansek R, Kirkwood B (2009) A randomized controlled trial of movement strategies compared with exercise for people with Parkinson's disease. *Movement Disorders*, 24:64–71

Morris ME, Martin C, Schenkman M (2010) Striding out with Parkinson disease: evidence based physical therapy for gait disorders. *Physical Therapy*, 90:280–8

Morris SL, Dodd KJ, Morris ME (2004) Outcomes of progressive resistance strength training following stroke: a systematic review. *Clinical Rehabilitation*, 18:27–39

Morris SL, Dodd KJ, Morris ME, et al (2009) Community-based progressive resistance strength training in traumatic brain injury: A multiple, single-system, trial. *Advances in Physiotherapy*, doi: 10.1080/14038190902856778

Moseley AM, Stark A, Cameron ID, et al (2005) Treadmill training and body weight support for walking after stroke. *Cochrane Database of Systematic Reviews*, Issue 4, Art No: CD002840. DOI: 10.1002/14651858. CD002840.pub2

Mostert S, Kesselring J (2002) Effects of a short-term exercise training program on aerobic fitness, fatigue, health perception and activity levels of subjects with multiple sclerosis. *Multiple Sclerosis*, 8:161–8

Pak S, Patten C (2008) Strengthening to promote functional recovery poststroke: an evidence-based review. *Topics in Stroke Rehabilitation*, 15:177–99

Pang TYC, Stam NC, Nithianantharajah J, et al (2006) Differential effects of voluntary physical exercise on behavioural and brain-derived neurotrophic factor expression in Huntington's disease transgenic mice. *Neuroscience*, 141:569–84

Paoloni M, Mangone M, Scettri P, et al (2009) Segmental muscle vibration improves walking in chronic stroke patients with foot drop: a randomized controlled trial. *Neurorehabilitation and Neural Repair*, 24:254–62

Pascual-Leone A, Dang N, Cohen L G, et al (1995) Modulation of muscle responses evoked by transcrannial magnetic stimulation during the acquisition of new fine motor skills. *Journal of Neurophysiology*, 74:1037–43

Paul R L, Merzenich M M, Goodman H (1972) Representation of slowly and rapidly adapting cutaneous mechanoreceptors of the hand in Brodmann;s area 3 and 1 of *Macaca mulatta*. *Braun Research*, 36:229–49

Pearce AJ (2000) Physiological studies in the human corticomotor system associated with dynamic and static movement. PhD thesis, University of Western Australia

Pearce AJ, Kidgell DJ (2009) Corticomotor excitability during precision motor tasks. *Journal of Science and Medicine in Sport*, 12:280–3

Pearce AJ, Kidgell DJ (2010) Comparison of corticomotor excitability during visuomotor dynamic and static tasks. *Journal of Science and Medicine in Sport*, 13:167–71

Pearce AJ, Thickbroom GW, Byrnes ML, et al (2000) Functional reorganisation of the corticomotor projection to the hand in skilled racquet players. *Experimental Brain Research*, 130:238–43

Petajan JH, Gappmaier E, White AT, et al (1996) Impact of aerobic training on fitness and quality of life in multiple sclerosis. *Annals of Neurology*, 39:432–41

Prange GB, Jannink MJA, Groothuis-Oudshoorn CGM, et al (2006) Systematic review of the effect of robot-aided therapy on recovery of the hemiparetic arm after stroke. *Journal of Rehabilitation, Research and Development*, 43:171–84

Ramaratnam S, Sridharan K (2002) Yoga for epilepsy. *Cochrane Database of Systematic Reviews*, Issue 1. Art No: CD001524. DOI: 10.1002/14651858.CD001524

Rao SM, Binder JR, Bandettini PA, et al (1993) Functional magnetic resonance imaging of complex human movements. *Neurology*, 43:2311–18

Rietberg MB, Brooks D, Uitdehaag BMJ, et al (2004) Exercise therapy for multiple sclerosis. *Cochrane Database of Systematic Reviews*, Issue 3, Art No: CD003980. DOI: 10.1002/14651858.CD003980.pub2

Rioult-Pedotti M-S, Donoghue JP (2002) Learning, retention and persistent strengthening of cortical synapses. *Society of Neuroscience*, 32:713

Rioult-Pedotti M-S, Donoghue JP (2003) The nature and mechanisms of plasticity. In: Boniface S, Ziemann U (eds) *Plasticity in the Human Nervous System: Investigations with Transcranial Magnetic Stimulation*. Cambridge: Cambridge University Press, pp 1–25

Rioult-Pedotti M-S, Friedman D, Donoghue JP (2000) Learning-induced LTP in neocortex. *Science*, 290:533–6

Rossini PM, Caltagirone C, Castriota-Scandberg A, et al (1998) Hand motor cortical area reorganisation in stroke: a study with fMRI, MEG and TMS maps. *Neuroreport*, 9:2141–6

Rothwell JC (1994) *Control of Human Voluntary Movement* (2nd ed). London: Chapman and Hall

Saunders DH, Greig CA, Young A, et al (2004) Physical fitness training for stroke patients. *Cochrane Database of Systematic Reviews*, Issue 1, Art No: CD003316. DOI: 10.1002/14651858.CD003316.pub3

Scandalis TA, Bosak A, Berliner JC, et al (2001) Resistance training and gait function in patients with Parkinson's disease. *American Journal of Physical Medicine and Rehabilitation*, 80:38–43

Sharp SA, Bouwer BJ (1997) Isokinetic strength training of the hemiparetic knee: effects on function and spasticity. *Archives of Physical Medicine and Rehabilitation*, 74:1192–8

Shores EA, Marosszeky JE, Sandanam J, et al (1986) Preliminary validation of a clinical scale for measuring the duration of PTA. *Medical Journal of Australia*, 144:569–72

Smith GV, Silver KHC, Goldberg AP, et al (1999) 'Task-orientated' exercise improves hamstring strength and spastic reflexes in chronic stroke patients. *Stroke*, 30:2112–18

Sorra KE, Harris KM (1998) Stability in synapse number and size at 2 hr after long-term potentiation in hippocampal area CA1. *Journal of Neuroscience*, 18:658–71

Subramanian SK, Massie CL, Malcolm, MP, et al (2009) Does provision of extrinsic feedback result in improved motor learning in the upper limb poststroke? A systematic review of the evidence. *Neurorehabilitation and Neural Repair*, 24:113–24

Teixeira-Salmela LF, Olney SJ, Nadeau S, et al (1999) Muscle strengthening and physical conditioning to reduce impairment and disability in chronic stroke survivors. *Archives of Physical Medicine and Rehabilitation*, 80:1211–18

Thickbroom GW, Byrnes ML, Walter S, et al (2006) Motor cortex reorganisation in Parkinson's disease. *Journal of Clinical Neuroscience*, 13:639–42

Thickbroom GW, Mastaglia FL (2009) Plasticity in neurological disorders and challenges for non-invasive brain stimulation (NBS). *Journal of Neuroengineering and Rehabilitation*, 6:4. Online. Available: http://jneuroengrehab.com/content/6/1/4 (accessed 17 Feb 2009)

Thickbroom GW, Sacco P, Kermode AG, et al (2006) Central motor drive and perception of effort during fatigue in multiple sclerosis. *Journal of Neurology*, 253:1048–53

Toni B, Buchs P-A, Nikonenko I, et al (1999) LTP promotes formation of multiple spin synapses between a single axon terminal and a dendrite. *Nature*, 402:421–5

Toole T, Hirsch MA, Forkink A, et al (2000) The effects of a balance and strength training program on equilibrium in Parkinsonism: a preliminary study. *Neurorehabilitation*, 14:165–74

Traversa R, Cicinelli P, Bassi A, et al (1997) Mapping of motor cortical reorganisation after stroke. A brain stimulation study with focal magnetic pulses. *Stroke*, 28:110–17

van Hedel H, Murer C, Dietz V, et al (2007) The amplitude of lower leg motor evoked potentials is a reliable measure when controlled for torque and motor task. *Journal of Neurology*, 254:1089–98

Wasserman EM (2005) Individual differences in the response to transcranial magnetic stimulation. In: Hallett M, Chokroverty S (eds) *Magnetic Stimulation in Clinical Neurophysiology*. Philadelphia: Elsevier, pp 303–10

Wassermann EM (2002) Safety and side-effects of transcranial magnetic stimulation and repetitive transcranial magnetic stimulation. In: Pascual-Leone AP, Davey NJ, Rothwell J, Wasserman EM Puri B K (eds) *Handbook of Transcranial Magnetic Stimulation*. New York: Oxford University Press, pp 39–49

Wevers L, van de Port I, Vermue M, et al (2009) Effects of task-oriented circuit class training on walking competency after stroke: a systematic review. *Stroke*, 40:2450–9

Williams GP, Morris ME (2009) High-level mobility outcomes following acquired brain injury: a preliminary evaluation. *Brain Injury*, 23:307–12

Wilson SA, Thickbroom GW, Mastaglia FL (1993) Transcrannial magnetic stimulation mapping of the motor cortex in normal subjects: the representation of two intrinsic hand muscles. *Journal of the Neurological Sciences*, 118:134–44

Yang Y-R, Wang R-Y, Lin K-H, et al (2006) Task-oriented progressive resistance strength training improves muscle strength and functional performance in individuals with stroke. *Clinical Rehabilitation*, 20:860–70

Chapter 6

Exercise as therapy in metabolic syndrome and polycystic ovary syndrome

Itamar Levinger and Nigel Stepto

Assumed concepts

This chapter is based on the assumption that readers will have some understanding of:

- metabolic conditions that alter glucose control, particularly metabolic syndrome (MetS), type 2 diabetes mellitus (T2DM), and polycystic ovary syndrome (PCOS)
- principles of exercise training, particularly aerobic exercise training and resistance exercise training.

INTRODUCTION

Obesity, metabolic syndrome (MetS), polycystic ovary syndrome (PCOS) and type 2 diabetes mellitus (T2DM) can all lead to cardiovascular disease and premature death. As such, they should be targeted vigorously in order to keep the metabolic factors within desirable ranges (Hanefeld & Schaper 2005). The treatment for metabolic conditions/diseases encompasses three main parts: diet; exercise and/or physical activity; and pharmacological interventions (Hanefeld & Schaper 2005; Moran et al 2009; Pi-Sunyer 2006). This chapter will highlight the role exercise should play as a therapy in metabolic conditions/diseases.

Note: part of this chapter is based on the literature review from Itamar Levinger's PhD thesis.

The mechanisation and computerisation of home and work environments has led to many people adopting sedentary lifestyles (Martinez-Gonzalez et al 1999; Martinez 2000; Pi-Sunyer 2002). It has been reported that physical inactivity is a major risk factor threatening global health (Murray & Lopez 1996). This is probably due to the direct association between physical inactivity and obesity (Cameron et al 2003; Grundy et al 1999; Martinez-Gonzalez et al 1999; Martinez et al 1999), T2DM (Helmrich et al 1991; Hu et al 2004; Hu et al 1999) and heart disease (Fletcher et al 1996; Haskel 1984; Smith et al 1995) and negative associations with insulin sensitivity and glucose tolerance. In contrast, increases in exercise capacity may protect people from premature death, where even small improvements in physical fitness are associated with significantly lower mortality even without changes in body fatness (Erikssen

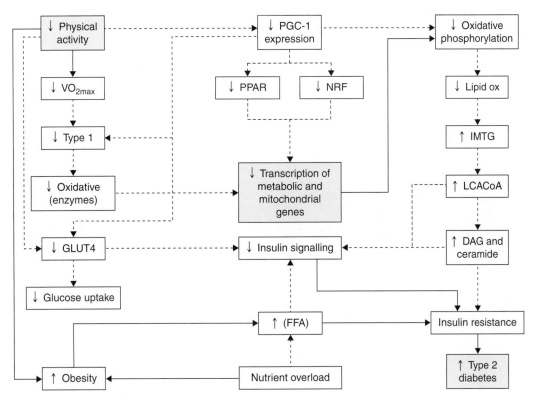

Figure 6.1 Proposed model by which physical inactivity directly contributes to the cascade of events leading to decreased transcription of metabolic and mitochondrial genes, decreased oxidative phosphorylation in skeletal muscle, accretion of muscle lipid and the expression of the metabolic phenotype associated with insulin resistance and type 2 diabetes

Key: VO2max, whole-body maximal oxygen uptake; PCG-1, peroxisomal proliferator activator receptor coactivator; NRF, nuclear respiratory factor; FAT/CD36, fatty acid transporters; FFA; free fatty acids; IMTG, muscle triacylglycerol; LCACoA, long-chain acyl CoA; DAG, diacylglycerol. [Reproduced with permission from Hawley JA (2004) Exercise as a therapeutic intervention for the prevention and treatment of insulin resistance. *Diabetes/Metabolism Research and Reviews*, 20(5):383–93]

et al 1998; Wing et al 2007). Hawley (2004) suggested a model (see Figure 6.1) to describe the relationship between reductions in physical activity and the development of obesity, insulin resistance and T2DM. According to the model, reductions in physical activity lead to a reduction in aerobic power and alterations to skeletal muscle structure and metabolism, in turn leading to reductions in lipid oxidation and glucose uptake and increased muscle triglyceride and free fatty acid (FFA) content. These muscle alteration may increase insulin resistance and cause T2DM (Hawley 2004).

It is accepted that exercise training should be included as an integral part of weight management for treatment for obese people and those with

MetS, PCOS and T2DM (American College of Sports Medicine [ACSM] 2000; American Diabetes Association 1999; Creviston & Quinn 2001; Eriksson 1999; Hagberg et al 2000; Hu et al 1999; Moran et al 2009).

EXERCISE TRAINING AS MULTIPLE THERAPEUTIC MEDICATION

People with metabolic risk factors and metabolic diseases are often prescribed a range of medications. These medications include medications to enhance weight loss and improve dyslipidaemia, increase insulin sensitivity and decrease insulin resistance, however, appropriately tailored exercise training can reduce the need for such pharmacotherapy and treat dyslipidaemia and insulin resistance with no side-effects.

Pharmacotherapy versus exercise for obesity and dyslipidaemia

The range of pharmacological options for obesity includes three main modes of action: modification of appetite (less food intake); increased thermogenesis (increase energy expenditure); and inhibition of nutrient absorption from the gastrointestinal tract (Alemany et al 2003; Bray 2001; Das & Chakrabarti 2006; Fernandez-Lopez et al 2002; Pi-Sunyer 2006).

The mechanism of action and the metabolic benefits from sibutramine, orlistat, and phentermine are presented in Table 6.1. The overall weight reduction with these medications is lower than 5kg over 2 years (Davidson et al 1999; Hansen et al 1998, 1999; James et al 2000; Li et al 2005; Maggio & Pi-Sunyer 1997; Sjostrom et al 1998; Walsh et al 1999; Yamamoto et al 2000) and they may or may not effect lipid profiles and glucose control (Davidson et al 1999; Drent et al 1995; Halford 2004; Sjostrom et al 1998). It appears that the anti-obesity medications may enhance short-term weight loss. However, these medications may have limited long-term benefits (Alemany et al 2003; Astrup & Lundsgaard 1998; Bray 2001; Fernandez-Lopez et al 2002) and there is lack of evidence for the effect of these drugs for changing long-term prognosis from obesity-related disease and quality of life (QoL) (Li et al 2005). In addition, these drugs have some severe side-effects including nausea and dry mouth (Hanotin et al 1998; James et al 2000), fatty/oily stools, increased defecation, oily spotting, liquid stools, flatus with discharge, abdominal pain and a reduction in the levels of vitamin D and E (Davidson et al 1999; Drent et al 1995; Li et al 2005; Sjostrom et al 1998) that in turn may lower QoL and may lead people to stop using them.

Exercise training also has been shown to enhance weight loss by up to 4kg over 14 months (Caballero 2003; Despres et al 1991). It is important to acknowledge that not all studies have reported a significant reduction in body mass following exercise interventions. Measuring absolute body mass or body mass index (BMI) may not be the most appropriate method to assess positive (or negative) alterations in body composition following training. Exercise

training may reduce fat mass and increase lean body mass (Caballero 2003; Despres et al 1991) with no absolute body mass change in many populations, including people who are overweight (Olson et al 2007), and those with clusters of risk factors or established diabetes (Castaneda et al 2002; Harris & Holly 1987; Hurley et al 1988; Levinger et al 2007; Stone et al 1991). As body mass measurement includes both lean and fat mass, fat loss may be accompanied by muscle gain.

Favourable changes to body composition after resistance training (RT) may lead to improved glucose homeostasis, and this is probably related to increased muscle mass (Eriksson et al 1997; Sanchez & Leon 2001). Another important factor is that unlike medication, exercise training has no long-term adverse effects. In other words, a person who is involved in exercise on a regular basis (RT or aerobic training) will have all the benefits the medications can offer without the side-effects of the medications.

Maintaining normal lipid levels is an important goal in clinical practice in order to prevent the development of coronary artery disease (Deedwania et al 2006; Expert Panel on Detection Evaluation and Treatment of High Blood Cholesterol In Adults 2001; Schuster et al 2004; Wood 1998). Statins prevent the formation of cholesterol by inhibiting the conversion of 3-hydroxy-3-methylglutaryl coenzyme A (HMG-CoA) to mevalonate (Endres & Laufs 2004). Treatment with statins has anti-atherosclerotic effects (Matsuo et al 2005) and can modify lipid profiles in individuals with dyslipidaemia and MetS (Ballantyne et al 2003; Deedwania et al 2006; Hanefeld & Schaper 2005; Schuster et al 2004). In addition, statins (such as atorvastatin), can improve insulin sensitivity in insulin-resistant individuals (Huptas et al 2006). In some cases statins may have adverse effects including myositis (painful myalgia), gastrointestinal disturbance and abnormal liver transaminases (see Table 6.1).

Similar to statins, exercise training may improve lipids profile. Both aerobic training (Couillard et al 2001) and RT (Cauza et al 2005; Honkola et al 1997; Hurley et al 1988; Rice et al 1999) reduce total cholesterol, low density lipoprotein (LDL) and/or triglyceride and increase high density lipoprotein (HDL) levels

Table 6.1 Comparison of sibutramine, orlistat, phentermine, statins and exercise when used as mono-therapy

Drug / Effect	Sibutramine	Orlistat	Phentermine	Statins	Exercise
Mechanism of action	Adrenaline and serotonin reuptake inhibitor, ↓ appetite	Gastrointestinal lipase inhibitor	Serotonin reuptake inhibitor, ↓ appetite	Inhibiting the conversion of HMG-CoA to mevalonate	
Weight loss	↓	↓	↓	↔	↓
Trig level	↔↓	↔↓	↔↓	↓	↓
HDL cholesterol level	↔	↔	↔	↑	↑
LDL cholesterol	↔↓	↓	↔↓	↓	↓
Glucose control	↔↑	↑	↔	↔↑	↑
Side-effects	↑Adrenaline secretion, HR, BP and plasma glucose level. Also, nausea and dry mouth	Fatty/oily stools, ↑ defecation, oily spotting, liquid stools, flatus with discharge, abdominal pain and ↓ in vitamin D and E	Palpitation, Tachycardia, hypertension and gastro-intestinal effects	Myositis (painful myalgia), gastrointestinal disturbance, abnormal liver transaminases	---------

(Eriksson et al 1998). See Chapter 11, case study 3, for an account of combined drug, exercise, and dietary intervention for weight reduction.

Pharmacotherapy versus exercise for type 2 diabetes

The effects of five T2DM medications: sulfonylureas, repaglinide, metformin, troglitazone and acarbose are presented in Table 6.2. From the five medications listed in the table, the two most frequently prescribed medications for individuals with T2DM are sulfonylureas and metformin (DeFronzo & Goodman 1995; Goodarzi & Bryer-Ash 2005; Tripathi & Srivastava 2006).

The mechanism of action and the benefits from the diabetic medications are presented in Table 6.2. Despite benefits such as a reduction in HbA1c

(between 0.5–2% points) and fasting glucose (between 1.1 ad 4 mmol/L) levels, approximately 75% of people treated with those drugs will not achieve long-term normalisation of glucose levels (DeFronzo 1999). In addition, some drugs such as sulfonylureas and repaglinide can increase body mass. Metformin is a biguanide type of medication and is the preferred medication for overweight individuals with T2DM, because it can lead to weight loss and improve lipid profiles (Campbell & Howlett 1995; DeFronzo 1999; Fontbonne et al 1996; Goodarzi & Bryer-Ash 2005; Tripathi & Srivastava 2006). Similar to sulfonylureas, only ~25% of the patients on metformin find that their T2DM is effectively managed with this drug. As such, the effectiveness of these drugs as a mono-therapy is relatively short-lived and combination

Table 6.2 Comparison of sulfonylureas, repaglinide, metformin, troglitazone, acarbose and exercise when used as mono-therapy

Effect \ Drug	Sulfonylureas and repaglinide	Metformin	Troglitazone	Exercise
Mechanism of action	↑ insulin secretion	↓ hepatic glucose production, ↑ muscle insulin sensitivity	↓ hepatic glucose production, ↑ muscle insulin sensitivity	↓ hepatic glucose production, ↑ muscle insulin sensitivity
FPG	↓	↓	↓	↓
HbA1c	↓	↓	↓	↓
Trig level	↔	↓	↓	↓
HDL cholesterol level	↔	↔↑	↑	↑
LDL cholesterol	↔	↓	↑	↓
Body mass	↑	↓	↑	↓
Plasma insulin	↑	↓	↓	↔↓
Adverse events	Hypoglycaemia	Gastrointestinal disturbance, lactic acidosis (very rare)	Anaemia, hepatic toxicity, irreversible hepatic failure (rare)	--------------

Note: FPG, fasting plasma glucose; Trig, triglyceride; HDL, high density lipoprotein; LDL, low density lipoprotein. Based on DeFronzo (1999).

therapies are needed in order to achieve long-term glucose control (Turner et al 1999). In addition these drugs have some severe side-effects that may affect QoL (see Table 6.2).

There is increased evidence that both aerobic training (Borghouts & Keizer 2000; Christ-Roberts et al 2004; Christ et al 2002; Colwell 2003; Couillard et al 2001; Dela et al 1995; Houmard et al 2004; Koivisto & DeFronzo 1984; Kraus et al 2002; Marcell et al 2005; Rinder et al 2004; Sciacqua et al 2003) and RT (Castaneda et al 2002; Dunstan et al 2002) can reduce HbA1c (up to 1.2% points) and fasting glucose level (up to 1.5mmol/L). Aerobic exercise can improve beta cell function, insulin secretion and muscle insulin sensitivity (Bloem & Chang 2008). Similarly, it has been reported that RT can improve insulin sensitivity, insulin resistance and glucose homeostasis in healthy people (Dela & Kjaer 2006; Hurley et al 1988; Poehlman et al 2000), and also people who are overweight with or without MetS or T2DM (Albright et al 2000; Dela & Kjaer, 2006; Maiorana et al 2001; Shaibi et al 2006). Exercise also increases the activity of some insulin-signalling molecules, including insulin receptor substrate (IRS-1) associated with PI3-kinase (Krisan et al 2004), and glycogen synthase protein (Holten et al 2004) which may lead to greater flux of glucose to muscle cells and increase muscle capacity to store muscle glycogen (Holten et al 2004). Exercise improves glucose control; the improvement in glucose metabolism may be related to increased GLUT4 level and activity in skeletal muscles (Christ-Roberts et al 2004; Christ et al 2002; Dela et al 1994; Ferrier et al 2004; Lemieux et al 2005; Tomas et al 2002) and the increased activation of glycogen synthase (Bak et al 1989; Christ-Roberts et al 2004; Lemieux et al 2005) and glycogen storage (Borst & Snellen, 2001; Chibalin et al 2000; Dela et al 1995).

Lifestyle modification including increased physical activity should be the first treatment for individuals with insulin resistance and T2DM. As described above, exercise training can offer similar benefits for individuals with elevated glucose level as do diabetic medications without the side-effects. The addition of pharmacotherapy should be considered if lifestyle modifications fail to maintain adequate blood glucose levels See Chapter 16, case study 1, for an account of using exercise concurrent with metformin for diabetes control.

POLYCYSTIC OVARY SYNDROME (PCOS)

PCOS is an endocrine condition affecting 5–10% of women of reproductive age (Azziz et al 2004). The diagnostic criteria for PCOS include: hyperandrogenism (increased production of androgen, a male sex hormone, in women); oligo- or anovulation; and the presence of polycystic ovaries on ultrasound (Rotterdam ESHRE/ASRM-sponsored consensus workshop group 2004). PCOS has serious clinical effects including reproductive manifestations (hirsutism, infertility and pregnancy complications; Boomsma et al 2006), metabolic complications (insulin resistance, MetS, impaired glucose tolerance and T2DM) and CV complications (Apridonidze et al 2005; Hart et al 2004; Legro et al 1999; Meyer et al 2005; Paradisi et al 2001; Solomon 1999) and psychological effects such as poor self-esteem and anxiety (Jones et al 2008). It is estimated that 40–60% of women with PCOS are overweight or obese (Balen et al 1995; Goldzieher & Axelrod, 1963; Kiddy et al 1990) with greater abdominal or visceral adiposity compared to weight-matched controls (Yildirim et al 2003). In addition, many women with PCOS (40–70%) have insulin resistance and the insulin resistance is independent of the obesity level (DeUgarte et al 2005; Dunaif et al 1989; Ovalle & Azziz 2002; Toprak et al 2001). Insulin resistance is a key factor in the aetiology of PCOS through insulin affecting the stimulation of ovarian androgen production and decreasing hepatic sex hormone binding globulin (SHBG) production leading to increased free androgens (Diamanti-Kandarakis & Papavassiliou 2006).

Pharmacotherapy versus exercise in PCOS

PCOS was traditionally considered as a gynaecological and/or reproductive disorder usually treated with the oral contraceptive pill to address the biochemical and clinical hyperandrogenism. However, this treatment strategy also increased insulin resistance and the risk of cardiovascular disease, especially when a high-dose oral contraceptive pill was used (Meyer et al 2007).

Currently, PCOS treatment is focused on a reduction of body fat and insulin resistance, all features of the MetS. That, in turn, may lead to a reduction in hyperandrogenism. Available anti-obesity and anti–insulin resistance medications are orlistat, metformin, sibutramine and rimonabant (Bray 2001). Table 6.3 summarises the effect of those drugs in relation to PCOS. Metformin may have positive effects on ovulation and pregnancy rates (Lord et al 2003). Sibutramine added to a reduced energy diet resulted in more spontaneous pregnancies and greater decreases in body weight, triglycerides (Sabuncu et al 2003), lipoprotein ApoA, and androgens (Lindholm et al 2007), compared with diet alone (Florakis et al 2007; Lindholm et al 2007) or ethinyl-estradiol plus cyproterone acetate (Sabuncu et al 2003). Orlistat plus diet reduced weight, waist to hip ratio and insulin resistance in obese women with or without PCOS, but androgens decreased only in women with PCOS (Diamanti-Kandarakis et al 2007; Panidis et al 2007).

A small number of studies have examined the effects of lifestyle interventions including exercise, diet and behavioural modification on women with PCOS (Clark et al 1995, 1998; Huber-Buchholz et al 1999). Weight loss is associated with reductions in androgens, increases in steroid hormone binding globulin (SHBG) and improvements in metabolic profile including improvement in glucose control, and reduction in plasminogen activator inhibitor-1, diastolic blood pressure and insulin resistance (Clark et al 1995; Huber-Buchholz et al 1999). Weight loss was also associated with improvement in menstrual function and ovulation (Clark et al

Table 6.3 Comparison of metformin, orlistat rimonabant, sibutramine and exercise when used as a therapy in PCOS on hormonal profiles and reproductive features

Drug Effect	Metformin	Orlistat	Rimonabant	Sibutramine	Exercise
SHBG	↔↑	↔↑	↔	↑	↔↑
T	↓	↓	↓	↔↓	↔↓
FAI	↓	↓	↓	↓	↔↓
Reproductive outcomes	↑O & ↑P	NA	NA	↑P	↑O & ↑P

Note: FAI, free androgen index; FPG, fasting plasma glucose; O, ovulation; P, pregnancy rate; SHBG, sex hormone binding globulin; T, testosterone; NA, not assessed.

1995; Clark et al 1998; Huber-Buchholz et al 1999) and spontaneous or assisted-reproduction pregnancies (Clark et al 1995; Clark et al 1998; Huber-Buchholz et al 1999).

Exercise, when incorporated in these lifestyle studies, was usually unstructured or unsupervised. Structured exercise as a fundamental lifestyle component may improve efficacy, feasibility, sustainability and clinical outcomes in PCOS (Palomba et al 2008; Vigorito et al 2007). Because exercise improves insulin sensitivity independent of weight loss, it offers significant potential benefits in PCOS (Bruner et al 2006; Erikssen et al 1998; Wing et al 2007).

There are few studies that investigated the effects of exercise on women with PCOS and even fewer randomised controlled trials (RCTs). To date, none have investigated the role of RT in PCOS. Palomba et al (2008) reported a non-randomised trial comparing exercise (30 minute bicycle ergometer, three times per week, at 60–70% VO_{2max}) to dietary energy restriction in two groups of 20 women with PCOS. Ovulation and pregnancy rates in the exercise group (65% and 6.2%) notably exceeded those in the dietary control group (25% and 1.7%). In a 3-month RCT a bicycle exercise training regimen improved insulin resistance and reduced BMI in women with PCOS (non-exercising control group; Vigorito et al 2007). Others reported no improvements in

insulin resistance with diet versus diet and exercise (Bruner et al 2006; Randeva et al 2002), however, those two studies have small sample sizes (n = 12 and n = 21).

It should be noted that current literature on the effects of exercise on women with PCOS is limited, and the few studies that have been published have some limitations including small sample sizes, short intervention, and they are not randomised controlled. Additionally, many studies investigating treatments often includes multiple interventions such as the use of caloric restriction or hormone therapy with exercise (Clark et al 1995; Clark et al 1998; Huber-Buchholz et al 1999). This makes interpreting the effect of exercise difficult. However, when all studies are considered it is now recommended that in PCOS, especially when complicated by obesity, a holistic lifestyle intervention should be adopted as an initial treatment strategy (Moran et al 2009). This strategy should include increased physical activity in some form of structured exercise training regimen. Although exercise alone does not generally induce large or rapid weight loss in PCOS women, it certainly provides many clinical benefits such as lowering cardiovascular disease risk, insulin resistance and enhances reproductive potential. These benefits come without the side-effects that are associated with pharmacotherapy (See Tables 6.1, 6.2 and 6.3). Importantly, exercise programs can be continued throughout pregnancy, where most medications must be stopped because they are contraindicated due to lack of safety information for use during early pregnancy (Lord et al 2003; Sathyapalan et al 2008). See Chapter 16, case studies 3 and 4, for accounts of using exercise in PCOS including during pregnancy.

OTHER THERAPEUTIC EFFECTS OF EXERCISE TRAINING

As highlighted above, pharmacological treatment usually targets a specific disorder or condition, but exercise training has positive effects on almost all systems in the body. In that regard, exercise training by itself can be regarded as 'multi-pill' intervention. The positive effects of exercise training are not limited for assisting in improving metabolic risk factors such as obesity, glucose levels, and poor lipids profile but also may have positive effects on functional capacities and QoL. Although this chapter highlights the role exercise (both aerobic and resistance exercises) can play as a multi-pill for metabolic conditions, it should be acknowledged that aerobic exercise and resistance exercise may offer different benefits which, if both methods of exercise are combined, may offer better adaptation to training and higher metabolic benefits (see Table 6.4).

Exercise training and aerobic power

Exercise training increases VO_{2peak} (Christ-Roberts et al 2004; Lee et al 2005; Ligtenberg et al 1997; Marcell et al 2005; Trovati et al 1984; Watkins et al 2003) and it is widely accepted that aerobic training is the most effective training mode to improve aerobic fitness (Belman & Gaesser 1991; Kohrt et al 1991; Makrides et al 1990). There is also a body of evidence supporting the application of RT to improve VO_{2peak}. The mechanism may include favourable alterations to muscle morphology in response to RT. RT may have the effect of shifting skeletal muscle phenotype towards a higher proportion of slow, oxidative muscle fibre types, improve oxidative enzyme activity and increase capillary density. These changes may increase the potential for oxygen delivery to, and consumption by, muscle (Frontera et al 1990; Hepple et al 1997), and offer an explanation for improvements in VO_{2peak} and exercise duration following RT (Ades et al

1996; Hagerman et al 2000; Staron et al 1989). An improvement in aerobic fitness is clinically important as it has been shown that an increase in VO_{2peak} is a strong predictor of all-cause mortality in both clinical and non-clinical populations (Blair et al 1996). In addition, epidemiology studies have shown that VO_{2peak} is a significant predictor for mortality (Sui et al 2007) and T2DM (Sui et al 2008) independent of fatness level. As such, an increase in VO_{2peak} should be an important goal in interventions for individuals with metabolic diseases.

Exercise training, muscle strength, capacity for activities of daily living, and quality of life

Elderly individuals and those with metabolic conditions characterise low muscle strength (Willey & Fiatarone-Singh 2003; Yki-Jarvinen & Koivisto 1983). Older adults with T2DM exhibit greater reduction in leg muscle strength and leg muscle lean mass (both approximately 50%) over 3 years, compared to non-diabetic individuals (Park et al 2007), and increased muscle strength is important for the performance of activities of daily living (ADL) in individuals with MetS and T2DM (Kraemer et al 2001; Levinger et al 2007; Maiorana et al 2002; Pollock et al 2000). Study by Levinger et al (2007) has reported that 10 weeks of RT improved all-body (sum of seven exercises) muscle strength (by 25%), the capacity to perform ADL (~10%) and QoL as measured by self-perception of physical (~13%) and mental (~8%) health dimensions of the SF-36 in individuals with clusters of metabolic risk factors. Furthermore, the change in muscle strength after training was negatively associated with time to perform ADL tasks (r = 0.53, p<0.01) and with the changes in both physical (r = 0.59, p<0.01) and mental (r = 0.45, p = 0.02) aspects of the SF-36. Changes in the capacity to perform ADL and QoL were independent of changes in body fat levels or aerobic capacity (Levinger et al 2007). These data highlight the importance of exercise training for people with metabolic conditions as it shows that exercise may not only improve clinical measurements but also functional capacity and QoL. Others also reported that an increase in muscle strength can lower disability in the elderly (Brandon et al 2000; Fiatarone et al 1994; Pennix et al 2001).

Table 6.4 The effects of aerobic and strength training on selected functional and clinical variables

Exercise	Aerobic	Resistance
Bone mineral density	↑↑	↑↑
Body composition		
%Fat	↓↓	↓
LBM	↔	↑↑
Strength	↔	↑↑↑
Glucose metabolism		
Insulin response to glucose challenge	↓↓	↓↓
Basal insulin levels	↓	↓
Serum lipids		
HDL	↑↑	↑↔
LDL	↓↓	↓↔
Resting heart rate	↓↓	↔
Stroke volume	↑↑	↔
Blood pressure at rest		
Systolic	↓↓	↔↓
Diastolic	↓↓	↓↔
VO_2max	↑↑↑	↑
Endurance time	↑↑↑	↑↑
Physical function	↑↑	↑↑↑
Basal metabolism	↑	↑↑

Note: LBM, lean body mass; HDL, high density lipoprotein; LDL, low density lipoprotein. ↓↔ refers to reduction or no change. ↑↔ refers to increase or no change.

(Source: adapted from Pollock & Vincent 1996)

CONCLUSION

Exercise training should be an important part of any intervention for individuals with metabolic diseases. In contrast to pharmacological therapy, which is designed to target a specific metabolic disorder, exercise can offer a wide range of metabolic benefits. These metabolic benefits are in a similar magnitude to the pharmacological therapy but without the side-effects and/or adverse effects associated with pharmacotherapy treatment. In addition, exercise has positive effects on functional capacities, the capacity to perform ADL and QoL. All are important goals for interventions for specific populations in general and those with metabolic disease in particular. It appears that exercise is a 'multi-therapeutic-pill'.

Practical considerations

The research data continually demonstrate health and therapeutic benefits of exercise for people with metabolic diseases. Clients, when commencing exercise therapy, will often have a number of co-morbidities and be taking a combination of medications. There is very little information on the interactions of exercise with these medications, and it is therefore important that, when exercise training is prescribed at an appropriate level for these people, regular medical reviews of medications should be undertaken in conjunction with referring physicians. In these reviews discussions should include recommendations on doses and the timing of medications with respect to the exercise training. Finally, one should also be cognisant that in providing exercise therapy for people with metabolic disorders that a lifestyle approach should be taken and issues such as changes in diet, mental state and socioeconomic backgrounds need to be considered for long-term success in treatment.

Summary of key lessons

- Exercise is a multifaceted 'pill' for metabolic syndrome.
- Exercise is as effective as pharmacotherapy.
- Generally there are no side-effects from exercise training.
- Exercise has benefits and implications beyond pathophysiology and is therefore likely to have better health outcomes.
- Clinical exercise practitioners will see clients on multiple medications, and care must be taken to ensure appropriate medical revisions are made with respect to pharmacotherapy and exercise training.

REFERENCES

Ades PA, Ballor DL, Ashikaga T, et al (1996) Weight training improves walking endurance in healthy elderly persons. *Annals of Internal Medicine*, 124(6):568–72

Albright A, Franz M, Hornsby G, et al (2000) American College of Sports Medicine position stand. Exercise and type 2 diabetes. *Medicine and Science in Sports and Exercise*, 32(7):1345–60

Alemany M, Remesar X, Fernandez-Lopez JA (2003) Drug strategies for the treatment of obesity. *IDrugs*, 6(6): 566–72

American College of Sports Medicine (ACSM) (2000) Exercise and type 2 diabetes: position stand of the American College of Sports Medicine. *Medicine and Science in Sports and Exercise*, 32(7):1345–60

American Diabetes Association (1999) Diabetes mellitus and exercise. *Diabetes Care*, 22:S49–S53

Apridonidze T, Essah PA, Iuorno MJ, et al (2005) Prevalence and characteristics of the metabolic syndrome in women with polycystic ovary syndrome. *Journal of Clinical Endocrinology & Metabolism*, 90(4):1929–35

Astrup A, Lundsgaard C (1998) What do pharmacological approaches to obesity management offer? Linking pharmacological mechanisms of obesity management agents to clinical practice. *Experimental and Clinical Endocrinology and Diabetes*, 106 (Suppl 2):29–34

Azziz, R, Woods KS, Reyna R, et al (2004) The prevalence and features of the polycystic ovary syndrome in an unselected population. *J Clin Endocrinol Metab*, 89(6):2745–9

Bak JF, Jacobsen UK, Jorgensen FS, et al (1989) Insulin receptor function and glycogen synthase activity in skeletal muscle biopsies from patients with insulin-dependent diabetes mellitus: effects of physical training. *Journal of Clinical Endocrinology and Metabolism*, 69(1):158–164

Balen AH, Conway GS, Kaltsas G, et al (1995) Polycystic ovary syndrome: the spectrum of the disorder in 1741 patients. *Hum Reprod*, 10(8):2107–2111

Ballantyne CM, Stein EA, Paoletti R, et al (2003) Efficacy of rosuvastatin 10 mg in patients with the metabolic syndrome. *American Journal of Cardiology*, 91(5A): 25C–27C; discussion 28C

Belman MJ, Gaesser, GA (1991) Exercise training below and above the lactate threshold in the elderly. *Medicine and Science in Sports and Exercise*, 23(5):562–8

Blair SN, Kampert JB, Kohl HW 3rd, et al (1996) Influences of cardiorespiratory fitness and other precursors on cardiovascular disease and all-cause mortality in men and women. *The Journal of the American Medical Association*, 276(3):205–10

Bloem CJ, Chang AM (2008) Short-term exercise improves beta-cell function and insulin resistance in older people with impaired glucose tolerance. *Journal of Clinical Endocrinology and Metabolism*, 93(2):387–92

Boomsma CM, Eijkemans MJ, Hughes EG, et al (2006) A meta-analysis of pregnancy outcomes in women with polycystic ovary syndrome. *Human Reproduction Update*, 12(6):673–83

Borghouts LB, Keizer HA (2000) Exercise and insulin sensitivity: a review. *International Journal of Sports Medicine*, 21(1):1–12

Borst SE, Snellen HG (2001) Metformin, but not exercise training, increases insulin responsiveness in skeletal muscle of Sprague-Dawley rats. *Life Sciences*, 69(13):1497–507

Brandon LJ, Boyette LW, Gaasch DA, et al (2000) Effects of lower extremity strength training on functional mobility in older adults. *Journal of Aging and Physical Activity*, 8214–27

Bray GA (2001) Drug treatment of obesity. *Review Endocrrine Metabolic Disorder*, 2(4):403–18

—— (2007) Medical therapy for obesity — current status and future hopes. *Med Clin North Am*, 91(6):1225–53, xi

Bruner B, Chad K, Chizen D (2006) Effects of exercise and nutritional counseling in women with polycystic ovary syndrome. *Applied Physiology Nutrition and Metabolism*, 31(4):384–91

Caballero AE (2003) Endothelial dysfunction in obesity and insulin resistance: a road to diabetes and heart disease. *Obesity Research*, 11(11):1278–89

Cameron A.J, Welborn TA, Zimmet PZ, et al (2003) Overweight and obesity in Australia: the 1999–2000 Australian diabetes, obesity and lifestyle (AusDiab) *Medical Journal of Australia*, 178:427–32

Campbell IW, Howlett HC (1995) Worldwide experience of metformin as an effective glucose-lowering agent: a meta-analysis. *Diabetes/Metabolism Reviews*,11 (Suppl 1):S57–S62

Castaneda C, Layne JE, Munoz-Orians L, et al (2002) A randomized controlled trial of resistance exercise training to improve glycemic control in older adults with type 2 diabetes. *Diabetes Care*, 25:2335–41

Cauza E, Hanusch-Enserer U, Strasser B, et al (2005) The relative benefits of endurance and strength training on the metabolic factors and muscle function of people with type 2 diabetes mellitus. *Archives of Physical Medicine and Rehabilitation*, 86(8):1527–33

Chibalin AV, Yu M, Ryder JW, et al (2000) Exercise-induced changes in expression and activity of proteins involved in insulin signal transduction in skeletal muscle: differential effects on insulin-receptor substrates 1 and 2. *Proceedings of the National Academy of Sciences of the United States of America*, 97(1):38–43

Christ-Roberts CY, Pratipanawatr T, Pratipanawatr W, et al (2004) Exercise training increases glycogen synthase activity and GLUT4 expression but not insulin signaling in overweight nondiabetic and type 2 diabetic subjects. *Metabolism*, 53(9):1233–42

Christ CY, Hunt D, Hancock J, et al (2002) Exercise training improves muscle insulin resistance but not insulin receptor signaling in obese Zucker rats. *Journal of Applied Physiology*, 92(2):736–44

Clark A.M, Ledger W, Galletly C, et al (1995) Weight loss results in significant improvement in pregnancy and ovulation rates in anovulatory obese women. *Human Reproduction*, 10(10):2705–12

Clark AM, Thornley B, Tomlinson L, et al (1998) Weight loss in obese infertile women results in improvement in reproductive outcome for all forms of fertility treatment. *Human Reproduction*, 13(6):1502–5

Colwell JA (2003) Delaying the onset of type 2 diabetes. In *Diabetes*. Philadelphia: Hanley & Belfus, pp 107–96

Couillard C, Despres JP, Lamarche B, et al (2001) Effects of endurance exercise training on plasma HDL cholesterol levels depend on levels of triglycerides: evidence from men of the Health, Risk Factors, Exercise Training and Genetics (HERITAGE) Family Study. *Arteriosclerosis, Thrombosis, and Vascular Biology*, 21(7):1226–32

Creviston T, Quinn L (2001) Exercise and physical activity in the treatment of type 2 diabetes. *Nursing Clinics of North America*, 36(2):243–71, vi

Das SK, Chakrabarti R (2006) Antiobesity therapy: emerging drugs and targets. *Current Medicinal Chemistry*, 13(12):1429–60

Davidson MH, Hauptman J, DiGirolamo M, et al (1999) Weight control and risk factor reduction in obese subjects treated for 2 years with orlistat: a randomized controlled trial. *Journal of the American Medical Association*, 281(3):235–42

Deedwania P, Barter P, Carmena R, et al (2006) Reduction of low-density lipoprotein cholesterol in patients with coronary heart disease and metabolic syndrome: analysis of the Treating to New Targets study. *Lancet*, 368(9539):919–28

DeFronzo RA (1999) Pharmacologic therapy for type 2 diabetes mellitus. *Annals of Internal Medicine*, 131(4):281–303

DeFronzo RA, Goodman AM (1995) Efficacy of metformin in patients with non-insulin-dependent diabetes mellitus. The Multicenter Metformin Study Group. *The New England Journal of Medicine*, 333(9):541–9

Dela F, Kjaer M (2006) Resistance training, insulin sensitivity and muscle function in the elderly. *Essays in Biochemistry*, 42:75–88

Dela F, Larsen JJ, Mikines KJ, et al (1995) Insulin-stimulated muscle glucose clearance in patients with NIDDM. Effects of one-legged physical training. *Diabetes*, 44(9):1010–20

Dela F, Ploug T, Handberg A, et al (1994) Physical training increases muscle GLUT4 protein and mRNA in patients with NIDDM. *Diabetes*, 43(7):862–5

Despres JP, Pouliot MC, Moorjani S, et al (1991) Loss of abdominal fat and metabolic response to exercise training in obese women. *American Journal of Physiology*, 261 (2 Pt 1):E159–E167

DeUgarte CM, Bartolucci AA, Azziz R (2005) Prevalence of insulin resistance in the polycystic ovary syndrome using the homeostasis model assessment. *Fertil Steril*, 83(5):1454–60

Diamanti-Kandarakis E, Katsikis I, Piperi C, et al (2007) Effect of long-term orlistat treatment on serum levels of advanced glycation end-products in women with polycystic ovary syndrome. *Clin Endocrinol (Oxf)*:66(1):103–9

Diamanti-Kandarakis E, Papavassiliou AG (2006) Molecular mechanisms of insulin resistance in polycystic ovary syndrome. *Trends Mol Med*, 12(7):324–32

Drent ML, Larsson I, William-Olsson T, et al (1995) Orlistat (Ro 18-0647):a lipase inhibitor, in the treatment of human obesity: a multiple dose study. *International Journal of Obesity and Related Metabolic Disorders*, 19(4):221–6

Dunaif A, Segal KR, Futterweit W, et al (1989) Profound peripheral insulin resistance, independent of obesity, in polycystic ovary syndrome. *Diabetes*, 38(9):1165–74

Dunstan DW, Daly RM, Owen N, et al (2002) High-intensity resistance training improves glycemic control in older patients with type 2 diabetes. *Diabetes Care*, 25(10):1729–37

Endres M, Laufs U (2004) Effects of statins on endothelium and signaling mechanisms. *Stroke*, 35(11 Suppl 1):2708–11

Erikssen G, Liestol K, Bjornholt J, et al (1998) Changes in physical fitness and changes in mortality. *Lancet*, 352:759–62

Eriksson J, Taimela S, Eriksson K, et al (1997) Resistance training in the treatment of non-insulin-dependent diabetes mellitus. *International Journal of Sports Medicine*, 18(4):242–6

Eriksson J, Tuominen J, Valle T, et al (1998) Aerobic endurance exercise or circuit-type resistance training for individuals with impaired glucose tolerance? *Hormone and Metabolic Research*, 30(1):37–41

Eriksson JG (1999) Exercise and the treatment of type 2 diabetes mellitus. *Sports Medicine*, 27(6):381–91

Expert Panel on Detection Evaluation and Treatment of High Blood Cholesterol In Adults (2001) Executive Summary of The Third Report of The National Cholesterol Education Program (NCEP) Expert Panel on Detection, Evaluation, And Treatment of High Blood Cholesterol In Adults (Adult Treatment Panel III) *JAMA*, 285(19):2486–97

Fernandez-Lopez JA, Remesar X, Foz M, et al (2002) Pharmacological approaches for the treatment of obesity. *Drugs*, 62(6):915–44

Ferrier KE, Nestel P, Taylor A, et al (2004) Diet but not aerobic exercise training reduces skeletal muscle TNF-alpha in overweight humans. *Diabetologia*, 47(4):630–7

Fiatarone MA, O'Neill EF, Ryan ND, et al (1994) Exercise training and nutritional supplementation for physical frailty in very elderly people. *The New England Journal of Medicine*, 330:1769–75

Fletcher GF, Balady G, Blair SN, et al (1996) Statement on exercise: benefits and recommendations for physical activity programs for all Americans. *Circulation*, 94:857–62

Florakis D, Diamanti-Kandarakis E, Katsikis I, et al (2007) Effect of hypocaloric diet plus sibutramine treatment on hormonal and metabolic features in overweight and obese women with polycystic ovary syndrome: a randomized, 24-week study. *Int J Obes* (Lond) 32:692–9

Fontbonne A, Charles MA, Juhan-Vague I, et al (1996) The effect of metformin on the metabolic abnormalities associated with upper-body fat distribution. BIGPRO Study Group. *Diabetes Care*, 19(9):920–6

Frontera WR, Meredith CN, O'Reilly KP, et al (1990) Strength training and determinants of VO_2 in older men. *Journal of Applied Physiology*, 68(1):329–33

Goldzieher JW, Axelrod LR (1963) Clinical and biochemical features of polycystic ovarian disease. *Fertil Steril*, 14:631–53

Goodarzi MO, Bryer-Ash M (2005) Metformin revisited: re-evaluation of its properties and role in the pharmacopoeia of modern antidiabetic agents. *Diabetes, Obesity and Metabolism*, 7(6):654–65

Grundy SM, Blackburn G, Higgins M, et al (1999) Physical activity in the prevention and treatment of obesity and its comorbidities: evidence report of independent panel to assess the role of physical activity in the treatment of obesity and its comorbidities. *Medicine and Science in Sports and Exercise*, 991:493–500

Hagberg JM, Park JJ, Brown MD (2000) The role of exercise training in the treatment of hypertension. *Sports Medicine*, 30(3):193–206

Hagerman FC, Walsh SJ, Staron RS, et al (2000) Effects of high-intensity resistance training on untrained older men. I. Strength, cardiovascular, and metabolic responses. *Biological Sciences*, 55A(7):B336–B346

Halford JC (2004) Clinical pharmacotherapy for obesity: current drugs and those in advanced development. *Current Drug Targets*, 5(7):637–46

Hanefeld M, Schaper F (2005) Treatment for the metabolic syndrome. In: Byrne CD, Wild S (eds) *The Metabolic Syndrome*. West Sussex: John Wiley & Sons Ltd, pp 381–406

Hanotin C, Thomas F, Jones SP, et al (1998) Efficacy and tolerability of sibutramine in obese patients: a dose-ranging study. *International Journal of Obesity and Related Metabolic Disorders*, 22(1):32–8

Hansen DL, Toubro S, Stock MJ, et al (1998) Thermogenic effects of sibutramine in humans. *American Journal of Clinical Nutrition*, 68(6):1180–6

—— (1999) The effect of sibutramine on energy expenditure and appetite during chronic treatment without dietary restriction. *International Journal of Obesity and Related Metabolic Disorders*, 23(10):101624

Harris KA, Holly RG (1987) Physiological response to circuit weight training in borderline hypertensive subjects. *Medicine and Science in Sports and Exercise*, 19(3):246–52

Hart R, Hickey M, Franks S (2004) Definitions, prevalence and symptoms of polycystic ovaries and polycystic ovary syndrome. *Best Pract Res Clin Obstet Gynaecol*, 18(5):671–83

Haskel WL (1984) Cardiovascular benefits and risk of exercise: the scientific evidence. In: Strauss R (ed) *Sport Medicine*. Philadelphia: WS Saunders Company, pp 57–76

Hawley JA (2004) Exercise as a therapeutic intervention for the prevention and treatment of insulin resistance. *Diabetes/Metabolism Research and Reviews*, 20(5):383–93

Helmrich SP, Ragland DR, Leung RW, et al (1991) Physical activity and reduced occurrence of non-insulin-dependent diabetes mellitus. *The New England Journal of Medicine*, 325:147–52

Hepple RT, Mackinnon SLM, Goodman JM, et al (1997) Resistance and aerobic training in older men: effects on VO_2peak and capillary supply to skeletal muscle. *Journal of Applied Physiology*, 82(4):1305–10

Hoeger KM, Kochman L, Guzick DS (2004) *Impact on androgen and cardiovascular risk parameters by treatment of overweight adolescents with polycystic ovary syndrome (PCOS): A randomized 24-week pilot study.* Paper presented at the 60th Annual Meeting of the American Society for Reproductive Medicine

Holten MK, Zacho M, Gaster M, et al (2004) Strength training increases insulin-mediated glucose uptake, GLUT4 content, and insulin signaling in skeletal muscle in patients with type 2 diabetes. *Diabetes*, 53:294–305

Honkola A, Forsen T, Eriksson J (1997) Resistance training improves the metabolic profile in individuals with type 2 diabetes. *Acta Diabetologica*, 34:245–8

Houmard JA, Tanner CJ, Slentz CA, et al (2004) Effect of volume and intensity of exercise training on insulin sensitivity. *Journal of Applied Physiology*, 96:101–6

Hu FB, Lindstrom J, Valle TT, et al (2004) Physical activity, body mass index, and risk of type 2 diabetes in patients with normal and impaired glucose regulation. *Archives of Internal Medicine*, 164(8):892–6

Hu FB, Sigal RJ, Rich-Edwards JW, et al (1999) Walking compared with vigorous physical activity and risk of type 2 diabetes in women: a prospective study. *The Journal of The American Medical Association*, 282:1433–9

Huber-Buchholz, MM, Carey DG, Norman RJ (1999) Restoration of reproductive potential by lifestyle modification in obese polycystic ovary syndrome: role of insulin sensitivity and luteinizing hormone. *Journal of Clinical Endocrinology and Metabolism*, 84(4):1470–4

Huptas S, Geiss HC, Otto C, et al (2006) Effect of atorvastatin (10 mg/day) on glucose metabolism in patients with the metabolic syndrome. *American Journal of Cardiology*, 98(1):66–9

Hurley BF, Hagberg JM, Goldberg AP, et al (1988) Resistive training can reduce coronary risk factors without altering VO_2max or percent body fat. *Medicine and Science in Sports and Exercise*, 20(2):150–4

James WP, Astrup A, Finer N, et al (2000) Effect of sibutramine on weight maintenance after weight loss: a randomised trial. STORM Study Group. Sibutramine Trial of Obesity Reduction and Maintenance. *Lancet*, 356(9248):2119–25

Jones GL, Hall JM, Balen AH, et al (2008) Health-related quality of life measurement in women with polycystic ovary syndrome: a systematic review. *Human Reproduction Update*, 14(1):15–25

Kiddy DS, Sharp PS, White DM, et al (1990) Differences in clinical and endocrine features between obese and non-obese subjects with polycystic ovary syndrome: an analysis of 263 consecutive cases. *Clin Endocrinol (Oxf)*, 32(2):213–20

Kohrt WM, Malley MT, Coggan AR, et al (1991) Effects of gender, age, and fitness level on response of VO2max to training in 60–71 year olds. *Journal of Applied Physiology*, 71(5):2004–11

Koivisto VA, DeFronzo RA (1984) Exercise in the treatment of type II diabetes. *Acta Endocrinologica*, 262(Suppl):107–111

Kraemer WJ, Mazzetti SA, Nindl BC, et al (2001) Effect of resistance training on women's strength/power and occupational performances. *Medicine and Science in Sports and Exercise*, 33(6):1011–25

Kraus WE, Houmard JA, Duscha BD, et al (2002) Effects of the amount and intensity of exercise on plasma lipoproteins. *The New England Journal of Medicine*, 347(19):1483–92

Krisan A.D, Collins DE, Crain AM, et al (2004) Resistance training enhances components of the insulin signaling cascade in normal and high-fat-fed rodent skeletal muscle. *Journal of Applied Physiology*, 96(5):1691–700

Lee S, Kuk JL, Davidson LE, Hudson R, et al (2005) Exercise without weight loss is an effective strategy for obesity reduction in obese individuals with and without type 2 diabetes. *Journal of Applied Physiology*, 99:1220–5

Legro RS, Kunselman AR, Dodson WC, et al (1999) Prevalence and predictors of risk for type 2 diabetes mellitus and impaired glucose tolerance in polycystic ovary syndrome: a prospective, controlled study in 254 affected women. *J Clin Endocrinol Metab*, 84(1):165–9

Lemieux AM, Diehl CJ, Sloniger JA, et al (2005) Voluntary exercise training enhances glucose transport but not insulin signaling capacity in muscle of hypertensive TG(mREN2)27 rats. *Journal of Applied Physiology*, 99(1):357–62

Levinger I, Goodman C, Hare DL, et al (2007) The effect of resistance training on functional capacity and quality of life in individuals with high and low numbers of metabolic risk factors. *Diabetes Care*, 30(9):2205–10

Li Z, Maglione M, Tu W, et al (2005) Meta-analysis: pharmacologic treatment of obesity. *Annual of Internal Medicine*, 142(7):532–46

Ligtenberg PC, Hoekstra JB, Bol E, et al (1997) Effects of physical training on metabolic control in elderly type 2 diabetes mellitus patients. *Clinical Science*, 93(2):127–35

Lindholm A, Bixo M, Bjorn I, et al (2007) Effect of sibutramine on weight reduction in women with polycystic ovary syndrome: a randomized, double-blind, placebo-controlled trial. *Fertil Steril*, 89:1221–8

Lord JM, Flight IHK, Norman RJ (2003) Metformin in polycystic ovary syndrome: systematic review and meta-analysis. *Bristish Medical Journal*, 327:951–6

Maggio CA, Pi-Sunyer FX (1997) The prevention and treatment of obesity. Application to type 2 diabetes. *Diabetes Care*, 20(11):1744–66

Maiorana A, O'Driscoll G, Cheetham C, et al (2001) The effect of combined aerobic and resistance exercise training on vascular function in type 2 diabetes. *Journal of the American College of Cardiology*, 38:860–6

Maiorana A, O'Driscoll G, Goodman C, et al (2002) Combined aerobic and resistance exercise improves glycemic control and fitness in type 2 diabetes. *Diabetes Research and Clinical Practice*, 56:115–23

Makrides L, Heigenhauscr GJ, Jones NL (1990) High-intensity endurance training in 20- to 30- and 60- to 70-year-old healthy men. *Journal of Applied Physiology*, 69(5):1792–8

Marcell TJ, McAuley KA, Traustadottir T, et al (2005) Exercise training is not associated with improved levels of C-reactive protein or adiponectin. *Metabolism*, 54(4):533–41

Martinez-Gonzalez MA, Martinez JA, Hu FB, et al (1999) Physical inactivity, sedentary lifestyle and obesity in the European Union. *International Journal of Obesity*, 23(11):1192–201

Martinez JA (2000) Body-weight regulation: causes of obesity. *Proceedings of the Nutrition Society*, 59: 337–45

Martinez JA, Kearney JM, Kafatos A, et al (1999) Variables independently associated with self-reported obesity in the European Union. *Public Health Nutrition*, 2(1A):125–33

Matsuo T, Iwade K, Hirata N, et al (2005) Improvement of arterial stiffness by the antioxidant and anti-inflammatory effects of short-term statin therapy in patients with hypercholesterolemia. *Heart Vessels*, 20(1):8–12

Meyer C, McGrath BP, Teede HJ (2005) Overweight women with polycystic ovary syndrome have evidence of subclinical cardiovascular disease. *J Clin Endocrinol Metab*, 90(10):5711–16

—— (2007) Effects of Medical Therapy on Insulin Resistance and the Cardiovascular System in Polycystic Ovary Syndrome. *Diabetes Care*, 30(3):471–8

Moran LJ, Pasquali R, Teede HJ, et al (2009) Treatment of obesity in polycystic ovary syndrome: a position statement of the Androgen Excess and Polycystic Ovary Syndrome Society. *Fertility and Sterility*, in press

Murray CJL, Lopez AD (1996) Evidence-based health policy lessons from the global burden of disease study. *Science*, 274:740–3

Olson TP, Dengel DR, Leon AS, et al (2007) Changes in inflammatory biomarkers following one-year of moderate resistance training in overweight women. *International Journal of Obesity*, 31(6):996–1003

Ovalle F, Azziz R (2002) Insulin resistance, polycystic ovary syndrome, and type 2 diabetes mellitus. *Fertil Steril*, 77(6):1095–105

Palomba S, Giallauria F, Falbo A, et al (2008) Structured exercise training program versus hypocaloric hyperproteic diet in obese polycystic ovary syndrome patients with anovulatory infertility: a 24-week pilot study. *Human Reproduction*, 23(3):642–50

Panidis D, Farmakiotis D, Rousso D, et al (2007) Obesity, weight loss, and the polycystic ovary syndrome: effect of treatment with diet and orlistat for 24 weeks on insulin resistance and androgen levels. *Fertil Steril*, 89:899–906

Paradisi G, Steinberg HO, Hempfling A, et al (2001) Polycystic ovary syndrome is associated with endothelial dysfunction. *Circulation*, 103(10):1410–15

Park SW, Goodpaster BH, Strotmeyer ES, et al (2007) Accelerated loss of skeletal muscle strength in older adults with type 2 diabetes: the health, aging, and body composition study. *Diabetes Care*, 30(6):1507–12

Pennix BW, Messier SP, Rejeski J, et al (2001) Physical exercise and the prevention of disability in activities of daily living in older persons with osteoarthritis. *Archives of Internal Medicine*, 161(19):2309–16

Pi-Sunyer FX (2002) The obesity epidemic: pathophysiology and consequences of obesity. *Obesity Research*, 10(Suppl 2):97S–104S

—— (2006) Use of lifestyle changes treatment plans and drug therapy in controlling cardiovascular and metabolic risk factors. *Obesity*, 14 (Suppl 3):135S–142S

Poehlman ET, Dvorak RV, DeNino WF, et al (2000) Effects of resistance training and endurance training on insulin sensitivity in nonobese, young women: a controlled randomized trial. *Journal of Clinical Endocrinology and Metabolism*, 85(7):2463–8

Pollock ML, Franklin BA, Balady GJ, et al (2000) Resistance exercise in individuals with and without cardiovascular disease: benefits, rationale, and prescription an advisory from the committee on exercise, rehabilitation, and prevention, council on clinical cardiology, American Heart Association. *Circulation*, 101–828–33

Pollock ML, Vincent KR (1996) Resistance training for health. *The President's Council on Physical Fitness and Sport Research Digest*, 2(8):December

Randeva HS, Lewandowski KC, Drzewoski J, et al (2002) Exercise decreases plasma total homocysteine in overweight young women with polycystic ovary syndrome. *Journal of Clinical Endocrinology and Metabolism*, 87(10):4496–501

Rice B, Janssen I, Hudson R, et al (1999) Effects of aerobic or resistance exercise and/or diet on glucose tolerance and plasma insulin levels in obese men. *Diabetes Care*, 22:684–91

Rinder MR, Spina RJ, Koenig CJ, et al (2004) Comparison of effects of exercise and diuretic on left ventricular geometry, mass, and insulin resistance in older hypertensive adults. *American Journal of Physiology — Regulatory Integrative and Comparative Physiology*, 287:R360–R368

Rotterdam ESHRE/ASRM-Sponsored PCOS consensus workshop group (2004) Revised 2003 consensus on diagnostic criteria and long-term health risks related to polycystic ovary syndrome (PCOS). *Human Reproduction*, 19:41–7

Sabuncu T, Harma M, Nazligul Y, et al (2003) Sibutramine has a positive effect on clinical and metabolic parameters in obese patients with polycystic ovary syndrome. *Fertil Steril*, 80(5):1199–204

Sanchez OA, Leon AS (2001) Resistance exercise for patients with diabetes mellitus. In: Graves JE, Franklin B (eds) *Resistance Training for Health and Rehabilitation* Champaign, IL: Human Kinetics, pp 295–319

Sathyapalan T, Cho L, Kilpatrick ES, et al (2008) A comparison between rimonabant and metformin in reducing biochemical hyperandrogenaemia and insulin resistance in patients with polycystic ovary syndrome: a randomised open labelled parallel study. *Clinical Endocrinology*, 69–931–5

Sciacqua A, Candigliota M, Ceravolo R, et al (2003) Weight loss in combination with physical activity improves endothelial dysfunction in human obesity. *Diabetes Care*, 26:1673–8

Schuster H, Barter PJ, Stender S, et al (2004) Effects of switching statins on achievement of lipid goals: Measuring Effective Reductions in Cholesterol Using Rosuvastatin Therapy (MERCURY I) study. *American Heart Journal*, 147(4):705–13

Shaibi GQ, Cruz ML, Ball GD, et al (2006) Effects of resistance training on insulin sensitivity in overweight Latino adolescent males. *Medicine and Science in Sports and Exercise*, 38(7):1208–15

Sjostrom L, Rissanen A, Andersen T, et al (1998) Randomised placebo-controlled trial of orlistat for weight loss and prevention of weight regain in obese patients. European Multicentre Orlistat Study Group. *Lancet*, 352(9123):167–72

Smith SD, Blair SN, Criqui MH, et al (1995) Preventing heart attack and death in patients with coronary disease. *Circulation*, 92(1):2–4

Solomon CG (1999) The epidemiology of polycystic ovary syndrome. Prevalence and associated disease risks. *Endocrinol Metab Clin North Am*, 28(2):247–63

Staron RS, Malicky ES, Leonardi MJ, et al (1989) Muscle hypertrophy and fast fiber type conversions in heavy resistance-trained women. *European Journal of Applied Physiology*, 60:71–9

Stone MH, Fleck SJ, Triplett NT, et al (1991) Health and performance related potential of resistance training. *Sports Medicine*, 114(4):210–31

Sui X, Hooker SP, Lee IM, et al (2008) A prospective study of cardiorespiratory fitness and risk of type 2 diabetes in women. *Diabetes Care*, 31(3):550–5

Sui X, LaMonte MJ, Laditka JN, et al (2007) Cardiorespiratory fitness and adiposity as mortality predictors in older adults. *The Journal of the American Medical Association*, 298(21):2507–16

Tomas E, Zorzano A, Ruderman NB (2002) Exercise effects on muscle insulin signaling and action exercise and insulin signaling: a historical perspective. *Journal of Applied Physiology*, 93(2):765–72

Toprak S, Yonem A, Cakir B, et al (2001) Insulin resistance in nonobese patients with polycystic ovary syndrome. *Horm Res*, 55(2):65–70

Tripathi BK, Srivastava AK (2006) Diabetes mellitus: complications and therapeutics. *Medical Science Monitor*, 12(7):RA130–RA147

Trovati M, Carta Q, Cavalot F, et al (1984) Influence of physical training on blood glucose control, glucose tolerance, insulin secretion, and insulin action in non-insulin-dependent diabetic patients. *Diabetes Care*, 7(5):416–20

Turner RC, Cull CA, Frighi V, et al (1999) Glycemic control with diet, sulfonylurea, metformin, or insulin in patients with type 2 diabetes mellitus: progressive requirement for multiple therapies (UKPDS 49) *The Journal of the American Medical Association*, 281:2005–2012

Vigorito C, Giallauria F, Palomba S, et al (2007) Beneficial effects of a three-month structured exercise training program on cardiopulmonary functional capacity in young women with polycystic ovary syndrome. *J Clin Endocrinol Metab*, 92(4):1379–84

Walsh KM, Leen E, Lean ME (1999) The effect of sibutramine on resting energy expenditure and adrenaline-induced thermogenesis in obese females. *International Journal of Obesity and Related Metabolic Disorders*, 23(10):1009–15

Watkins LL, Sherwood A, Feinglos M, et al (2003) Effects of exercise and weight loss on cardiac risk factors associated with syndrome X. *Archives of Internal Medicine*, 163:1889–95

Willey KA, Fiatarone-Singh MA (2003) Battling insulin resistance in elderly obese people with type 2 diabetes: bring on the heavyweights. *Diabetes Care*, 26(5):1580–9

Wing RR, Jakicic J, Neiberg R, et al (2007) Fitness, fatness, and cardiovascular risk factors in type 2 diabetes: look ahead study. *Medicine and Science in Sports and Exercise*, 39(12):2107–16

Wood D (1998) European and American recommendations for coronary heart disease prevention. *European Heart Journal*, 19 (Suppl A):A12–19

Yamamoto M, Shimura S, Itoh Y, et al (2000) Anti-obesity effects of lipase inhibitor CT-II, an extract from edible herbs, Nomame Herba, on rats fed a high-fat diet. *International Journal of Obesity and Related Metabolic Disorders*, 24(6):758–64

Yildirim B, Sabir N, Kaleli B (2003) Relation of intra-abdominal fat distribution to metabolic disorders in nonobese patients with polycystic ovary syndrome. *Fertil Steril*, 79(6):1358–64

Yki-Jarvinen H, Koivisto VA (1983) Effects of body composition on insulin sensitivity. *Diabetes*, 32: 965–9

Chapter 7

Exercise as therapy for clients requiring special care

Melainie Cameron and Geraldine Naughton

INTRODUCTION AND ASSUMED CONCEPTS

Exercise is good for us. Almost all of us. Almost all of the time. But one size does not fit all. In this chapter we have drawn together scientific evidence supporting the judicious use of exercise for therapeutic purposes in people needing special care, particularly children, frail and elderly people, and people with chronic, complex diseases, permanent impairments, or terminal diseases. We have not repeated more general evidence presented in earlier chapters, but assume that readers will, by this stage of the book, have come to understand the health benefits of exercise on most body systems. Also, the fundamental principles and evidence-base behind strength training programs for young people have recently been revised and provide compulsory reading prior to any intervention with children and adolescents, independent of starting level (Faigenbaum et al 2009).

In this chapter we consider the evidence for exercise as a management strategy in chronic disease. Because several chronic conditions fall under other classifications used in this text, we cross-reference this chapter with others in this section (eg: type 2 diabetes mellitus [T2DM] is classified as a metabolic condition and is considered in Chapter 6). Also, we have omitted athletes from this chapter — working with athletes is covered in detail in Chapter 8. Athletes are particularly accustomed to engaging in exercise, thus the special care required when working with athletes is markedly different

from the special care necessitated by working with vulnerable populations.

CHILDREN

The first two decades of life are characterised by unprecedented growth and development. The stages of growth and development are specifically known as infancy, childhood, adolescence and early adulthood. The order of development is common for all people but the timing and the tempo through the stages varies markedly, particularly around the adolescent years.

Primitive reflex movements of newborn infants such as grasping and sucking provide the movements for survival in the earliest months of life. Reflexes make way for more deliberate movement patterns such as lifting, touching, pushing and pulling that essentially build the neurological and musculoskeletal pathway for crawling and walking. Most children develop movement skills through play. Play is the most developmentally appropriate form of movement from birth well into childhood.

Once a child is independently mobile, movement becomes one of the vital processes by which children explore, negotiate and learn about the world. Play is said to be the 'currency' of childhood. Movement in infancy and early childhood supports structural growth of the musculoskeletal and cardiovascular systems and contributes to general child health. Mastery of fundamental movement skills involves 'locomotion' such as running and jumping, and 'manipulation'

Note: parts of this chapter are based on the literature review from Melanie Cameron's PhD thesis.

such as throwing and kicking. Mastery is usually achieved by the early years of primary skills with lots of opportunities to practice, vary, play and build on existing skills. Structured activity such as swimming or dance lessons should compliment (and not replace) several hours of free play activity, preferably outdoors, spread throughout the day. Active outdoor play is preferred. Relatively more opportunities to use large muscle groups (gross motor skills) exist outdoors compared with indoors.

During the middle years of primary school, children's fundamental movement skills coincide with the more mature, 'abstract' thinking skills. Abstract thinking allows children to follow instructions, understand rules and work well with others in more challenging movement tasks such as modified sports. Simplified versions of all popular sporting codes are available for children of all abilities, to encourage enjoyable participation. Towards the later years of primary school, children should be familiar with many sports and physical activities.

Movement in adolescence has the capacity to focus on skill refinement, and sport specialisation is recommended in most sports around mid-adolescence after the peak of the adolescent growth spurt. However, some adolescents may simply prefer to be physically activity as a means of keeping, or making friends. Early pubertal maturation in boys is often synonymous with advanced physical activity skills, but the opposite is generally true for girls. Programs need to be inclusive of physical activity abilities. The option that is not so healthy is dropping out of physical activity. Health benefits are possible from physical activity at any age, but particularly in these first two formative decades of life. The link with chronic disease consistently exists with a lack of physical activity. Preferences, habits and autonomy become apparent over these first two decades of life. Regrettably physical activity declines the greatest during adolescent years. For some adolescents, competition that is so evident in physical activity is empowering. Others can be disempowered by competition. Specifically, a lack of unlikely success from physical activity (independent of effort), a threat of potentially embarrassing performances, and/or the attraction of less active interests can become barriers that need to be overcome by young people needing to be more physically active. The value of individual

efforts, social opportunities from being active and a growing belief in self-determination need to supersede comparisons of physical abilities with others at this particular time when inequality in body size, shape, skills, experience, and resources are difficult for many adolescents to understand.

Weight management and health promotion in childhood

The pandemic of childhood obesity has distorted many adults' understanding of exercise prescription and neglected the more critical need for developmental appropriateness. Movement experiences of overweight or obese children should be presented as opportunities for success, not punishment, for future gain or past errors.

Success of media-based programs of rapid and exceptional weight loss have provided extraordinary attention to aggressive interventions. Scientific literature also has examples of adolescents with metabolic syndrome capable of 9kg weight loss after 10 weeks of school-based interval, high intensity training. In addition to weight loss, health gains were observed in total cholesterol, low density lipoprotein (LDL) and glycosylated haemoglobin (HbA1c) (Coppen et al 2008). Studies prescribing intensive interval training protocols have also produced impressive results. The prescribed intervals have been as high as four lots of 4 minute interval training at 90% of maximum heart rate, separated by 3 minutes at 70% of maximum heart rate, twice per week for 3 months (Tjonna et al 2009). Recruitment and compliance may, however, generate impregnable barriers among adolescent populations removed from the laboratory environment.

Thus, profoundly healthful improvements are possible, but are they probable in the real world? Paediatric weight management specialists may suggest that a more ethically salient question surrounding scientific experiments and popular weight loss programs should focus on the sustainability of effects in everyday life.

Independent of health, the elephant in the corner of contemporary society is the health risks carried by our inactive younger generation. It is acknowledged that physical activity is not the only means to address the consequences of an inactive lifestyle at a young age. For example, most children leading undesirably sedentary lives can equally improve health by being fundamentally willing to change over a prolonged period, and embrace changes to nutrition simultaneously with physical activity increases. Furthermore, compared with either intervention alone, physical activity and balanced nutrition produced the most significant reductions in cardiovascular diseases risk factors and HOMA-IR index in adolescent boys with obesity (Ounis et al 2008). Subsequently, physical activity is not the only means to improve health. In fact, it is unlikely to be successful alone. However, physical activity will always be part of a multidisciplinary long-term sustainability plan, including cognitive behavioural therapy (CBT) in paediatric weight management clinics (Luttikhuis et al 2009). The evidence for pharmacotherapy as an addition to CBT in overweight adolescents (not children) currently lacks long-term results.

Recommended multidisciplinary interventions for overweight and obese young people appear dose responsive (Kelly & Melnyk 2008). Interventions offering one consultation per month are less likely to be as successful as those in which contact is initially quite intensive. No one prescription can effectively support all children and adolescents with weight management issues. Daily opportunities for activity need to replace less active times or options. Physical activity needs to be prescribed on an individual basis, around tasks that are developmentally appropriate and family friendly. For example, parents and carers of pre-schoolers can add more opportunities to play and replace times spent in a stroller with more time for walking. Children and adolescents may need a play buddy; a person who drives the incentive to play or help with regular exercise. Adolescents who don't relate to sport should experience what is possible through activities such as walking, dancing, or perhaps part-time manual commitments such as community service or employment involving movement. To support the all-important goal of sustainability, activities need to be low-cost and convenient. Supportive environments also rely on encouragement, interest, and efforts from families and significant others in the lives of overweight or obese young people wanting to make changes.

Simply apportioning the responsibility of childhood obesity to any one sector is ineffective. Parents, doctors, governments and schools working in isolation, cannot make a difference to childhood obesity. For example, a meta-analysis spanning the period from 1986 to 2006 included 51 studies of school-based interventions in children 7–19 years (Shaya et al 2008). Most of the studies involved physical activity programs, and some also included behavioural change strategies. Persistent sustainable results were rarely apparent. Therefore the efficacy of school-based interventions alone is insufficient from a long-term health perspective. The role of many members of society such as teachers lies largely in prevention. Treatment is a specialist service that may require a multi-agency, multi-dimensional support. Nevertheless, all adults in our society who make decisions involving young people have an obligation to nurture child health.

Obesity can be classified as a behaviour of addiction. Subsequently, recommended treatments require motivational enhancing and CBT for changing behaviour. Part of the appeal of the addiction-based treatment strategies is the capacity to incorporate realistic discourse about the major issues of physical activity and nutritional balance.

Disease management in childhood

Physical activity remains dominant in statements and recommendations about preventive and long-term management of chronic disease in childhood. Also, physical activity remains within the first line of treatment for cardiovascular and musculoskeletal health issues. Unequivocally, physical activity has a cardio-protective role (Balagopal 2006) and needs to occur in a supportive and sustainable family health context during childhood. Physical activity is developmentally appropriate, has the capacity to be effective retrospectively and prospectively, and is generally free and accessible. Independent of ability and health, physical activity in the form of play can be beneficial to children.

Positive effects of physical activity for cardiovascular and musculoskeletal health, functional capacity, and quality of life (QoL) are found in systematic reviews, randomised controlled trials (RCTs) and cross-sectional studies of children with cerebral palsy, spinal cord injury, cystic fibrosis and asthma. The pathophysiology of chronic conditions that can occur early in childhood is markedly different but the role of physical activity remains fundamental to healthy development and improvement in the musculoskeletal, neurophysiological, endocrine and cardiovascular systems.

Cardiovascular disease

Even in childhood, the pathophysiology of cardiovascular disease is complex and includes cytokines, autoantibodies, responses to physical activity and nutrition and perhaps carefully prescribed medications. Approximately half of the children of a parent with premature cardiovascular disease have a primary dyslipidaemia, but screening is not always rigorous (Kwiterovich 2008).

Cardiovascular risk decreases have been observed in obese children only when multidimensional treatments have resulted in weight loss over a prolonged period of time (Reinehr et al 2006).

Physical activity remains a strong component in the treatment of young patients at risk of cardiovascular disease. However, independent of compliance, some children will require drug therapy. In cases of a poor response to treatment, tertiary referrals to specialist services are essential. Prescription guidelines for activity remain most relevant within developmentally appropriate activities and within the capacity of families and carers to manage on a daily basis.

Metabolic disease

Among children and adolescents with type 1 diabetes, the benefits of exercise can only outweigh the risks in well-managed conditions. Essentially, monitoring involves regular modification to insulin doses before, during, and following activity (Riddell & Iscoe 2006). Feeling included (not different) is a challenge for young people with type I diabetes and coaches and teachers are among the people who can make a difference to how physical activity is perceived in children and adolescents with this condition.

The increasing prevalence of a diagnosis of type 2 diabetes early in life is disturbing. The benefits of physical activity to children with type 2 diabetes may include improved glucose control, lean body mass, blood lipid profiles, and psychological wellbeing (Vivian 2006). Daily and sustainable physical activity remains fundamental to treatment, but again, physical activity needs to coincide with other treatments from cognitive behavioural therapists, educators, social workers, and dietitians to optimise and sustain blood glucose management (Berry et al 2006).

Similarly, gradually increasing physical activity is highly recommended along with other weight management strategies for the one-third of females with polycystic ovary syndrome (PCOS) who also have metabolic syndrome (Essah et al 2007; see Chapters 6 and 16 for further discussion of PCOS and metabolic syndrome).

Cancers

Survivors of childhood cancers are among the growing number of young people for whom advice about physical activity and balanced nutrition needs to be acted upon and requires careful monitoring.

Medications fundamental to the struggle for survival create a challenge between oncological efficiency and potential cardiac effects. Specifically, often medications effective for cancer can advance cardiovascular disease later in life, if lifestyle management strategies are not in place (Alvarez et al 2007). Although the research remains preliminary, promising effects of home-based activity and nutrition program were found compared with usual maintenance therapy in children aged 4–10 years who had survived cancer (Moyer-Mileur et al 2009).

Human immunodeficiency virus

Child human immunodeficiency virus (HIV) survivors are also predisposed to a lipodystrophic syndrome and are in need of strategic and ongoing healthy lifestyle choices (Alves et al 2008). Physical activity can play a major role in insulin sensitisation and lipid reduction in these children.

Also worth a mention are the very important social opportunities that exercise offers for health education and the re-engagement of chronically ill children in activities of daily living. For example, Grassroots Soccer, part of the Fédération Internationale de Football Association (FIFA) Football for Hope movement, uses soccer-skills training as a forum for HIV education and prevention among children in countries with very high infection rates. Similarly, Camp Quality offer recreational camping programs for children and teenagers with cancer, engaging campers in rigorous physical activities including abseiling, boating, skiing, and water sports. Camp Quality programs are paced to suit the functional capacity of young people with cancer, and provide safe environments for campers to enjoy physical activities typically available to healthy children and teenagers.

Respiratory disease

Cystic fibrosis rates among the most debilitating respiratory diseases for children and adolescents. A systematic review of the effectiveness of inspiratory muscle training on respiratory function markers of forced expiratory volume in one second (FEV_1) and forced vital capacity (FVC) in patients with cystic fibrosis identified only two studies out of 36 within the acceptable study quality criteria (Reid et al 2008). Somewhat understandably, the review concluded the evidence behind this practice was weak. More careful scrutiny or high and low responders to inspiratory muscle training was recommended. Broader outcomes such as exercise capacity, dyspnoea and psycho–social health remained unclear. Exercise prescription needs to be a broadly consulted, carefully managed, and highly monitored component of support in the lives of children with cystic fibrosis.

A counsellor led, home-based program of either 8 weeks of resistance training or aerobic activities was conducted with 67 children, aged 8–18, with cystic fibrosis (Orenstein et al 2004). Monthly visits followed the 8-week program for 1 year. Children in the aerobic group were given a stair-stepping machine, and the upper-body strength training group were given an upper-body-only weight-resistance machine. Training for both groups was associated with increased strength and physical work capacity but compliance due to medical barriers remained a major issue.

Musculoskeletal conditions

Physical activity capacity is significantly impaired by rheumatic diseases including juvenile idiopathic arthritis. The highly undesirable secondary outcome of reduced activity is sedentary behaviour. Reduced physical activity can impact on cardiovascular health, and low levels of weight-bearing activity in children with juvenile idiopathic arthritis may impact on bone mass and strength (Klepper 2008). Thus, progressive, weight-bearing and aerobic activity may become graded interventions in young people with inflammatory arthritic diseases.

A systematic review on the impact of exercise on juvenile idiopathic arthritis (Takken et al 2008) concluded there were favourable, but not significant effects of exercise were evident in QoL, functional ability and aerobic capacity in young people with this condition. Importantly exercise

was found not to exacerbate the condition. While short-term effects of exercise were promising, long-term impacts remained unclear.

An 83% point prevalence of musculoskeletal (ankle and lower back) pain was reported prior to an intervention in 30 elite gymnasts aged 10–14 years of age (Mirca et al 2008). Fifteen were assigned to usual training and the other 15 performed additional training, including a treatment of shortened muscle chains (known as active posture reduction), proprioceptive coordination training on a wobble board, and mobilisation and stretching on a medicine ball. No changes were reported in the pain scales for the control group. In contrast, the additional training group showed consistent decreases in the incidence of gymnasts with mild to severe lower back and ankle pain compared with baseline results.

Research on lower back pain in non-athletic paediatric populations has also been conducted. Lower back pain is likely to track into adulthood. An RCT of individualised therapy and exercise programs versus standardised self-training over 12 weeks in 45 children showed both groups improved in general health and functional measures over time (Ahlqwist et al 2008). However, the individualised group reduced perceptions of pain and performed better on the Roland & Morris Disability Questionnaire compared with the standardised care group. The authors believed individual assessment and an active treatment model were fundamental to reversing the impact of lower back pain in children.

Neurological conditions

Case studies and limited sample sizes characterise the research into the impact of physical activity on children challenged by neuromusculoskeletal conditions. Improved functional independence remains the single greatest function of most musculoskeletal research with children and adolescents. For example, a case study of an 18-year-old male with an incomplete spinal cord injury (C5/6) involved an intervention of walking, crawling and running (Schalow 2009). The intervention also included exercise on coordination dynamics therapy devices. After 3 years, the young male was walking, running and jumping and had regained full bladder control as well as eliminating medications. Evidence was quantified using electromyogram (EMG) during antagonistic action of muscles and the improvement of the mean stability of motor patterns.

Four children with spinal cord injury were part of a case series study to examine the effects of home-based stationary cycling with and without the aid of functional electrical stimulation (FES) over a 6-month period (Johnston et al 2008). Two children had passive stimulation to the cycling action and the other two cycled with the FES for 1 hour, three times per week. Data collected included: lower-limb bone mineral density, quadriceps and hamstring muscle volume; stimulated quadriceps and hamstring muscle strength and other cardiovascular-related measures of a fasting lipid profile; and heart rate and oxygen consumption during incremental upper extremity ergometry testing. Bone mineral, muscle volume, leg strength and resting heart rate improved in the two children with the stimulated cycling and one of the two children cycling and one child from the passive cycling. Fasting lipid results were inconclusive. The results showed home-based cycling with or without FES may be associated with health benefits for children with spinal cord injury.

Treadmill training was used to improve the soleus reflex modulation in seven children with cerebral palsy (Hodapp et al 2009). Gait velocity improvements were observed after 10 consecutive days of training for 10 minutes per day. Similar to children without cerebral palsy, complete suppression of the soleus H-reflex during the swing phase of walking was observed in this group of children. Heterogeneity of cerebral palsy conditions in children however, may limit the external validity of this study.

Chronic conditions

With life expectancies for children with disabilities extending into adulthood, community-based family friendly incentives are required to support healthy lifestyle needs. If disabilities challenge mobility in childhood, then prevention of secondary diseases related to inactivity, such as obesity, type 2 diabetes and respiratory conditions, becomes a salient issue.

A systematic review of the literature up to 2006 regarding children with cerebral palsy (CP) and exercise interventions was conducted (Verschuren et al 2008). The quality of methods of included studies was assessed as scientifically poor, but the

authors concluded that young people with CP are likely to benefit from progressive programs for lower limb muscle strength and/or cardiovascular fitness. A major criticism was that outcomes were not specific to the nature of the intervention and that poor attention was paid to important issues such as QoL. A small study of strength training in children with CP showed unexpected positive effects of self-concept highlighting that QoL measures are often of great importance to children with chronic conditions but overlooked by investigators (Dodd et al 2004). Refer to Chapter 15, case study 2, for a detailed account of the use of exercise to enhance and maintain QoL across the lifespan.

Well-designed progressive strength-training protocols for children with CP have involved 12 week programs, three sessions per week, each session having four of five exercises in a circuit and an exercise intensity based on 8 repetition maximum (8RM) efforts (Scholtes et al 2008). Testing can include gross motor function, walking, muscle strength and mobility. Adverse events can be checked with additional tests for spasticity and range of motion.

Sixteen young patients with spastic diplegia categorised as ambulatory without aids, were required to perform resistance training of 3 weekly sessions over 8 weeks (Eek et al 2008). Training included the use of conventional devices such as free weights, rubber bands, and their own body weight. At baseline, poor strength was identified mostly at the ankle. Following training, improvements were observed in gross motor function measures and gait-related gains in stride length without compromising velocity. Treadmill walking tests also showed improved hip extensor moment and power generation at takeoff.

Practical home options for regular physical activity have to be considered for children with chronic disabilities. Opportunities to succeed, improve, and extend movement possibilities remain a major developmental need. As often as possible, play is the most appropriate form of activity for young children. Exercise programs for older children are unlikely to be supported by fixed resistance training equipment in the home. Loose materials (eg: weighted balls) may be an alternative and, ideally, programs can remain effective and sustainable through creative engagement of children in play-based exercise.

Gender biases

Some gender-predominant and gender-specific conditions are affected by physical activity in childhood and adolescence. For example, chronic fatigue syndrome occurs in a three-to-one female to male ratio, and physical exertion is both a trigger for deterioration and, ironically, the principal treatment in some 'curative strategies' (full recovery remains illusive). There is some level of agreement that chronic fatigue syndrome manifests most in the combined presence of genetic polymorphisms and personality traits. Treatment strategies of graded exercise therapy and CBT offer a better prognosis for this condition in adolescents than adults (Wyller 2007).

Sadly, anorexia nervosa also occurs predominantly in young females. Deterioration of the condition may lead to hospitalisation of females in critical states of malnutrition for graded nutrition therapy. With hospitalisation there is also a risk of skeletal insults (eg: disuse osteopenia and increased fracture risk) due to the immobility (Di Vasta et al 2009). Even 5 days of hospitalisation provided evidence of imbalance in bone formation and bone resorption responses in a study of 28 females aged 13 to 21 years (Di Vasta et al 2009). Gentle weight-bearing activity may also need to be considered as a part of acute holistic anorexia management.

ELDERLY CLIENTS

Unlike childhood and adolescence, where numerical parameters are commonly agreed, albeit with some debate, the definition of 'elderly' is open to much greater conjecture. Does one become elderly simply by reaching a particular age? Recruitment to most research trials is based on such simplistic definitions, but perhaps this reliance on numerical age alone compromises the external validity of research among older people. What does it mean to be old? Is old an age, or a measure of function, or a state of mind?

Traditionally elderly clients are considered a special care population, based on the somewhat questionable belief that people of a certain age share common characteristics. In this section we contend that elderly people are quite unlikely to be a consistent population, at least for the purposes of exercise delivery. Any adult aged 70 years who has exercised daily for the past 40 years is likely to have a quite different exercise capacity and tolerance than an adult of the same age who has been sedentary for the same length of time. Factors that contribute to adults requiring special care are not age per se, but include chronicity of disease, chronicity of pain, pain behaviour, risk of falls, memory loss, and physiological frailty. Accepting that the likelihood of these problems developing increases with increasing age, we emphasise that exercise and physical activity can be enjoyed by, and beneficial for, people of all ages.

Chronicity

Although chronic disease is long-term disease, chronicity of disease is not simply persistence. Chronic disease differs from acute disease in that pathophysiological changes in tissues seem to serve little useful purpose. For example, the tissue temperature spikes of acute inflammation serve to destroy bacteria, but in chronic inflammation, temperature elevations are mild to moderate, may be localised rather than systemic, are unpleasant to experience, but do not reduce bacterial load (if indeed, there is any bacterial load at all). Also, some chronic diseases may appear less severe than acute disease, but do not resolve as expected when symptoms abate. In other conditions, pathological changes advance with time and chronic disease is necessarily severe disease. Some chronic diseases never resolve; clients are wedded to disease management 'till death do us part' (see Chapter 17, case study 1, for discussion of a chronic illness that persists until death). Because chronic diseases do persist, for months, years, or lifetimes, management is a more realistic expectation than is cure.

Chronic disease progression is physiologically similar to physical deconditioning: over time people with chronic diseases (cancer, chronic obstructive pulmonary disease, human immunodeficiency virus disease, diabetes mellitus, chronic renal disease) show impaired cardiac and vascular function, reduced muscle mass, strength/power, and exercise capacity, and increased percentage of body fat (Painter 2008). Most people with chronic disease also experience fatigue, leading to reductions in physical activity, and poor QoL. Because these people become more sedentary as disease progresses, some consequences of chronic disease may be due to inactivity.

Because chronic diseases take a protracted course, and all of us age over time, the effects of chronicity can become entwined with age-related decline. Further, many of the factors that reduce function and wellbeing in older age also complicate chronic disease. For example, some wearing out of synovial joints is expected with increasing age, and chronic rheumatoid arthritis can lead to considerable erosion of joint surfaces. These two processes, age and rheumatoid arthritis, may both contribute to the development of osteoarthritis in joints, and it is almost impossible for a clinician to make any etiological distinction in an elderly person with longstanding rheumatic joint disease. Neither is this distinction likely to be meaningful — an older client is older, the clock cannot be wound back — clinicians must accept that the processes of ageing can exacerbate chronic diseases.

Exercise, on the other hand, is a powerful medicine for buffering the physiological declines of increasing age. Further, the expected physiological and psychological responses to exercise are preserved in most chronic conditions, even well into advanced disease. People who do resistance training (eg: lift weights) experience muscle hypertrophy and become stronger, almost regardless of age or underlying disease (Maurer et al 1999). Similarly, people who undertake cardiovascular exercise such as distance running or aerobic dance improve their lung function, reduce their resting heart rate, lower their blood pressure, and decrease arterial resistance (de Jong et al 2003). These physiological changes occur even in people who have had heart disease, including open heart surgery such as coronary artery bypasses or valve replacements, although the speed of physiological improvement may be slower than in disease-free individuals (see Chapter 3). Similarly, Philbin et al (1995) demonstrated that even in elderly people with very advanced and severe osteoarthritis, regular tailored training programs led to improvements in cardiovascular fitness and muscle strength without exacerbation of arthritic symptoms.

Justifications for exercise in clients with chronic conditions

Painter (2008) argued four justifications for the use of regular exercise training in people with chronic diseases. These principles and examples of studies supporting these principles (RCTs and systematic reviews of RCTs) are outlined in Table 7.1.

Chronic pain

Pain is an unpleasant sensory and emotional experience associated with actual or potential tissue damage, or described in terms of such damage.

(Merskey & Bogduk 1994:209–14)

The International Association for the Study of Pain (IASP) definition of pain, cited above, is largely acceptable to both clinicians and researchers because it incorporates both physical and psychological experiences of pain, and includes pain perceived in the absence of tissue damage.

Kugelmann conducted a qualitative investigation of pain, and demonstrated that the experience of pain differs little according to cause, making it questionable to differentiate between biological and psychological pain. Perception and description of pain includes both sensory (physical) and affective (emotional, psychological) components, regardless of whether the precipitating factor is physical or psychological. 'Psychological and physical pain have similar phenomenological structures. Both are felt bodily … entail at least temporarily a disabling of a potentiality for action' (Kugelmann 2000:305). In this sense, hearts really do break, grief is gut-wrenching, and back pain is hellish. People experience emotional responses to physical pain and physical responses to emotional pain. Increasingly, clinicians are realising that it is futile to try to tease these aspects of pain apart, recognising that strategic pain management accounts for both the sensory and affective components of pain.

Pain is a subjective experience. Pain perception and description is influenced by age, disease, gender, health beliefs, self-efficacy, social expectation, and social roles (Melzack 1975, 1999; Payer 2000). It is also difficult to capture in surveys or questionnaires. Some qualitative representations of pain have provided more personal glimpses into this complicated phenomenon. Padfield (2003), a photographer, asked 25 people with chronic pain to construct visual representations of their pain, which she photographed. Participants also provided brief written explanations of their artwork as images of pain. A striking feature of Padfield's book (2003), *Perceptions of Pain*, is the diversity

Table 7.1 Examples of clinical trials providing support for exercise training in people with chronic conditions

Principle	Disease and research published	Summary of key findings
Exercise training will attenuate the physical deconditioning typically experienced upon diagnosis	Mild to moderate heart failure (primary or secondary) — systematic review with meta-analyses (Rees et al 2004)	VO_{2max} was measured in 24 studies (n = 848) and improved markedly with exercise (WMD 2.16 ml/kg/min, 95% CI 2.82 to 1.49). Similar significant improvements were seen in the exercising participants for measures of exercise duration (15 studies, n = 510), mean increase of 2.38 minutes (95% CI 2.85 to 1.92), and maximum work capacity (6 studies, n = 219), mean increase of 15.1 Watts (95% CI 17.7 to 12.6)
Exercise training may optimise function when used as adjunctive therapy to standard pharmacological or surgical treatments	Rheumatoid arthritis — RCT comparing high intensity exercise to usual care (de Jong et al 2003) Chronic fatigue syndrome — systematic review with meta-analysis (Edmonds et al 2004)	After 2 years the exercise group (n = 136) reported significantly better functional ability than the control group (n = 145) using the MACTAR Patient Preference Disability Questionnaire (p < .02) Participants receiving exercise therapy were less fatigued than those receiving the antidepressant fluoxetine at 12 weeks (WMD -1.24, 95% CI -5.31 to 2.83)
Exercise training may reduce secondary cardiovascular risk factors and attenuate other clinical consequences of the disease or treatment	Rheumatoid arthritis — systematic reviews (van den Ende et al 1998; Hurkmans et al 2009)	Aerobic exercise at 55–60% of maximal heart rate for 20 minutes, twice per week, for at least 6 weeks, was effective in increasing aerobic capacity and muscle strength in people with rheumatoid arthritis. This level of training produced no detrimental effects on disease progression
Improving physical functioning will optimise QoL and wellbeing	Knee pain, probably due to osteo-arthritis — RCT comparing home-based exercise to no exercise (Thomas et al 2002) Mild to moderate heart failure (primary or secondary) — systematic review with meta-analyses (Rees et al 2004)	Home-based exercise was consistently better than no exercise in controlling knee pain over 6, 12, and 18-month follow-ups Mean increased distance of 40.9 metres on the 6-minute walk test (8 studies, n = 282) among exercising participants

of images. Pain means markedly different things to different people. Because pain is both personal and of high priority, improvements of almost any size, in most aspects of pain, might be clinically important and individually meaningful. Clinicians monitoring pain are reminded that most pain scales are not useful for comparisons between individuals, but may allow measurement in an individual over time. Also, individuals who reframe their thinking about pain may experience considerable response shift in their reporting of pain and other aspects of wellbeing (Osborne et al 2006).

Exercise appears to be of benefit in reducing pain in chronic disease. As noted in Chapter 2, Thomas et al (2002) demonstrated in a clinical trial of 786 people, aged over 45 years, with self-reported knee pain, that home-based exercise was consistently better than no exercise in controlling pain over 6, 12, and 18-month follow-ups.

Pain behaviour

Pain and disability are poorly correlated. Avoidance of pain is a basic human response. Retraction from a painful stimulus is a reflex that is preserved even in some unconscious states. A particularly common pain behaviour of people with chronic pain is to avoid those activities that aggravate pain. Initially, this pain behaviour seems logical and reasonable, but avoidance of an activity may worsen a health complaint over the long term despite the short-term benefit of reduced pain.

Despite evidence that regular exercise may modulate pain, some people report pain when attempting physical activities. If daily activities are perceived to aggravate pain, negative self-talk and reluctance to exercise may follow. People in pain may say to themselves, 'It hurts just putting on my shoes. How will I ever go for a walk?' Exercise avoidance is a problematic pain behaviour because physical inactivity leads to further compromise of muscle strength, cardiovascular and respiratory fitness, bone mineral density, and self-confidence to exercise, and most disappointing of all, avoidance of activity might not resolve pain.

Multon et al (2001) tested the effects of stress management training on pain behaviours in 131 people with rheumatoid arthritis. Although participants in the intervention group reported reduced pain and reduced stress, their pain behaviours (eg: grimacing, active rubbing of muscles, sighing) did not differ significantly from the non-intervention or attention control groups. These results suggested that pain behaviours are not necessarily direct responses to pain, but more complex patterns of behaviours that may become ingrained over time.

Exercise clinicians have an important role in reframing clients' thinking about pain such that pain perceptions, related mood changes, and pain behaviours do not overly limit participation in exercise and hamper recovery. In particular, clinical exercise practitioners could emphasise that chronic pain is not synonymous with tissue level damage. Also, practitioners are cautioned to understand that pain perceptions are personal and diverse, and to avoid unhelpful judgment or dismissal of clients' pain.

Impairment, disability and handicap

Impairment is the physical and organic effects of illness. Impairment includes pain, loss of range of motion of joints, and atrophy and weakness of associated soft tissues. At simplest, impairment is the direct effects of the disease on the tissues of the individual. Impairment may continue for months or years. Over time, some therapies, and the behaviour of the client, may limit or exacerbate impairment.

Disability is a task-oriented measure. A person is disabled if unable to perform individual tasks considered to be within normal adult limits. For example, disabilities associated with arthritis of the small joints of the hands may include inability to turn door handles, open jars, turn on taps, hold or turn keys, type, write, and so forth, but may be overcome with the use of aids (eg: a rubber grip for opening jars).

Impairment and disability are linked, but not so closely, nor directly, as it first appears. The initial supposition is that impairment leads to disability; muscle weakness (impairment) means that I cannot carry heavy shopping bags (disability). Muscle tissue, however, is dynamic and responds to stressors. Muscle that is not stressed through use weakens; muscle that is stressed strengthens. Impairment may lead to disability, and disability may worsen impairment, which in turn, may promote further disability.

A downward spiral of worsening impairment and disability is a common theme across many chronic diseases. Regardless of the disease under investigation, impairment and disability are not always well correlated. Secondary psychological gain, catastrophising, and depression may promote disability in the absence of worsening physical impairment. Determination, strategic goal setting, and social support may promote increased function, or maintain current function, despite increasing impairment.

The distinction between impairment and disability in chronic pain syndromes has been well documented. Despite stable symptoms, progressively declining function is likely in some people with intractable musculoskeletal pain. Pincus and colleagues (2002) completed a systematic review of studies investigating the predictors of chronic disability in people with stable low back pain. These investigators found that psychological and social markers are consistently more accurate predictors of chronic disability than are measures of pain severity, quality, or type. Measures of current function are moderate predictors of future function. The most accurate markers for future disability are the psychosocial 'yellow flags' of depression and catastrophising. The vast majority of low back pain is non-specific; the pathophysiology is not well understood and cannot be demonstrated via imaging or laboratory tests. The basic pathophysiology of other chronic diseases may be better understood than is that of back pain, but there is room to consider that the findings of Pincus et al (2002) may apply to other chronic, painful conditions.

Risk of falls

Risk of falling increases both with increasing age, and in many chronic diseases, and therefore deserves special mention in this chapter. Further, falls can lead to injury and compromise confidence and self-efficacy, worsening functional decline.

There is a substantial body of evidence (43 clinical trials included in a single Cochrane review) examining exercise interventions for reducing risk and rate of falls in older adults living in the community (Gillespie et al 2009). In some trials exercise was a component of a broader falls prevention program, and in other trials exercise alone formed the intervention. The trials covered diverse exercise types, including gait and balance training, strength (resistance) training, flexibility exercises (stretching and range of motion exercises), tai chi and other three-dimensional and/or spatial exercises, endurance training, and generalised physical activity. This review provided high quality evidence that exercise programs targeting two or more exercise components (flexibility, strength, balance, endurance) are effective in reducing both rate of falls and overall number of people falling. Exercising in supervised groups, participating in tai chi, and carrying out individually prescribed exercises at home are all effective in reducing falls.

Evidence for population-based interventions, which may include advice to increase physical activity, for fall prevention among older adults is less substantial but still showed favourable outcomes (McClure et al 2005). Evidence for in-hospital falls prevention programs is unclear, but a systematic review of these trials is planned (Cameron et al 2005).

Cognitive and memory decline

Physical activity programs have multiple positive effects on cognition and mental health in older adults (Angevaren et al 2008; Barnes et al 2007; Netz et al 2005). A Cochrane review of 11 RCTs of aerobic physical activity programs for healthy older adults reported improvement in at least one aspect of cognitive function with the largest effects on cognitive speed, memory, auditory, and visual attention (Angevaren et al 2008). Improvements differed across studies and most comparisons were not significantly different, but even small improvements in key cognitive functions may be of importance and value to individuals. Similarly, another meta-analysis of 36 studies of physical activity on psychological wellbeing in healthy older adults derived an overall small positive effect size (Netz et al 2005).

Further, exercise appears to prevent cognitive decline. Several longitudinal cohort studies in healthy older adults have demonstrated that physical activity is associated with a 3- to 6-year delayed risk of developing dementia (Abbott et al 2004; Karp et al 2006; Larson et al 2006; Laurin et al 2001). High levels of physical activity in older adults without dementia are associated with a 30–50% reduction in the risk of cognitive decline and dementia (Barnes et al 2007). Anticipated cognitive decline may also be delayed in older adults with mild cognitive impairment (Scherder et al 2005).

Physical activity appears to delay the onset of dementia in older adults and slow down cognitive decline to prevent the onset of significant cognitive disability (Barnes et al 2007), but in adults with established dementia there is insufficient evidence to demonstrate beneficial effects of physical activity programs on dementia symptoms and cognitive functioning (Forbes et al 2008). That said, older adults with dementia are likely to experience the physical functional capacity gains derived from regular exercise, despite their reduced cognitive function (Forbes 2007).

Hospitalisation

Although we have argued that exercise is of benefit to most people, regardless of age or physiological frailty, the combination of advanced age and admission to hospital might be considered a unique combination of circumstances due specific attention. de Morton et al's (2007) Cochrane review of exercise for older patients in hospital located only nine clinical trials on this topic. This evidence was equivocal as to whether in-hospital exercise sessions for older people lead to any differences in function, harms (measured as falls, moves to intensive care units, and deaths), length of stay in hospital, or whether patients go home or to a nursing home or other care facility. Special care programs that included exercise components demonstrated slightly better results; trials of these more comprehensive interventions showed small reductions in length of hospital stay and cost of care, and a slight increase in the number of people discharged home rather than to nursing homes. Because there is no evidence that exercise increases harms among older people

when hospitalised, and small but meaningful improvements may be gained, we recommend that in-hospital exercise programs continue. Simultaneously, we caution clinicians against frustration by recognising that improvements gained from in-hospital exercise programs are likely to be modest.

CLOSING REMARKS

Evidence-based clinical practice involves the judicious application of scientific evidence to the peculiarities of a given clinical encounter. On one hand, all clients are individuals requiring special care, and yet, ethically all clients deserve the same standards of care. In this chapter we have attempted to balance these scales by acknowledging that clinical exercise service delivery may be somewhat more complicated when working with children, or with anyone who is chronically ill, physically frail, or impaired in their ability to make decisions, use clinical information, or undertake exercise alone.

Summary of key lessons

- Research providing an evidence base for exercise as therapy for clients requiring special care is limited and somewhat patchy.

- Recommendations for exercise among these clients may be based on case studies, case series, and small clinical trials, yet a body of evidence appears to confirm the widespread application of exercise among these more vulnerable clients.

REFERENCES

Abbott RD, White LR, Ross GW, et al (2004) Walking and dementia in physically capable elderly men. *JAMA*, 292:1447–53

Ahlqwist A, Hagman M, Kjelby-Wendt G, et al (2008) Physical therapy treatment of back complaints on children and adolescents. *Spine*, 30(20):E721–727

Alvarez JA, Scully RE, Mitter TL, et al (2007) Long-term effects of treatments for childhood cancers. Current Opinion in Pediatrics, 19(1):23–31

Alves C, Oliveira AC, Brites C (2008) Lipodystrophic syndrome in children and adolescents infected with the human immunodeficiency virus. *Brazilian Journal of Infectious Diseases*, 12(4):342–8

Angevaren M, Aufdemkampe G, Verhaar HJJ, et al (2008) Physical activity and enhanced fitness to improve cognitive function in older people without known cognitive impairment (Review). *Cochrane Database of Systematic Reviews*, Issue 2. DOI: 10.1002/14651858. CD005381.pub2

Balagopal P (2006) Physical activity and cardiovascular health in children. *Pediatric Annals*, 35(11):814–18

Barnes D, Whitmer R, Yaffe K (2007) Physical activity and dementia: the need for preventive trials. *Exercise and Sport Sciences Reviews*, 35(1):24–9

Berry A, Urban A, Grey M (2006) Management of type 2 diabetes in youth (part 2). *Journal of Pediatric Health Care*, 20(2):88–97

Cameron ID, Murray GR, Gillespie LD, et al (2005) Interventions for preventing falls in older people in residential care facilities and hospitals. *Cochrane Database of Systematic Reviews*, Issue 3. DOI: 10.1002/14651858. CD005465

Coppen AM, Risser JA, Vash PD (2008) Metabolic syndrome resolution in children and adolescents after 10 weeks of weight loss. *Journal of CardioMetabolic Syndrome*, 3(4):205–10

de Jong Z, Munneke M, Zwinderman AH et al (2003) Is a long-term high-intensity exercise program effective and safe in patients with rheumatoid arthritis? *Arthritis and Rheumatism*, 48, 2415–24

de Morton NA, Keating JL, Jeffs K (2007) Exercise for acutely hospitalised older medical patients. *Cochrane Database of Systematic Reviews*, Issue 1. DOI: 10.1002/14651858.CD005955.pub2

Di Vasta AD, Feldman HA, Quach AE, et al (2009) The effect of bed rest on bone turnover in young women hospitalized for anorexia nervosa: a pilot study. *Journal of Clinical Endocrinology & Metabolism*, 94(5):1650–5

Dodd KJ, Taylor NF, Graham HK (2004) Strength training can have unexpected effects on the self-concept of children with cerebral palsy. *Pediatric Physical Therapy*, 16(2):99–105

Edmonds M, McGuire H, Price J (2004) Exercise therapy for chronic fatigue syndrome. *Cochrane Database of Systematic Reviews*, Issue 3. DOI: 10.1002/14651858. CD003200.pub2

Eek MN, Tranberg R, Zugner R, et al (2008) Muscle strength training to improve gait function in children with cerebral palsy. *Developmental Medicine and Child Neurology*, 50(10):759–64

Essah PA, Wickham EP, Nestler JE, (2007) The metabolic syndrome in polycystic ovary syndrome. *Clinical Obstetrics & Gynecology*, 50(1):205–25

Faigenbaum, AD, Kraemer, WJ, Blimkie, CJR, et al (2009) Youth resistance training: Updated position statement paper from the National Strength and Conditioning Association. *Journal of Strength Conditioning Research*, 23(5): S60–S79

Forbes D (2007) An exercise programme led to a slower decline in activities of daily living in nursing home patients with Alzheimer's disease. *Evidence Based Nursing*, 10(3):89

Forbes D, Forbes S, Morgan DG, et al (2008) Physical activity programs for persons with dementia. *Cochrane Database of Systematic Reviews*, Issue 3. DOI: 10.1002/14651858.CD006489.pub2

Gillespie LD, Robertson MC, Gillespie WJ, et al (2009) Interventions for preventing falls in older people living in the community. *Cochrane Database of Systematic Reviews*, Issue 2. DOI: 10.1002/14651858.CD007146.pub2

Hodapp M, Vry J, Mall V, Faist M (2009) Changes in soleus H-reflex modulation after treadmill training in children with cerebral palsy. *Brain*. 132(Pt 1):37–44

Hurkmans E, van der Giesen FJ, Vliet Vlieland TPM, et al (2009) Dynamic exercise programs (aerobic capacity and/or muscle strength training) in patients with rheumatoid arthritis. *Cochrane Database of Systematic Reviews,* Issue 4. DOI: 10.1002/14651858.CD006853.pub2

Johnston TE, Smith BT, Oladeji O, et al (2008) Outcomes of a home cycling program using functional electrical stimulation or passive motion for children with spinal cord injury: a case series. *Journal of Spinal Cord Medicine*. 31(2):215–21

Karp A, Paillard-Borg S, Wang HX, et al (2006) Mental, physical and social components in leisure activities equally contribute to decrease dementia risk. *Dementia and Geriatric Cognitive Disorders*, 21:65–73

Kelly SA, Melnyk BM (2008) Systematic review of multicomponent interventions with overweight middle adolescents: implications for clinical practice and research. *Worldviews on Evidence-Based Nursing*. 5(3):113–135

Klepper SE (2008) Exercise in pediatric rheumatic diseases. *Current Opinion in Rheumatology*, 20(5):619–24

Kugelmann R (2000) Pain in the vernacular: Psychological and physical. *Journal of Health Psychology*, 5:305–13

Kwiterovich PO (2008) Recognition and management of dyslipidemia in children and adolescents. *Journal of Clinical Endocrinology and Metabolism*, 93:4200–49

Larson EB, Wang L, Bowen JD, et al (2006) Exercise is associated with reduced risk for incident dementia among persons 65 years of age and older. *Annals of Internal Medicine*, 144:73–81

Laurin D, Verreault R, Lindsay J, et al (2001) Physical activity and risk of cognitive impairment and dementia in elderly persons. *Archives of Neurology*, 58:498–504

Luttikhuis HO, Baur L, Jansen H, et al (2009) Interventions for treating obesity in children. *Cochrane Database of Systematic Reviews*. Issue 1: CD001872

Maurer BT, Stern AG, Kinossian B, et al (1999) Osteoarthritis of the knee: Isokinetic quadriceps exercise versus an educational intervention. *Archives of Physical Medicine and Rehabilitation*, 80:1293–9

McClure RJ, Turner C, Peel N, et al (2005) Population-based interventions for the prevention of fall-related injuries in older people. *Cochrane Database of Systematic Reviews*, Issue 1. DOI: 10.1002/14651858. CD004441.pub2

Melzack R (1975) The McGill Pain Questionnaire: Major properties and scoring methods. *Pain*, 1:277–9

Melzack R (1999) Pain and stress: a new perspective. In: Gatchel & Turk (eds):*Psychosocial Factors in Pain: Critical Perspectives*. New York: Guilford Press, pp 89–106

Merskey H, Bogduk N (1994) *Classification of chronic pain. Definitions of chronic pain syndromes and definition of chronic pain* (2nd ed). Seattle, WA: International Association for the Study of Pain

Mirca M, Eleonora S, Edy B, et al (2008) Pain syndromes in competitive level female gymnasts. Role of specific preventive-compensative activity. *Italian Journal of Anatomy & Embryology*, 113, 45–54

Moyer-Mileur LJ, Ransdell L, Bruggers CS (2009) Fitness of children with standard-risk acute lymphoblastic leukemia during maintenance therapy: response to a home-based exercise and nutrition program, *Journal of Pediatric Hematology/Oncology*, 31(4):259–66

Multon KD, Parker JC, Smarr KL, et al (2001) Effects of stress management on pain behavior in rheumatoid arthritis. *Arthritis Care and Research*, 45, 122–8

Netz Y, Wu MJ, Becker BJ, et al (2005) Physical activity psychological wellbeing in advanced age: a meta-analysis intervention studies. *Psychology and Aging*, 20:272–84

Orenstein DA, Hovell M, Mulvihill M (2004) Strength vs aerobic training in children with cystic fibrosis: a randomized controlled trial. *Chest*, 124, 1204–14

Osborne RH, Hawkins M, Sprangers MA (2006) Change of perspective: a measurable and desired outcome of chronic disease self-management intervention programs that violates the premise of preintervention /postintervention assessment. *Arthritis Rheumatism*, 55, 458–65

Ounis B, Elloumi O, Ben Chiekh M, et al (2008) Effects of two-month physical endurance and diet-restriction programmes on lipid profiles and insulin resistance in obese adolescent boys. *Diabetes and Metabolism*, 34(6 Pt 1):595–600

Padfield D (2003) *Perceptions of pain*. London: Dewi Lewis

Painter P (2008) Exercise in chronic disease: Physiological research needed. *Exercise and Sport Science Review*, 36:83–90

Payer L (2000) *Medicine & Culture* (revised ed). London: Gollancz

Philbin EF, Groff GD, Ries MD et al (1995) Cardiovascular fitness and health in patients with end-stage osteoarthritis. *Arthritis and Rheumatism*, 38:799–805

Pincus T, Burton K, Vogel S, et al (2002) A systematic review of psychological factors as predictors of chronicity/disability in prospective cohorts of low back pain. *Spine*, 27:E109–E120

Rees K, Taylor RS, Singh S et al (2004) Exercise based rehabilitation for heart failure. *Cochrane Database of Systematic Reviews*, Issue 3. DOI: 10.1002/14651858. CD003331.pub2

Reid WD, Geddes EL, O'Brien K et al (2008) Effects of inspiratory muscle training in cystic fibrosis: a systematic review. *Clinical Rehabilitation*, 22(10–11):1003–13

Reinehr T, De Sousa G, Toschke AM, et al (2006) Long-term follow-up of cardiovascular disease risk factors in children after an obesity intervention. *Amercian Journal of Clinical Nutrition*, 84(3):490–6

Riddell MC, Iscoe KE (2006) Physical activity, sport and pediatric diabetes. *Pediatric Diabetes*, 7, 60–70

Schalow G, Jaigma P, Belle VK (2009) Near-total functional recovery achieved in partial cervical spinal cord injury (50% injury) after 3 years of coordination dynamics therapy. *Electromyography & Clinical Neurophysiology*. 49(2–3):67–91

Scherder EJ, Van Paasschen J, Deijen JB, et al (2005) Physical activity and executive functions in the elderly with mild cognitive impairment. *Aging and Mental Health*, 9:272–80

Scholtes VA, Dallmeijier AJ, Ramechers EA, et al (2008) Lower limb strength training in children with cerebral palsy – a randomized controlled trial protocol for functional strength training based on progressive resistance exercise principles. *BMC Pediatrics*, 8(41)

Shaya FT, Flores D. Gbarayor CM, et al (2008) School-based interventions: a literature review. *Journal of School Health*, 78(4):189–96

Takken T, Van Brussel M, Engelbert RH, et al (2008) Exercise therapy in juvenile idiopathic arthritis (Cochrane Review) Issue 2. Art. No.: CD005954. DOI: 10.1002/14651858.CD005954.pub2

Thomas KS, Muir KR, Doherty M, et al (2002) Home based exercise programme for knee pain and knee osteoarthritis: Randomised controlled trial. *British Medical Journal*, 325, 752–7

Tjonna AE, Stolen TO, Bye A, et al (2009) Aerobic interval training reduces cardiovascular risk factors more than a multitreatment approach in overweight adolescents. *Clinical Science*, 116:317–26

van den Ende CHM, Vleit Vleiland TPM, Munneke M, et al (1998) Dynamic exercise therapy for treating rheumatoid arthritis. *Cochrane Database of Systematic Reviews,* Issue 4. DOI: 10.1002/14651858.CD000322.pub2

Verschuren O, Ketelaar M, Taaken T, et al (2008) Exercise programs for children with cerebral palsy: a systematic review of the literature. *American Journal of Physical Medicine and Rehabilitation*, 87(5):404–17

Vivian EM (2006) Type 2 diabetes in children and adolescents — the next epidemic? *Current Medical Research & Opinion*, 22(2):297–306

Wyller VB (2007) The chronic fatigue syndrome – an update. *Acta Neurologica Scandinavica*. (Suppl) 187:7–14

Chapter 8

Exercise as therapy for athletes

Alan Pearce and Mark Sayers

Assumed concepts

This chapter is based on the assumption that readers already understand key concepts and have some background knowledge of:

- models of planning and periods of training
- fundamental principles of exercise prescription, particularly with regard to progressive overload, specificity of training, and exercise selection
- fundamental principles of resistance training, particularly between concentric, eccentric, isotonic, isometric, and isokinetic training
- differences between power training and plyometrics.

INTRODUCTION

Defining someone as an 'athlete' usually implies that the individual has enhanced traits in the areas of skill, agility, strength and power, or endurance. However, the term 'athlete' is ubiquitous and can be used, justifiably, for any person who regularly trains and/or competes in any level of competition. Being a 'serious recreational athlete' may involve similar amounts of training and, therefore, bring about similar physical concerns to those who compete at the high performance levels. Moreover, many athletes (at all levels) attempt to balance training with school, university or work commitments (as only a minority of athletes are fortunate enough to be full-time professionals), thereby placing greater stress on themselves which may contribute to potential injuries.

The aim of this chapter is to introduce the reader, who may not be fully *au fait* with the demands of sport, to expectations of training and the challenges associated with those who train and compete at varying levels of athlete participation. Given the dearth of epidemiological injury studies currently available, this chapter will provide evidence from a generalist perspective, discussing extrinsic issues such as team management pressures (at the high performance level) and athlete compliance (at all levels), and concluding with an outline of the principles underpinning effective rehabilitation. It is assumed that clinical exercise practitioners would understand that rehabilitation should be performed with individualistic, specific and holistic intentions; specific case study examples are cited in Chapter 18.

THE ATHLETE AND CHARACTERISTICS OF TRAINING

Training for any sport or event involves two broad areas: improvements in specific performance qualities pertaining to the sport or event; and progressive understanding of the training requirements of that sport to best facilitate healthy improvement.

Athletic training encompasses five broad areas: skill (techniques and/or tactics of the sport); stamina; strength; speed; and suppleness (Dick 1985). In order to be successful, at any level the individual wishes to complete in, athletes need to train in each area. For some it may be balancing the training across all areas (eg: court or field sports such as badminton or rugby), whereas for others it may encompass heavy emphasis on one or two of these areas (eg: weightlifting or marathon running). Regardless of the sport, there are a number of theoretical models proposed that athletes must pass through in order to become elite (eg: Bayli & Hamilton 1996; Bayli & Hamilton 2003; Bompa & Haff 2009). These 'Long-Term Athlete Development' models were first instituted in Eastern Europe in the 1960s and formed the basis of the highly successful talent identification programs implemented by these countries. However, the continued internationalisation of sport has meant that the majority of countries who compete at major international competitions (eg: Olympics, World Cups, etc) have integrated long-term athlete developmental models into their national sporting structures. These models are based on research that has found high performance athletes take approximately 10 years of regular, structured training to reach optimal performance (Ericsson et al 1993). Istvan Bayli is widely acknowledged as the worldwide leader in this field with many countries adopting sporting systems based on his models (an excellent example can be found at www.canadiansportforlife.ca).

Clear limitations to these models are the assumption of early age introduction, relative to the sport, as well as development towards elite participation. However, many recreational athletes start a sport relatively late (eg: many take up triathlon in their 20s or 30s to overcome obesity issues) or simply enjoy the individual goal of training and achieving personal satisfaction, without interest in competition. The application of these long-term athlete development models to these individuals is therefore questionable. Regardless, serious recreational athletes still often undertake voluminous and intense exercise that can take a physical toll.

Developing athletes

Developing athletes usually refers to junior participants and those just recently out of junior competition levels and moving into the senior ranks (sometimes colloquially termed 'rookies'). Training loads may vary, depending on school–life balance, with the recommended ratio of training to competition being 60:40 in favour of training over competition, between the ages 11–16 years, alternating to a 40:60 ratio of training to competition from the ages 15–16 to 18 years (Bayli & Hamilton 1996). In terms of actual participating hours (which incorporates both training and competition), it is not uncommon to see developing athletes devoting anywhere between 10 and 25 hours per week (depending on the sport), whilst balancing school or work (eg: as an apprentice trades person). In some extreme cases, it is possible that the developing athlete has forgone school or work entirely and is competing 75% or more of the time and devoting at least 30 hours or more per week to sports-specific training.

Evidence has shown that younger athletes can adapt well to the same type of training routines as mature athletes (Arnheim & Prentice 2002). However, concerns raised regarding the developing athlete include: stresses placed on immature musculoskeletal structures, particularly with repetition training practices (such as tennis drills) as well as collision sports; as well as younger athletes having the same psychological understanding to work as adults (Arnheim & Prentice 2002).

Elite or professional athletes

Athletes in this category will be participating at the highest levels of international competition. In most cases training will be at a near full-time basis (minimum of 30 hours per week) with regular participation in competition. High level competition also typically brings the need for an increased focus on sports science, rehabilitation (from both injury and high training loads) and travel. The latter is a key issue for most high performance Australian athletes as competition in major events is held typically in the Northern Hemisphere, out of season with domestic competition, with the subsequent need to both travel long distances and tour for many weeks in succession. In addition to these stressors, elite athletes must also juggle promotional activities, media events and sponsorship deals into these extremely busy schedules. Many elite athletes are also involved in continuing education as part of 'preparation for life after sport' programs that are common within the sector. (Athlete Career and Education [ACE] are employed by the majority of high performance sports organisations and teams in Australia.) The total sporting load of non-professional elite athletes is similar to those of the professional athletes with the additional pressures of having to juggle training and competition commitments with part-time work or part- or full-time study. In some cases of minor sports a few elite athletes, in trying to balance their sport with work, have forgone cross-training activities (eg: strength and conditioning) to spend all available training time focused in their sport, in other words 100% training has been completed on the court (Pearce et al 2000).

Serious recreational athletes

Serious recreational athletes encompass the largest group of participants in regular activity. Therefore it is difficult to define the 'typical' recreational athlete in terms of training loads, the intensities of those training sessions, competitions competed and the level of those competitions. For some, their regular serious competition events may be at 'C' grade level (Open or 'A' grade being classified as elite), or some who may run 60–100 km or cycle 200–300 km per week without entering competitions. However, this group does differ to the average person who participates in general fitness activities in that the serious recreational athlete will devote their time training and (if applicable) competing towards specific goals centred around that one sport or event.

Usual common characteristics of these individuals involve balancing work, usually full-time, with training. Therefore, training will be scheduled around work hours, being before and/or after work. As discussed in the case studies in Chapter 18, a number of recreational athletes may also be participating in physically demanding work (eg: working in a factory moving heavy loads manually) which may also impact on their training in terms of recovery.

EVIDENCE OF EXERCISE MODALITY EFFICACY IN RESTORING THE ATHLETE TO FUNCTION

As described in the introduction, exercise prescription should follow an individualistic, specific, and holistic approach. The current literature (see review by Morrissey et al 1995) suggests a range of modalities in restoring muscular strength, endurance and power, and is described in general terms below. However, a paucity of rigorous evidence still exists as to their overall effectiveness in the rehabilitation setting, although limited data exists for their inclusion as clinical exercise modalities to be used by the exercise practitioner for rehabilitation exercise prescription. It should be noted that contraindications exists with the resumption of any exercise rehabilitation program and depend on the type of injury and the type of athlete. Prior to starting exercise rehabilitation programs, ill and injured athletes should undergo physical examinations and clinical assessments to ensure that they are ready to resume exercise.

Isometric exercise

Isometric exercises have been suggested to be performed during the early phase of rehabilitation, particularly following immobilisation; and may assist in developing strength where range of motion (ROM) exercise may be detrimental to the individual (Arnheim & Prentice 2002). It has been noted by Brandy (2008) that no evidence to date demonstrates the optimal duration for contraction times. Brandy and Lovelace-Chandler (1991) have suggested contraction times between 6 to 10 seconds in duration will induce gains in strength. However, well-known limitations in isometric training include benefits confined only to the static contraction time maintained (Morrissey et al 1995) and the joint angle trained (Kitai & Sale 1989).

Isokinetic dynamometry

A common practice in the rehabilitation process is isokinetic dynamometry. Here speed of movement is fixed with accommodating resistance to provide maximal resistance throughout the ROM (Perrin 1993). The advantages of isokinetic dynamometry is that movement speed for both concentric and eccentric phases can be controlled which indirectly influences resistance to the individual. However, isokinetic exercise is notably different to normal muscular function, and as a result many applied sports scientists are reluctant to use isokinetic dynamometry as a measurement or rehabilitation tool (Ashley & Weiss 1994; Mahler et al 1992; Murphy et al 1994; Viitasalo 1985). Similarly, Brandy (2008) has highlighted that this deficiency further emphasises the importance of integrating all means of open-chain resistance training in rehabilitation (see section on rehabilitation principles later in this chapter).

Progressive resistance training

Also known as isotonic exercise, progressive resistance training is the most common and well prescribed training method in both performance improvements and rehabilitation. There are a number of ways to provide resistance including free weights, resistance bands, a range of other apparatus or even an individual's own body weight. Altering the intensity (weight) or volume (repetitions and sets) will provide continual stimulus to challenge the physiological systems, and for further reading on strength training the reader is directed to Beachle and Earle (2008) and Brandy and Sanders (2008).

Plyometric exercises

Usually prescribed in the functional phase (see section on principles of rehabilitation later in this chapter), plyometric exercises aim to restore power which is a vital component of almost all sporting activities (Dick 1985). Plyometric exercises are open-chain exercises involving a stretch-shortening cycle whereby the muscle is eccentrically stretched to facilitate a subsequent concentric contraction (Kibler 2002; Arnheim & Prentice 2002). Although used more commonly for lower-extremity training, a number of studies have demonstrated benefits of plyometric exercises for upper-extremity power (eg: see Swanik et al 2002 and Schulte-Edelmann et al 2005). However, discussion on using plyometric exercises to augment power during rehabilitation appears to be limited to describing applications of data to the rehabilitation setting (Swanik et al 2002; Schulte-Edelmann et al 2005) and theoretical models rather than evidence based research (Davies & Matheson 2001).

Cardiorespiratory training

Cardiorespiratory training can become the neglected component of a rehabilitation program due to the focus on restoring musculoskeletal function. Although dependent on the site of injury, there are many opportunities to continue exercise to maintain or, at least attenuate the loss in, athletes' cardiorespiratory fitness through non-weight-bearing activities such as water therapy, cycling or arm ergometry.

EVIDENCE OF EXERCISE REHABILITATION FOR ATHLETIC POPULATIONS

Evidence about the effectiveness of exercise rehabilitation protocols for athletes currently remains predominantly anecdotal. For example, a Cochrane review on rehabilitation protocols for hamstring injuries concluded that current practice and widely published rehabilitation protocols cannot be either supported or refuted (Mason et al 2007). Similarly, Trees et al (2007) systematically reviewed evidence of exercise modalities as treatment post anterior cruciate ligament (ACL) reconstructions, finding no evidence to support one form of exercise intervention over another. Issues arising included the wide variety of exercise rehabilitation programs making systematic comparison difficult. More interestingly, studies reviewed did not compare the effectiveness of exercise to a control (no exercise) condition (Trees et al 2007). Similarly, a systematic review by Loudon et al (2008) on exercise therapy for those with functional ankle instability (FAI) concluded that exercise treatments such as balance, proprioceptive and strength exercises are effective for individuals with FAI. However, Loudon et al (2008) noted that a lack of large randomised controlled trials limits the application of these findings to practice. Moreover, studies generally investigated the effect of these interventions, limiting current knowledge.

The concepts of appropriately prescribed exercise loading and progression are further important issues that both need to be addressed and limit current knowledge on the effectiveness of exercise rehabilitation protocols. An example to illustrate the current lack of specificity in exercise rehabilitation guidelines has been provided by Kidgell et al (2007) who, in a preliminary study, aimed to investigate the efficacy of 'high-volume training' (HVT) versus 'low-volume training' (LVT) (Table 8.1) in progressive balance training on postural sway for adults with FAI. Participants, having at least presented with two ankle inversion injuries in the previous 18 months, completed

8-weeks of a balance training program consisting of up to 30 minutes duration, three times per week. LVT consisted of 40 repetitions of exercises for week 1, progressing to 90 repetitions by week 8. HVT consisted of 60 repetitions of exercises for week 1, progressing to 130 repetitions by week 8.

Following the training intervention both HVT and LVT provided improvements in postural sway, compared to the pre-test. Comparisons between groups in the effectiveness of training loads, showed an HVT provided a greater effect on postural sway (effect size d = 1.7) compared to the LVT (effect size d = 0.6) (see Cohen 1988 for a discussion of effect size). However, as there were no significant differences between groups, the data needs to be considered with caution. Research questions regarding the load of training do need to be addressed however.

Another key issue in providing evidence based support for the efficacy of rehabilitation programs concerns the absence of universal, systematic assessment protocols. In Australia the reliability and accuracy of sports science assessment has been the focus of the National Sports Science Quality Assurance (NSSQA) program. To date NSSQA has focused primarily on exercise physiology and strength and conditioning testing, and has yet to focus on assessment in rehabilitation settings. This has been a major stumbling block in exercise rehabilitation as the lack of consistency of assessment and reliance on subjective protocols makes it difficult to provide meaningful comparisons between subject populations. The end result has been a discipline that relies heavily on case study reporting, which although is a valid research tool, means that data collected on one individual or population must be viewed in the context in which it was collected.

The final area that needs to be considered when interpreting results from intervention research concern project design and the highly individualised responses that human participants have to exercise. It is common in this field to use quite small participant numbers due to the limited population

Table 8.1 Exercises and training loads prescribed between LVT and HVT

		Low-volume training		High-volume training	
	Exercise	Set	Reps/Time	Set	Reps/Time
Weeks 1 & 2	Single leg stance	2	20 sec	3	30 sec
	Controlled inversion/eversion	2	10	3	15
	Controlled plantarflexion/dorsiflexion	2	10	3	15
Weeks 3 & 4	Single leg stance	2	30 sec	4	40 sec
	Single leg squat	2	15	4	10
	4-point star	2	15	4	10
Week 5 & 6	Single leg stance	3	30 sec	4	45 sec
	1/4 squat to raise	4	10	4	20
	Single leg hip hike	4	10	4	20
Weeks 7 & 8	Single leg stance (eyes closed)	2	20 sec	3	30 sec
	4-point star (opposite leg)	4	12	4	20
	Single leg stance with distraction	4	12	4	20

(Source: adapted from Kidgell et al 2007)

of injured athletes available (fortunately). Research projects on 10–15 participants should be viewed with caution, due to lower statistical power, and more when participants come from across several sporting populations. For example, a study on acromioclavicular (AC) joint injury on a group of 12 international level rugby players will provide greater incite for exercise therapists working on that same population than a study on the same number of athletes, but taken from all sports, across amateur and professional levels. In addition, years of research has shown that even within the one population of athletes the individual responses to exercise can differ dramatically. Figure 8.1 shows the results of a training study (Sayers 1999) that aimed to increase explosive leg power in a group of high performance rowers. The mean for the group indicates that the majority of participants improved performance over the 10 week intervention period (effect sized = 0.55). However, within the group one athlete realised no benefit from the training program (non responder), while another athlete actually decreased performance considerably (negative responder). Results such as these are common in sports science assessment, particularly within high performance athletic populations, but are not typically presented in the literature. In fact

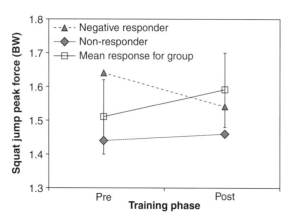

Figure 8.1 Diagram showing the changes in peak force (expressed as a function of body weight [BW]) during a squat jump exercise for a group of high performance rowers (n = 20)

Note: data shows the mean response for the group (±SD) together with individual values for: a negative responder who decreased squat jump peak force by 1SD; and a non-responder who realised minimal to no improvement in performance.

(Source: adapted from Sayers 1999)

some researchers even remove 'outliers' from the results, such as the non-responder from the data set. Clearly, from both a clinical and practical perspective the results from these individuals have great importance. In order to address issues such as these, researchers such as Stoové and Andersen (2003) have been exploring the statistical monitoring of individual changes, and the reader is referred to these papers for further exploration.

REHABILITATION PRINCIPLES FOR ATHLETES

It is well recognised that rehabilitation is the key to restoration of athletic function after injury (Kibler 2002). However the current lack of evidence-based research on exercise therapy interventions makes it is difficult to describe precisely the best practice protocols. Therefore we are limited to describing effective rehabilitation to a set of principles to guide the practitioner when designing and prescribing exercise as therapy.

Principle 1 — understanding anatomical, physiological and biomechanical functioning of the athlete

Kibler (2002) proposed that the goal of rehabilitation is to restore function to as near normal as possible. Although many clinical exercise practitioners will have a good understanding of anatomy and physiology, it is important that they acknowledge the limitations of their knowledge — particularly in relation to the training and rehabilitation of high performance athletes. An excellent example of this issue can be found in the conditioning of players from team sports such as rugby union. To the lay person it would probably appear that these players both run at maximum speed frequently and simply collide into the opposition using relatively linear running patterns. Accordingly the training of these players is dominated frequently by maximum speed training, with limited emphasis on agility. This notion was even supported by research on rugby union that simply tallied number and type of running events (Duthie et al 2003, 2005), with no consideration to outcome. These researchers showed that straight running formed the basis of most ball carries in the game. However, subsequent research has indicated that straight line running is associated rarely with positive game outcomes, and that some position groups almost never run at maximum speed, but achieve maximum acceleration frequently (Sayers 2008; Sayers & Washington-King 2005). The design of training programs that ignore these issues would have the potential to both decrease athletic performance, but also expose the athlete to injury. Clearly, clinical exercise practitioners need to have a sound awareness of the issues surrounding performance in sports before embarking on developing training programs.

Another important consideration is that anatomical and physiological functioning for the injured athlete is relative to the biomechanics of the activity — an area less studied by clinical exercise practitioners. For example, in badminton many would assume hitting the shuttle is driven by the wrist (and therefore prescribe exercise for the wrist and forearm), when it is in fact driven by force summation initiated by the legs (see Principle 4). Overhead forehand stroke production, although shown to incorporate pronation (Gowitzke 1979), is also the result of circumduction of the shoulder and internal rotation of the upper arm, facilitating pronation. Therefore exercise practitioners should consult sport-specific personnel if they are unsure of the requirements in lesser known or less understood sports.

Restoration of function will depend on the type of injury sustained which may be a consequence of the type of sport. In non contact sports, such as tennis, injuries are relatively mild, therefore good results and normal functioning can often be achieved within reasonable timeframes (Kibler 2002). In more physical sports, such as the football codes, rehabilitation from serious, long-term injuries must often follow a multistage protocol that sometimes even has the player returning to sport prior to achieving 'complete' recovery. In these situations the medical team and support staff must work closely together to provide an integrated plan that has the ultimate goal of returning the player to optimal athletic shape. Recovery from severe injuries such as Achilles tendon ruptures or anterior cruciate ligament (ACL) injuries provide excellent examples of injuries where the player may be able to return safely to the game and play with 6 months post operation (approximately) but will often take 12–18 months to regain full function in the injured limb (eg: ability to change directions rapidly in game contexts). Clearly, where possible, rehabilitation must continue beyond the resolution of symptoms to normal anatomical and physiological functioning, allowing for biomechanical efficacy.

Principle 2 — providing an holistic diagnosis

An important aspect of the rehabilitation process amongst athletes is the development of an accurate diagnosis. A key aspect of this is the maintenance of a database based on the regular screening of each athlete. This is particularly important in high performance athletes who, by their very nature rarely conform to 'established norms'. For example, high performance marathon runners often have very poor static and dynamic flexibility in their lower limbs. Similarly, track sprinters (particularly 200m and 400m runners) typically have a stride asymmetry that has resulted from the centripetal loads experienced whilst running the bends on the track. In addition, it is quite easy to tell what side a swimmer breathes on by simply looking at their posture. Despite these apparent 'conditions', these athletes are able to compete at the highest levels in their chosen sport without complications — the body simply adapts. There are numerous other examples of how high performance sport has affected the body shapes, and physical attributes of its competitors. Traditionally, the results from pre-screening testing on these athletes were used to try and 'change' these athletes to make them conform to the 'norms'. However, a more modern approach treats every athlete as an individual and considers the cause-effect nature of any condition before deciding on whether intervention is necessary. For example, would there be any point in making a multiple gold medallist freestyle swimmer with no real injury history learn how to bilaterally breathe, just to 'provide postural symmetry'? Similarly, goal kickers in the two rugby codes frequently present with limited hip ROM in their stabilising leg, a condition that exists as a result of the significant stabilising forces present in the stance leg during the kicking action. While it is clear that these asymmetries need to be monitored, it is also likely that they will always exist, regardless of attempts to 'remove' them.

Other factors that are overlooked frequently in the diagnosis process are centred on developing an understanding of the athlete's psychology, developmental state and compliance to change. High performance athletes are highly competitive in nature and are frequently very intrinsically focused. Therefore, when providing a diagnosis or screening the analyst should consider the implications of their findings. A standard issue to consider is whether the specific condition likely to impact on performance or result in injury? If the answer to both questions is no, then there is probably little point in reporting it and risk having the athlete focusing on something that has little relevance. The previous example of the postural asymmetry in a freestyle swimmer is an excellent example of such a situation. Similarly, there are always some athletes who struggle to develop skills and/or modify technique. It may be surprising for the reader, but this is also the case within high performance sport. The capacity of an athlete to change is considered rarely during diagnosis, but it is clearly a factor of some importance. Another issue for the practitioner to consider is: What are the expected benefits for the athlete, and how difficult are they going to be to adopt? Please note that we are not suggesting that analysts and medical support teams compromise standard ethical practice regarding diagnosis. Athlete injury prevention and performance enhancement are key concerns that should not be compromised.

The bottom line is that unless exercise practitioners understand where athletes have started from, it is extremely difficult to develop an accurate diagnosis based on how they present on any given day. Effective diagnoses must include both physiological and biomechanical components in addition to the traditional approach of providing anatomical diagnoses based on clinical symptoms. The advantage of functional based assessment is that it considers both what the athlete is capable of, and is also contextualised to the sport.

Principle 3 — programming and completing all phases of rehabilitation

It is well recognised that athletes find passive rehabilitation unrewarding, however, phases of rehabilitation must match the biological stages of healing and the tissue's ability to accept loads to provide optimal progress (Kibler 2002). These phases of rehabilitation should be communicated effectively to the athlete, with goals and performance indicators used to guide the athlete through each phase. The phases commonly used have been acute, recovery and functional phases (Amy & Micheo 2008; Kibler 2002; Micheo 2008). The acute phase is the presentation of clinical symptoms

for an injury, which may be a muscle tear, fracture or dislocation if acute; or the individual presents a chronic condition such as tendinitis or radiculopathy. Rehabilitation continues from the acute phase to the recovery phase where the goal is to provide graduated training stimulus to increase wound healing towards normal anatomical and physiological functioning. As noted in Principle 1, rehabilitation must continue beyond sequitur of symptoms which forms the functional phase. Being asymptomatic does not assume normal return to function as in this time subclinical maladaptations may have developed (Kibler 2002). The functional phase aims to address remaining sport-specific biomechanical deficits and use progressive overload allowing the athlete to return to training and competition.

Principle 4 — integration of biomechanics and motor control into the rehabilitation program

A key factor to consider relates to understanding the technical implications of injury and how this impacts upon the rehabilitation process. For example, injuries to distal segments (particularly during high speed movements) are linked frequently to actions proximal to the injury site. Biomechanical analyses of high speed sporting actions such as throwing have shown that the small movements that occur in the trunk contribute significantly to ball velocity (Hirashima et al 2002). The role that the deep trunk muscles play in transferring, and then stabilising force during multi-segment movements has received considerable attention in strength and conditioning (Kendrick 2003). However, it is important that these movements are contextualised into the relevant sporting movement to enhance their effectiveness. This raises an interesting and controversial issue regarding the role of open and close chain kinetic exercises in the rehabilitation process. Standard philosophy in physiotherapy dictates that open chain exercises are largely ineffective and that closed chain exercises should be used in rehabilitation (Kibler 2002). However, this practice has not been subjected to thorough analysis and may be ignoring the fact that many sporting actions are open chain in nature. This notion is supported by a Cochrane review (Heintjes et al 2003) systematically reviewing exercise for therapy patellofemoral pain syndrome. These authors show strong evidence that both open and closed kinetic chain exercise are equally effective. Moreover, recent data has demonstrated that open chain exercises resulted in less tibial translation in ACL deficient participants than closed chain exercises (Keays et al 2009). Therefore, although further research is necessary comparing closed and open kinetic chain exercises for rehabilitation, the role that inter and intra-muscular coordination plays in developing fluid, efficient movements can not be underestimated and so it appears obvious that open chain exercises must form part of the rehabilitation process.

Injury in distal segments may also occur as a result of the inefficient actions at joints earlier in the kinetic chain. In kicking, for example, failing to adopt an acute knee angle at the end of the backswing will result in greater total leg moment of inertia during the swing phase. A large, or obtuse knee angle during this phase places greater stress on the hip flexors and groin muscles, exposing them to potential injury risks. Accordingly, focusing rehabilitation on the hip flexors will not address the issue and so can lead to frustration for the athlete and trainer alike.

Principle 5 — use progressive loading and exercise progression

As shown in the preliminary study by Kidgell et al (2007), progressive overload provides a systematic plan in the prescription of exercise that demonstrates results. However, progression should also include choice of exercises as it is quite common to hear anecdotal accounts of athletes prescribed exercises too advanced to perform in the recovery and functionality phases. This can result in frustration in the athlete's slow rehabilitation or worse, reoccurrence of injury through poor biomechanical efficiency. While uncommon, the latter situation no doubt arises as support staff are placed under increasing pressures (both internal and external) to return high performance athletes to the playing arena following shorter and shorter rehabilitation times. Another, equally frustrating situation arises when athletes are returned to sport without due consideration for a thorough rehabilitation program that integrates all aspects of sporting performance. For example, recent research has shown that the presence of decision making elements in an agility task results in completely different movement patterns than pre-planned conditions (Wheeler & Sayers 2009). This research showed that some of the movement patterns associated with pre-planned agility tasks are not representative of reactive, match based situations where players must respond to stimuli from the opposition. Importantly, some of the pre-planned movement patterns would not be considered to be related to effective performance (Sayers 2000; Sayers 2008; Sayers & Washington-King 2005).

Principle 6 — evaluate the progression of the rehabilitation

Historically, resumption of activity implies an 'all clear' to the athlete based on the satisfactory performance in skill, agility, strength and power, and endurance (and confidence), with deficiencies attended to promptly (Purdam et al 1992). What determines when an athlete can return to sport or fitness activities, similar to exercise therapy prescription, is based on anecdotal evidence and clinical experience. Despite limitations of benchmarking, the principle of assessment should be utilised to provide an objective measure of rehabilitation progression as well as a record for potential future occurrences (although, as discussed in Principle 5, many professionals are under increased pressure from team management to give the 'all clear' to their elite athletes sooner, resulting in recurring injury).

The use of rating scales may assist the exercise practitioner with the assessment of pain associated with progression of rehabilitation. Williamson & Hoggart (2005) reviewed the reliability and validity of three rating scales for pain: visual analogue scale (VAS), verbal rating scale (VRS) and the numerical rating scale (NRS). These authors found that all three scales measured were valid, reliable and appropriate for use in clinical practice. However, the VAS was found to provide more practical difficulties than the VRS or the NRS. The NRS was shown to have good sensitivity and, moreover, generate quantitative data that could be statistically analysed. Alternatively, for simplicity patients preferred the VRS, but the authors found it lacked sensitivity and the data it produced could be misleading to the practitioner.

Functional progression is also a tool used commonly to evaluate rehabilitation. However, similar to prescription of exercise, testing is mainly anecdotal due to the individualised nature of the injury and rehabilitation. Some authors (eg: Arnheim & Prentice 2002) have provided suggestions for functional testing, however, quantifying improvement is rarely discussed and still conducted on an ad-hoc basis.

CONCLUSION

Currently, evidence points towards prescribing exercise that is individualised, specific and uses an integrated or holistic approach. The clinical exercise practitioner needs to be aware of their own limitations when it comes to understanding the specific sporting requirements of the athletes who they deal with. This extends to the training requirements which will differ between developing, elite (or high performance) and serious recreational athletes. A 'one size fits all' approach is not appropriate in rehabilitating athletes, with practitioners aiming to prescribe specific exercise based on principles described in this chapter. Issues that still require research include effectiveness of different exercise prescription programs, and, although more difficult in a research design sense, testing the effectiveness of various modalities in athletic populations recovering from injury.

Summary of key lessons

- Although developing athletes can tolerate high volumes of training, this sub-group of athletes need to be monitored, with considerations focusing on repetition, collision and psychological aspects of training.

- Recreational athletes can undertake training loads and volumes well above the 'average' person, and their commitment to their sport is similar to that of elite athletes (while balancing full-time work).

- Appreciate the specific characteristics of a sport and the training culture that surrounds it. Ask athletes questions on what their sport entails in both the competitive and training environments.

- Where possible, apply scientific reasoning and use of evidence to clinical work with athletes. In particular, test and re-test athletes' performance using reliable, valid measures that are both sport-specific and sensitive to small changes in athletic performance.

- If changes to training are required to reduce the likelihood of re-injury, introduce small but effective changes so that athletes will comply by altering their training behaviours toward good practice.

REFERENCES

Amy E, Micheo W (2008) Anterior cruciate ligament tear. In: Frontera WR, Silver JK, Rizzo Jr TD (eds) *Essentials of Physical Medicine and Rehabilitation* (2nd ed). Philadelphia: Sauders Elsevier, pp 307–14

Arnheim DD, Prentice WE (2002) Essentials of Athletic Training (5th ed). Boston: McGraw-Hill

Ashley CD, Weiss LW (1994) Vertical jump performance and selected physiological characteristics of women. *Journal of Strength and Conditioning Research*, 8:5–11

Bayli I, Hamilton A (1996) The concept of long-term athlete development. *Strength and Conditioning Coach*, 3:5–6

Bayli I, Hamilton A (2003) Long-term athlete development update: trainability in childhood and adolescence. *Faster, Higher, Stronger*, 20:6–8

Beachle TR, Earle RW (2008) *Essentials of Strength Training and Conditioning* (3rd ed). Champaign Illinois: Human Kinetics

Bompa T, Haff G (2009). *Periodization: Theory and Methodology of Training* (5th ed). Champaign Illinois: Human Kinetics

Brandy WD (2008) Open-chain resistance training. In: Brandy WD, Sanders B (eds) *Therapeutic Exercise* (2nd ed). Baltimore: Lippincott Williams & Williams, pp 103–36

Brandy WD, Lovelace-Chandler V (1991) Relationship of peak torque to peak work and peak power of the quadriceps and hamstrings muscles in a normal sample using an accommodating resistance measurement device. *Isokinetic Exercise Science*, 1:87–91

Brandy WD, Sanders B (2008) *Therapeutic Exercise* (2nd ed). Baltimore: Lippincott Williams & Williams

Cohen J (1988) Statistical power analysis for the behavioural sciences. Erlbaum: Hillsdale

Davies GJ, Matheson JW (2001) Shoulder plyometrics. *Sports Medicine and Arthroscopic Review*, 9:1–18

Dick F (1985) *From Senior to Superstar*. Ottawa: CAC, Sports

Duthie G, Pyne D, Hooper S (2003) Applied physiology and game analysis of rugby union. *Sports Medicine*, 33:973–91

Duthie G, Pyne D, Hooper S (2005) Time motion analysis of 2001 and 2002 Super 12 rugby. *Journal of Sports Sciences*, 23:523–30

Ericsson KA, Krampe RT, Tesch-Romer C (1993) The role of deliberate practice in the acquisition of expert performance. *Psychological Review*, 100:363–406

Gowitzke B (1979) Biomechanical principles applied to badminton stroke production. In: Terauds J (ed.) *Science in Racquet Sports*. California: Academic Publishers, pp 7–15

Hirashima M, Kadota H, Sakurai S et al (2002) Sequential muscle activity and its functional role in the upper extremity and trunk during overarm throwing. *Journal of Sports Sciences*, 20:301–31

Heintjes EM, Berger M, Bierma-Zeinstra SMA et al (2003) Therapy for patellofemoral pain syndrome. *Cochrane Database of Systematic Reviews*, Issue 4

Keays S L, Sayers M, Mellifont D, et al (2009) Measuring anterior tibial translation in anterior cruciate ligament deficient and healthy individuals during open chain knee extension and closed chain wall squat exercises [abstract]. *Australian Journal of Physiotherapy*, 55:23

Kendrick R (2003) Injury prevention and motor control. In: Reid M, Quinn A, Crespo M (eds) *Strength and Conditioning for Tennis*. Londo: International Tennis Federation, pp 175–85

Kibler WB (2002) Rehabilitation principles of injuries in tennis. In: Renström PAFH (ed.) *Tennis*. Oxford: Blackwell Science, pp 262–77

Kidgell DJ, Castricum TJ, Pearce AJ et al (2007) The effects of a high volume versus low volume balance training program on postural sway. *Journal of Science and Medicine in Sport*, 10 (Dec Supp):84

Kitai TA, Sale DG (1989) Specificity of joint angle in isometric training. *European Journal of Applied Physiology and Occupational Physiology*, 58:744–8

Loudon JK, Santos MJ, Franks L et al (2008) The effectiveness of active exercise as an intervention for functional ankle instability: a systematic review. *Sports Medicine*, 38:553–63

Mahler P, Mora C, Gremion C et al (1992) Isotonic muscle evaluation and sprint performance. *Excel*, 8:139–45

Mason DL, Dickens VA, Vail A (2007) Rehabilitation for hamstring injuries. *Cochrane Database of Systematic Reviews*, Issue 1

Micheo W (2008) Rehabilitation of shoulder injury in the throwing athlete. *Critical Reviews Physical and Rehabilitation Medicine*, 20:65–75

Morrissey MC, Harman EA, Johnson MJ (1995) Resistance training modes: specificity and effectiveness. *Medicine and Science in Sports and Exercise*, 27:648–60

Murphy AJ, Wilson GJ, Pryor JF (1994) Use of the iso-inertial force mass relationship in the prediction of dynamic human performance. *European Journal of Applied Physiology and Occupational Physiology*, 69:250–7

Pearce AJ, Thickbroom GW, Byrnes ML et al (2000) Functional reorganisation of the corticomotor projection to the hand in skilled racquet players. *Experimental Brain Research*, 130:238–43

Perrin D (1993) *Isokinetic Exercise and Assessment*. Champaign Illinois: Human Kinetics

Purdam CR, Fricker PA, Cooper B (1992) Principles of treatment and rehabilitation. In: Bloomfield J, Fricker PA, Fitch KD (eds) *Textbook of Science and Medicine in Sport*. Oxford: Blackwell Scientific, pp 218–34

Sayers M (2000) Running techniques for field sport players. *Sports Coach*, 23:26–7

—— (2008) Development of an offensive evasion model for training high performance rugby players. In: Reilly T, Korkusuz F (eds) *Science in Football*. New York: VI Routledge, pp 215–20

Sayers M, Washington-King J (2005) Characteristics of effective ball carries in Super 12 rugby. *International Journal of Performance Analysis in Sport*, 5:92–106

Sayers MGL (1999) The influence of dynamic strength on rowing performance. Unpublished Doctoral Thesis, Royal Melbourne Institute of Technology

Schulte-Edelmann JA, Davies GJ, Kernozek TW et al (2005) The effects of plyometric training of the posterior shoulder and elbow. *Journal of Strength and Conditioning Research*, 19:129–34

Stoové MA, Andersen MB (2003) What are we looking at, and how big is it? *Physical Therapy in Sport*, 4:93–7

Swanik KA, Lephart SM, Swanick CB et al (2002) The effects of shoulder plyometric training on proprioception and selected muscle performance characteristics. *Journal of Shoulder and Elbow Surgery*, 11:579–86

Trees AH, Howe TE, Grant M, et al (2007) Exercise for treating anterior cruciate ligament injuries in combination with collateral ligament and meniscal damage of the knee in adults. *Cochrane Database of Systematic Reviews Issue*, 3

Viitasalo JT (1985) Measurement of force-velocity characteristics for sportsmen in field conditions. In: Winter DA, Norman RW, Wells RP, Hayes KC, Patla EA (eds) *Biomechanics IX-A*. Champaign: Human Kinetics, pp 96–101

Wheeler KW, Askew CD, Sayers MG (2009) Effective attacking strategies in rugby union. *European Journal of Sport Science*, 10:237–42

Williamson A, Hoggart B (2005) Pain: a review of three commonly used pain rating scales. *Issues in Clinical Nursing*, 14:798–804

Chapter 9

Occupational rehabilitation

Melainie Cameron

INTRODUCTION AND ASSUMED CONCEPTS

We spend approximately one-quarter of our lives at work. After allowing for non-working periods of childhood and retirement, and daily activities such as sleeping, eating, and dressing, most of the remaining time is spent in work. It is not surprising then, that the injuries and diseases that occur at work are largely consistent with injuries and diseases that occur commonly outside of work. Certainly, some occupations have particular injury risks, but mostly, we are injured or become sick at work in much the same ways as we do elsewhere. If this claim is reasonable, why include a chapter on occupational injuries?

In most Western countries a substantial body of legislation covers people who are injured or develop diseases in the course of their work. The involvement of third parties (insurers, unions, governments) complicates injury recovery and disease management. This chapter is devoted to the ways in which people with occupational injuries and diseases think and behave differently to people injured outside of work. I have not repeated descriptions of common occupational injuries, but recommend that readers review Chapters 2 to 7. It is beyond the scope of this chapter to include specific details of any particular employee compensation systems, which vary between regions. Rather, practitioners working in occupational health and rehabilitation are expected to maintain current knowledge of the relevant legislation for their regions.

Note: this chapter is drawn from work undertaken by Melanie Cameron during her collaboration with Jardine Lloyd Thompson.

Our choice of language reveals a good deal of what we believe and the values we hold. For example, as a healthcare practitioner I refer to the people I serve as *clients* rather than patients. I choose this word deliberately, in an attempt to balance the power in the relationship. Patient comes from the same Greek root word as passive, implying that ill or injured people are recipients of healthcare rather than participants in it.

In this chapter, however, I refer to people with work-related injuries as employees, regardless of whether they are attending work or not attending work. I avoid the terms worker, claimant, injured person and patient because these labels somewhat downgrade people's status as employees. Because occupational rehabilitation may involve layers of service delivery, to individuals, businesses, unions, and governing authorities, the term client is confusing. At various stages in the process of service delivery, each of these entities may be a client.

EMPLOYEE COMPENSATION SYSTEMS AND SELF-MANAGEMENT

People who become ill or are injured at work may find themselves asking 'Who's the boss?' Not literally, 'Who is my employer?' but rather 'Who is in charge now that I am injured? Who takes care of me (at work) when I am ill? Who gives advice? Who tells me what to do, and when? Who makes decisions? Who pays?' For most injured employees, these questions crop up very soon after the initial illness or injury incident.

When people are ill or injured unrelated to their work, the answers to these questions seem clearer and are derived more easily. For example, if

I sprain my wrist while gardening at home, largely I take charge of my own care. I might recruit help, asking my teenage child to put away the garden tools, and my partner to help me find the ice pack, but the decisions are my own. I am the boss. I decide when, or whether, I will see my doctor about this injury. I decide to continue gardening today or not. I choose when I resume gardening, or whether I employ a gardener to finish the job on my behalf. I might discus returning to gardening with my doctor, but I do not need his or her agreement and certification to go back to planting bulbs. I can choose to accept or ignore my doctor's advice, or to seek a second opinion. Whatever I decide, I do so knowingly, and I bear the costs.

Employee compensation is a form of legislated compassion, a safety net to catch people who through injury or illness related to work incur healthcare expenses and may be unable to continue working. Employee compensation systems cover medical expenses and replace a portion of wages according to formulae. Although the existence of such legislative protection is far superior to the alternative (no protection, risk of destitution through concurrent medical expenses and loss of income), there is a considerable bureaucracy that accompanies this legislation, and the weight of 'the system' can bear down on injured employees, leaving them feeling disempowered. Similarly, treating practitioners and employers may feel that they are somewhat at the mercy of the system, rather than free to make their own decisions.

> Self-management:
> involves [the client] engaging in activities that protect and promote health, monitoring and managing of symptoms and signs of illness, managing the impacts of illness on functioning, emotions and interpersonal relationships and adhering to treatment regimes.
>
> (Gruman & Von Korff 1996:1)

Clients who are self-managing effectively are empowered to take charge of their own health. They are able to gather and use health information, select appropriate health interventions, track their own health progress, and take responsibility for personal health promotion by engaging in health-promoting behaviours and avoiding health-damaging behaviours.

At present, occupational injury management and return to work is a highly structured, managed care process in which employees have limited autonomy to make decisions about their own healthcare, rehabilitation or return to work. There is substantial evidence that self-management is a fine approach to healthcare delivery among people with chronic illnesses and complex health problems that returns equal or better outcomes than other systems of service delivery (Cronan et al 1997; Lorig et al 1981; Lorig & Holman 1989; Lorig et al 1989; Lorig et al 1993). Often occupational injury management and return to work is an expensive and time-consuming process. Evidence from other areas of healthcare demonstrates that people who manage their own care can expect increased self-efficacy, and reduced pain, fatigue and anxiety (Lorig et al 1981; Lorig & Holman 1989; Lorig et al 1989; Lorig et al 1993), and that the direct and indirect costs of care may be reduced when applied under a self-management model (Cronan et al 1997; Lorig et al 1993).

As explained in Chapter 2, exercise and physical activity are important components of injury or disease self-management. In Australia, the Victorian Workcover Authority (VWA) recommends, in the *Clinical Framework* for the delivery of health services to injured employees, an approach that is consistent with self-management principles and good clinical exercise service delivery that:

(a) includes measures of clinical effectiveness
(b) applies a biopsychosocial model of healthcare delivery assessed using physical and psychological outcome measures
(c) focuses on empowering employees
(d) focuses on occupational injury management and return to work.

(VWA 2004)

Self-management is an intuitively logical model of service delivery in occupational injury management and return to work, but may be difficulty to enact because of the overbearing nature of some compensation systems.

STAGES OF CHANGE

Prochaska and DiClemente (1983, 1998) developed a transtheoretical model of change to explain the stages a person moves through to change health behaviours. The stages of change, in chronological order, are: pre-contemplation; contemplation; preparation; action; and maintenance. This model has been used as the basis for developing interventions to effect health behaviour change, both ceasing health-damaging behaviours (eg: smoking, heroin addiction) and commencing health-promoting behaviours (eg: regular exercise).

Kerns and Rosenberg (2000) identified that group based client-driven therapies may fail to engage a portion of the targeted population, and are associated with high drop-out and relapse rates. They found that in a group of people with chronic pain, the Pain Stages of Change Questionnaire (Kerns et al 1997) could be used to discriminate between those who would complete a course of client-driven treatment, and those who would not. Kerns and Rosenberg suggested that increased commitment to self-management for chronic pain improved the probability of therapeutic success. That is, people who were further along in the stages of change were more likely to continue with self-management, and those people in early stages of change were likely to drop out. People in early stages of change are unlikely to participate in client-driven therapies. For example, these clients are likely to respond to an invitation to join an exercise class with comments such as 'That's not something I have thought about before,' or 'I'll consider it and let you know'. Information gathering and deliberation need to occur before these clients will be prepared to undertake the life change of commencing a client-driven therapy.

Li-Tsang et al (2007), using the Chinese Lam's Assessment of Employment Readiness, investigated the psychological aspects of return to work among injured employees in Hong Kong. They determined that pre-contemplation and contemplation sub-scores were important predictive factors in determining return to work. Put simply, injured employees who are not psychologically ready to return to work are unlikely to do so, or do so well.

IDENTIFICATION OF CLIENTS UNLIKELY TO CHANGE

Readiness to change is a key predictor of whether self-management approaches will be successful. People in the pre-contemplation and contemplation stages of change are unlikely to engage in or persist with self-management activities including exercise. There is little purpose in prolonged discussion of exercises or goal setting with clients in these stages. Practitioners are likely to experience frustration as they attempt to motivate clients in the non-believer pre-contemplation stage to change behaviours. In response to a suggestion that an employee return to work, possibly on light or altered duties, that employee may demonstrate pre-contemplation and non-belief by arguing that he/she is not ready to return to work, or that his/her injury is permanent. A pre-contemplation, non-believing employer may state that altered duties are not available in this workplace, and a treating practitioner of the same mindset may simply refuse to negotiate an early return to work plan.

Presenteeism

Presenteeism is a social scientific label used to describe employees attending work while sick. Presentees are expected to be less productive at work than their healthy peers, and consequently, presenteeism has come to mean non-productive attendance at work (Schultz & Edington 2007). The underlying tone is that presenteeism is undesirable because employees satisfy the expectation that they are present at work while accomplishing little. I contend, however, that this attitude to presenteeism is sometimes unhelpful.

It appears that employers, and in some sectors, trade unions, do not routinely recognise that work can be used to promote health, rather insisting that employees are 100% healthy before returning to work. Also, employers may fear that allowing recovering employees to return to work might be interpreted as management taking a soft line on non-productive work attendance. Trade unions may criticise early return to work as discriminatory because recovering employees are treated differently to healthy employees, and argue that this practice increases the likelihood of dissent and discontent between staff members.

Alternately, I recommend that an amount of presenteeism (unproductive work time) be tolerated amongst injured workers early in their return to work. Most injured employees could return to work quite early if: (a) healthcare practitioners recognise that, for the most part, work is healthy for adults; (b) employers are prepared to accommodate employees with lighter or limited duties; and (c) all stakeholders shared the understanding that employees recovering from injury are likely and expected to be less productive than their colleagues.

By way of comparison, consider injured athletes who return to some training before they have completely recovered, and with guidance from healthcare practitioners and support from coaches, gradually increase their training load to increase fitness (Petitpas et al 1999). Over time, with progressions in training, and supported by strong therapeutic relationships, injured athletes recover and regain pre-injury capabilities. In the same way, injured employees can return to modified work duties before they have completely recovered. Injured employees are likely to be more tired and less productive than their peers early in the return to work period. Employers tolerating some presenteeism at this stage may be helpful because early return to modified work duties, followed by gradual increases in work requirements, can serve as a form of physical rehabilitation training for injured employees, allowing them to progressively regain pre-injury function. Graduated return to work can be ideal work-hardening training, and I recommend that employers be strongly encouraged to support early return to work plans.

At first blush, employers' expectation that employees are fully fit for work may seem reasonable, but in refusing to provide safe, modified duties consistent with injured employees' current physical capacities, employers and unions refuse employees the opportunity to train specifically for increases in work capacity. In employees with musculoskeletal injuries, early return to work greatly increases the likelihood that injured employees will complete functional restoration (work-hardening) training, and conversely absence from work predicts non-return to work (Proctor et al 2005; Hewitt et al 2007). Employers who refuse early return to work make an important mistake, and in so doing, increase the likelihood that their employees will not return to work at all. Further, refusing early return to work may be discriminatory because it withholds from injured employees the other social, mental, and spiritual benefits of work. Occupational rehabilitation managers are well placed to educate employers, return to work coordinators, and trade unions as to the diverse benefits of work, including the physical training effects that occur with graduated return to work.

COMPLEX SYSTEMS AND EMPLOYEES' SENSE OF CONTROL

Most people do not start working life intending to seek employee compensation for a workplace injury or work-related illness. Rather, employees who are injured or become ill at work find themselves thrust into systems of employee compensation that they have not explored, and for the most part, do not understand. Confusion disempowers people because it undermines sense of control. If we do not understand the parameters in which we can operate, then it becomes difficult to make meaningful decisions.

Sense of control in healthcare is a widely researched health construct. Studies of locus of control investigate the assumption that people who believe they have control over their own health are more likely to engage in health-promoting behaviours and consciously avoid health-damaging ones. Health locus of control is attributed to beliefs about health control along three dimensions; that is, the extent to which individuals believe that their health: (a) results from their own actions (internal locus of control); (b) is under the control of other powerful people such as doctors (powerful others locus of control); and (c) due to fate (chance locus of control; Wallston et al 1978; Norman et al 1998).

Norman et al (1998) explored locus of control in a stratified sample of 11 632 people representative of the general population of Wales (UK). They identified weak, statistically significant, correlations of each of the health locus of control dimensions with health behaviours. The strongest correlation observed was a negative relationship between chance locus of control and health-promoting behaviours (r = -0.16, p < 0.01). It is plausible that clients with strong chance locus of control, who see their health as being under the influence of erratic external forces, might not undertake client-driven positive health behaviours (eg: regular exercise). Alternatively, they might commence such an activity but discontinue it within a few weeks and attribute responsibility to an external force such as the weather or another person's attitude.

Several subtypes of control appear to be of importance in people with chronic illness or injury: behaviour, cognitive, informational, and decisional control (Sarafino 2002). Behavioural control is the ability or opportunity to take action, a sense of being able to 'do something' about illness or injury. Cognitive control is the ability to use thoughts to consciously modify the stressful effects of injury. Informational control is the ability to gain knowledge, and decisional control is the ability to choose among possible actions. It appears that health locus of control is malleable, and that increasing injured employees' informational, decisional, and behavioural control will somewhat internalise their health loci of control.

PERCEPTIONS OF HEALTH AT WORK

According to the World Health Organization (WHO 1948:100), 'health is a state of complete physical, mental and social wellbeing and not merely the absence of disease or infirmity'. This definition, originally adopted by the WHO in 1948 and unamended since, has been both criticised and applauded because it includes subjective assessment as an aspect of health. Should I really be considered healthy (or sick) simply because I feel that I am?

There is now a considerable body of evidence to confirm that the WHO was far-sighted when including subjective wellbeing as part of health in the 1948 definition. Health is not entirely subjective; but thoughts, moods, and health beliefs correlate with some health behaviours and with the likelihood of becoming ill or sustaining injuries. Athletes who have high levels of anxiety about competition have more injuries and more severe injuries (Levallee & Flint 1996). People who believe that the benefits of healthy promotion activities outweigh the costs are likely to engage in such activities (Becker & Rosenstock 1984).

What individuals say about their health gives a surprisingly accurate representation of their health behaviour. For example, self-report questionnaires to measure health offer some of the best representations of functional status and disease activity in people with arthritis (Pincus et al 1989, 1994; Mason et al 1992). They are better predictors of work disability (Wolfe & Hawley 1998), mortality, disability, and chronicity (Pincus et al 1994) than traditional medical tests. Callahan et al (1992) found that a functional status questionnaire (Modified Health Assessment Questionnaire [MHAQ]; Pincus et al 1983) was the best measure in a series of physical, radiographic, laboratory, and self-report tests to identify whether someone with rheumatoid arthritis is working or not. People receiving work disability payments (ie: currently not working) had worse scores on almost all arthritis assessments, including joint count, radiographs, blood tests, and grip strength, than people in paid employment, but the results of physical, radiographic, and laboratory tests added no explanatory power to the information gleaned from the MHAQ.

FUNCTIONAL CAPACITY EVALUATIONS

Functional capacity evaluations are structured assessment procedures to determine employees' physical capacities (what someone can do) at a point in time. Although widely used in occupational rehabilitation, formal functional capacity evaluations have important limitations and are associated with false beliefs, anxieties, and misunderstandings. Not all functional capacity tests are work-specific; rather, activities tested in a functional capacity evaluation are somewhat similar to activities required in work (eg: lifting, pushing, pulling, standing tolerance). The component tasks of functional capacity evaluations do not always match well with the work tasks of individuals (Kuijer et al 2006). More, testing environments do not always replicate work environments, which may be noisier and less controlled than clinical testing sites. These assessments may cause considerable distress for employees who experience performance anxiety associated with feeling judged, and for employees who do not see clearly the relationship between functional capacity tests and their work. Also, results of functional capacity evaluations are open to misuse, sometimes fuelled by false beliefs that physical performance is static or that functional capacity evaluations are objective measures of performance or predictive measures of ability.

As discussed previously, a sense of control over health is an important aspect of human wellbeing. Under most employee compensation schemes, employees can, at some stage, be compelled to undertake functional capacity evaluations and other medical assessments. Typically, communication about functional capacity evaluations includes emphasis on employees being compelled to attend or participate, and withdrawal of financial support for non-attendance. Although this communication may be factual, it does little to afford informational control to employees. Further, in this situation employees have little decisional control, and behavioural control is associated with punishment.

Human physical performance is not static. Usually, physical function improves with training, and declines with disuse or disease. Even in people with long term illness or injury, physical training can limit decline. Based on this premise, functional capacity evaluations are point in time measures only. Permanent impairment determinations should not be based on functional capacity evaluations, because the variables assessed in these evaluations are, by definition, variable. People who engaged in exercise training can expect that their performance in functional capacity evaluations will improve over time. Conversely, people who remain sedentary can expect functional capacity decline due to disuse, increasing age, and (where applicable) illness or injury. At most, functional capacity evaluations serve as baseline measures from which improvements and declines may be monitored.

Functional capacity evaluations are physical performance tests, but they are not objective measures of physical performance. These tests are (at least partly) influenced by employees' cultural backgrounds, health beliefs, perceived wellbeing including self-reported pain, and duration of injury (Asante et al 2007; Gross & Battie 2005a; Reneman et al 2006; Schiphorst Preuper et al 2008). For example, Reneman et al (2006) compared Dutch, Swiss, and Canadian employees' performances on a standardised functional capacity evaluation, and identified that across all components of the test, and particularly in maximum lifting measures, Dutch employees performed better than Swiss or Canadian employees. These between-group differences were statistically significant, and because they persisted after controlling for confounders, cannot be explained by variance in clinical presentation or baseline pain. Reneman et al suggested that cultural perceptions of work, health, and employee compensation influenced performance.

In contrast, expectations of how test results will be used, and beliefs (accurate or otherwise) about employee compensation policies, do not appear to influence functional capacity evaluation test performance (Gross & Battie 2005a). It would seem to be a matter of natural justice that employees are informed about how the results of functional capacity evaluations could be used. Because this information does not seem to influence test performance, there is no good reason to withhold it. Further, being less than fully informed in this matter may contribute to employees' anxiety and distress.

Functional capacity evaluations have limited predictive utility regarding likelihood of return to work (Gross et al 2004), and almost no predictive validity for recurrence of complaint (Gross & Battie 2004, 2005b, 2006). Readiness to return to work appears to be a product of complex psychological variables rather than based on physical performance alone (Li-Tsang et al 2007).

RELATIONSHIP AND COMMUNICATION AS MOTIVATION

In counselling psychology, 'the quality of the counselling relationship has proved to be the most significant factor in facilitating treatment adherence and positive counselling outcomes' (Petitpas et al 1999:344). A collaborative relationship between the client and the therapist, working together to improve the psychological functioning (health) of the client, is sometimes called a 'working alliance'. The quality of the working alliance influences treatment outcomes, partly because a strong working alliance is an important factor in a client persisting with treatment through a plateau or setback.

Rogers (1967) argued that therapeutic relationships are based on three facilitative conditions: acceptance, genuineness and empathy. Acceptance, sometimes called unconditional positive regard, means that parties in a therapeutic relationship are accepted as they are, for who they are. Genuineness means being aware of, and honest about, feelings in a relationship, so that verbal and non-verbal communication are aligned. Empathy is understanding other parties' points of view. Rogers claimed that these facilitative conditions could be helpful across a range of situations, including therapeutic relationships between practitioners and clients, business relationships, education, and in the resolution of social problems.

Healthcare providers are likely to have considerable training and experience in the development of therapeutic relationships (Mauksch et al 2008), but other parties in the employee compensation system (employees, employers, unions, insurers) may not. Because communication and relationships are not unidirectional, all parties can contribute to improved communication. Further, communication is internal as well as external: self-talk may be used to reinforce goals of rehabilitation.

EVIDENCE-BASED HEALTHCARE

Evidence-based healthcare is not blind faith in scientific numbers; a growing body of scientific literature confirms that the quality of the human encounter is a key component of health service delivery that accounts for a considerable portion of the variance in clinical outcomes. In evidence-based healthcare interventions offered are firmly underpinned by current science, and delivered with due consideration of clients' needs and practitioners' experience. For the management of some common conditions such as back pain, arthritis, knee pain, and neck pain, evidence-based clinical guidelines have been developed and published (see Appendix 2). Clinical guidelines (sometimes region specific) are public domain documents that are widely available to both healthcare practitioners and members of the public. Most regions in which injured employees can be eligible for compensation have highly regulated healthcare systems that impose an expectation of evidence-based care delivery upon treating practitioners. For example, the Victorian Workcover Authority (in Australia) is explicit in the expectation that treating practitioners deliver evidence-based healthcare to injured employees in Victoria, Australia (VWA 2004). It is reasonable to expect treating practitioners to be familiar with evidence-based clinical guidelines within their field of practice.

Despite expectation, practice of evidence-based healthcare is not universal. McGuirk and Bogduk (2007) assessed the application of evidence-based guidelines among compensable employees with acute back pain. Via a prospective audit, employees in a health service who presented with acute low back pain were offered the option of usual care from their general practitioner or care provided by a staff specialist who practiced according to evidence-based guidelines. Evidence-based care was elected by 65% of injured employees, and when compared with those who chose usual care, these employees had less time off work, spent less time on modified duties, and had fewer recurrences. Also, many more of these employees (70%) resumed normal

duties immediately, and fewer developed chronic pain, than those who chose usual care (McGuirk & Bogduk 2007).

Public health campaigns can be used to reinforce evidence-based healthcare message, alter health beliefs, and change health delivery by prompting health 'consumers' to request evidence-based practices. A widespread media campaign to alter beliefs about back pain, and align these beliefs with scientific evidence, ran in Victoria (Australia) from September 1997 until December 1999. Immediately following the campaign both community and practitioners' beliefs about back pain were largely consistent with scientific evidence, and there was a concurrent decline in the number of employee compensation claims for back pain. When compared with demographically identical groups in New South Wales (neighbouring state used as control), scientifically consistent beliefs about back pain were sustained among the Victorian community 3 years and 4.5 years after the cessation of the media campaign (Buchbinder & Jolley 2005, 2007).

Although evidence-based public health education campaigns are powerful tools for changing widespread health beliefs, influence on health behaviour at work may be limited. The Working Backs Scotland public education campaign brought about considerable change in public health beliefs, but despite an occupational focus in this campaign, rates of new compensation claims and absences from work due to back pain among employees of the Royal Mail in Scotland were comparable with the those across the remainder of the United Kingdom (Waddell et al 2007). It is inadequate to rely on public health education alone to drive demand for evidence-based healthcare.

A wealth of healthcare information is available via the internet. Some of this information is of very high quality and useful for supporting evidence-based healthcare, but many people are unable to make full use of this information. Dart (2008) surveyed three subsections of the Australian population (high socioeconomic, low socioeconomic, university) to determine the utilisation, importance, trust, and future preference for the internet as a source of health information. Fewer respondents in the low socioeconomic group accessed online health information than in the other two groups. In all groups use and ascribed importance of online health information was consistent with home internet availability and the frequency of internet use, but was not related to age alone. Unsurprisingly, the internet was a particularly important source of health information for the university sample. Seventy percent of those who accessed online health information did not bring this information to their doctors, and most respondents (all groups) reported that they did not trust the internet for health information (Dart 2008).

CONCLUSION

Clinical exercise practitioners are ideally placed to assist clients with work-related injuries or illnesses to return to function, and in some cases, return to their pre-injury employment. Although exercise testing may be used to determine clients' capacity for some types of work, I caution against using exercise in reductionist and punitive ways, particularly if the test tasks are not work specific. Functional capacity testing is most useful when used as a measure of physical fitness parameters (eg: muscle strength, endurance, power, etc) at a point in time and informs both client and practitioner of directions for future training. As well as the obvious physiological utility of physical activity and specific exercise in injury rehabilitation, the stages of change involved in return to work are comparable to the stages of change associated with the adoption of physical activity and other health-promoting behaviours. Accordingly, re-engagement in physical activity can become a metaphor for clients' return to function, to work, and to the fullness of life.

Summary of key lessons

- Understand the employee compensation systems that apply to your region, and as far as possible, be ready to explain systems to clients. Clients may feel overwhelmed by complex employee compensation systems and clear explanations can increase clients' informational control of their occupational injury or illness.

- Encourage early and graduated return to work as a component of work hardening training. Clients and employers may resist early return to work or resent the unproductive work time that may occur at this stage. Practitioners can support early return to work by explaining the importance of engagement in work, and assisting employers in identifying suitable duties for injured employees.

- As far as possible, deliver evidence-based healthcare. In particular, use functional capacity testing to set training goals and inform exercise selection. Do not use functional capacity tests to forecast expected return to work or likelihood of injury recurrence because predictive validity for these outcomes is poor.

REFERENCES

Asante AK, Brintnell ES, Gross DP (2007) Functional self-efficacy beliefs influence functional capacity evaluation. *Journal of Occupational Rehabilitation*, 17:73–82

Becker MH, Rosenstock IM (1984) Compliance with medical advice. In: Steptoe A, Mathews A (eds) *Healthcare and human behavior*. London: Academic Press

Buchbinder R, Jolley D (2005) Effects of a media campaign on back beliefs is sustained 3 years after its cessation. *Spine*, 30:1323–30

—— (2007) Improvements in general practitioner beliefs and stated management of back pain persist 4.5 years after the cessation of a public health media campaign. *Spine*, 32:E156–162

Callahan LF, Bloch DA, Pincus T (1992) Identification of work disability in rheumatoid arthritis — physical, radiographic, and laboratory variables do not add any explanatory power to demographic and functional variables. *Journal of Clinical Epidemiology*, 45:127–38

Cronan T A, Groessl E, Kaplan RM (1997) The effects of social support and health education interventions on healthcare costs. *Arthritis Care and Research*, 10:99–110

Dart J (2008) The internet as a source of health information in three disparate communities. *Australian Health Review*, 32:559–69

Gross DP, Battie MC, Cassidy JD (2004) The prognostic value of functional capacity evaluation in patients with chronic low back pain: Part 1: Timely return to work. *Spine*, 29:914–19

Gross DP, Battie MC (2004) The prognostic value of functional capacity evaluation in patients with chronic low back pain: Part 2: Sustained recovery. *Spine*, 29: 920–4

—— (2005a) Factors influencing functional capacity evaluations in workers' compensation claimants with low back pain. *Physical Therapy*, 85:315–22

—— (2005b) Predicting timely recovery and recurrence following multidisciplinary rehabilitation in patients with compensated low back pain. *Spine*, 30:235–40

—— (2006) Does functional capacity evaluation predict recovery in workers' compensation claimants with upper extremity disorders? *Occupational and Environmental Medicine*, 63:404–10

Gruman J, Von Korff M (1996) *Indexed Bibliography on Self-management for People with Chronic Disease.* Washington DC: Center for Advancement in Health

Hewitt JA, Hush JM, Martin MH, et al (2007) Clinical prediction rules can be derived and validated for injured Australian workers with persistent musculoskeletal pain: an observational study. *Australian Journal of Physiotherapy*, 53: 269–76

Kerns RD, Rosenberg R (2000) Predicting responses to self-management treatments for chronic pain: Application of the pain stages of change model. *Pain*, 84:49–55

Kerns RD, Rosenberg R, Jamison RN, et al (1997) Readiness to adopt a self-management approach to chronic pain: The Pain Stages of Change Questionnaire (PSOCQ). *Pain*, 72:227–34

Kuijer W, Brouwer S, Reneman MF, et al (2006) Matching FCE activities and work demands: an explorative study. *Journal of Occupational Rehabilitation*, 16:469–83

Levallee L, Flint F (1996) The relationship of stress, competitive anxiety, mood state, and social support to athletic injury. *Journal of Athletic Training*, 31:296–9

Li-Tsang CW, Chan HH, Lam C, et al (2007) Psychological aspects of injured workers' returning to work in Hong Kong. *Journal of Occupational Rehabilitation*, 17:279–88

Lorig K, Holman H (1989) Long-term outcomes of an arthritis self-management study: effects of reinforcement efforts. *Social Science Medicine*, 29:221–4

Lorig K, Kraines RG, Holman H (1981) A randomized prospective controlled study of the effects of health education for people with arthritis. *Arthritis & Rheumatism*, 24(Suppl 4), S90

Lorig K, Mazonson P, Holman H (1993) Evidence suggesting that health education for self-management in patients with chronic arthritis has sustained health benefits while reducing healthcare costs. *Arthritis & Rheumatism*, 36:439–46

Lorig K, Seleznick M, Lubeck D, et al (1989) The beneficial outcomes of the arthritis self-management course are inadequately explained by behavior change. *Arthritis & Rheumatism*, 32:91–5

Mason JH, Anderson JJ, Meenan RF, et al (1992) The Rapid Assessment of Disease Activity in Rheumatology (RADAR) Questionnaire — validity and sensitivity to change of a patient self-report measure of joint count and clinical status. *Arthritis and Rheumatism*, 35:156–62

Mauksch LB, Dugdale DC, Dodson S, et al (2008) Relationship, communication, and efficiency in the medical encounter: Creating a clinical model from a literature review. *Archives of Internal Medicine*, 168:1387–95

McGuirk B, Bogduk N (2007) Evidence-based care for low back pain in workers eligible for compensation. *Occupational Medicine*, 57:36–42

Norman P, Bennett P, Smith C, et al (1998) Health locus of control and health behavior. *Journal of Health Psychology*, 3:171–80

Petitpas AJ, Giges B, Danish SJ (1999) The sport psychologist-athlete relationship: Implications for training. *The Sport Psychologist*, 13:344–57

Pincus T, Brooks RH, Callahan LF (1994) Prediction of long-term mortality in patients with rheumatoid arthritis according to simple questionnaire and joint count measures. *Annals of Internal Medicine*, 120:26–34

Pincus T, Mitchell JM, Burkhauser RV (1989) Substantial work disability and earnings losses in individuals less than age 65 with osteoarthritis: Comparisons with rheumatoid arthritis. *Journal of Clinical Epidemiology*, 42:449–57

Pincus T, Summey JA, Soraci SA, et al (1983) Assessment of patient satisfaction in activities of daily living using a modified Stanford Health Assessment Questionnaire. *Arthritis and Rheumatism*, 26:1346–53

Prochaska JO, DiClemente CC (1983) Stages and processes of self-change of smoking: toward an integrative model of change. *Journal of Consulting and Clinical Psychology*, 51:390–5

—— (1998) Towards a comprehensive, transtheoretical model of change: States of change and addictive behaviors. In: Miller WR, Heather N (eds) *Applied Clinical Psychology* (2nd ed). New York: Plenum Press

Proctor T, Mayer T, Theodore B, et al (2005) Failure to complete a functional restoration program for chronic musculoskeletal disorders: A prospective 1-year outcome study. *Archives of Physical Medicine and Rehabilitation*, 86: 1509–15

Reneman MF, Kool J, Oesch P, et al (2006) Material handling performance of patients with chronic low back pain during functional capacity evaluation: A comparison between three countries. *Disability Rehabilitation*, 28:1143–9

Rogers C (1967) The necessary and sufficient conditions of therapeutic personality change. *Journal of Consulting Psychology*, 21:95–103

Sarafino EP (2002) *Health Psychology* (4th ed). New York: John Wiley

Schiphorst Preuper HR, Reneman MF, Boonstra AM, et al (2008) Relationship between psychological factors and performance-based and self-reported disability in chronic low back pain. *European Spine Journal*, 17:1448–56

Schultz AB, Edington DW (2007) Employee health and presenteeism: A systematic review. *Journal of Occupational Rehabilitation*, 17:547–79

Victorian Workcover Authority (VWA) (2004) *Clinical Framework for the Delivery of Health Services to Injured Workers*. Victorian Workcover Authority, Melbourne, Australia

Waddell G, O'Connor M, Boorman S, et al (2007) Working Backs Scotland: a public and professional health education campaign for back pain. *Spine*, 32:2139–43

Wallston KA, Wallston BS, DeVellis R (1978) Development of Multidimensional Health Locus of Control (MHLC) Scales. *Health Education Monographs*, 6:160–70

Wolfe F, Hawley DJ (1998) The long-term outcomes of rheumatoid arthritis: work disability: a prospective 18 year study of 823 patients. *The Journal of Rheumatology*, 25:2108–17

World Health Organization (WHO) (1948) Preamble to the Constitution of the World Health Organization as adopted by the International Health Conference, New York, 19–22 June 1946; signed on 22 July 1946 by the representatives of 61 States and entered into force on 7 April 1948

Clinical tales

Chapter 10

Setting the tone: practitioner self-care

Melainie Cameron, Mark B Andersen, Helen Webb and Dennis Hemphill

INTRODUCTION

We have chosen to tell our stories. Each of us is a practitioner in some health-related discipline. We have learned over our working lives that we do not have all the answers. We are human, and frail. We make mistakes, get things wrong, over-extend ourselves, and make errors of judgment. In time we have come to the view that caring for ourselves first allows us to deliver better care, and makes us more competent practitioners. We present these cases as studies in methods of practitioner self-care.

In this chapter we include neither 'assumed concepts' nor a 'summary of the key lessons' of the chapter. Rather, we tell personal stories and encourage readers to take from them whatever they wish. We offer some discussion questions to encourage practitioners, regardless of age and experience, to draw from our stories lessons for themselves.

MELAINIE

I am an osteopath and an exercise scientist. In the third year of my osteopathic studies, precisely as I was learning about arthritides, my mother was diagnosed with progressive systemic sclerosis. This event was formative for me; the beginning of my interest in arthritic diseases. Arthritides are chronic illnesses, common in musculoskeletal practice, and many respond favourably to exercise interventions, making them an ideal interest area around which to build a clinical career. Desire for further enquiry led me to research. After my clinical training, I moved into research degrees. My doctoral degree comprised a series of studies on the effects of exercise and manual therapy on quality of life

in people with arthritides. My doctoral research supervisor was not even slightly surprised that I might want to investigate a topic of personal importance. In his words, 'If it's not one thing, it's your mother'.

My interest in arthritides was of my mother born, but that baby began to grow up. While writing a book chapter for physical and manual therapists on the psychological effects of chronic arthritides, a publication from my PhD, I was diagnosed with rheumatoid arthritis. *Physician heal thyself* rang loud and clear in my ears. Unfortunately, it is one thing to understand the theories and principles of good arthritis care and quite another to live them out.

As for many people with arthritides, my journey from symptoms to diagnosis had been long and hard won. I first experienced pain and swelling in the small joints of my hands, and in my right shoulder and elbow, when I was an undergraduate student osteopath. Numerous visits to osteopaths, chiropractors, physiotherapists, and general medical practitioners left me without any firm diagnosis. Unlike some patients, I was never dismissed or told that the pain was 'all in my head', but I didn't get any answers either. Symptoms would subside, and both my practitioners and I would think everything was fine.

The American College of Rheumatology classification criteria for arthritides are strict (Arnett et al 1988). Scientifically these criteria are excellent; high specificity and sensitivity, with low false positive and false negative rates. Arthritides are, for the most part, chronic diseases that evolve over time. Inflammatory arthritic diseases are typified by flares that peak and ebb; people may appear healthy between flares. Clients with incompletely evolved and unsustained disease presentations may wait in 'diagnostic darkness' because they do not yet meet the criteria for disease classification.

I knew from my research that I was not alone in this experience — many people with arthritic diseases report protracted diagnostic processes — but I still felt alone. Without a diagnostic label, I was unable to explain to my family, friends, or colleagues, and, of great frustration to an academic, I could take no refuge in books because I didn't know which of over a hundred arthritides to investigate.

Eventually one medical practitioner had the courage to say to me:

> I think you probably have an arthritis, mostly likely rheumatoid arthritis, but you know that you don't meet the diagnostic criteria, so I can't officially use that label. We just need to wait and see what happens. If it is arthritis then you will meet the diagnostic criteria eventually. And if we're really lucky, it will burn itself out before that happens.

He prescribed some anti-inflammatories, and asked me to see him again if my symptoms didn't clear up. His honesty about diagnostic difficulty was refreshing, and I felt slightly less alone.

More, he was right. Seven years after the first symptoms had sent me running off to a doctor, I had an episode of morning stiffness, joint pain and swelling that lasted longer than 6 weeks, affected more than three types of joints including the small joints of my hands and wrists, and was accompanied by some tiny, but clear, joint surface erosions visible on plain film radiographs. I had rheumatoid arthritis.

I tell myself that I am fortunate. I have had the pleasure of working with doctors who believed me. Also, I seem to have mild disease; I am completely well between flares, and have not had any apparent progression of joint erosions since diagnosis. So far, I have not needed to take disease modifying anti-rheumatic drugs, and I am grateful to have avoided the side-effects and ongoing monitoring of those powerful medications.

There have also been costs. I am an academic. My osteopathic colleagues tell me that from my undergraduate days they identified me as cut for academe, but for me the transition from manual therapy practice to academic life was a road marked by grief. I might be good at academic work, I might be a skilful teacher, but I also delight in clinical practice. I loved working with my clients, and I enjoyed the relief that manual therapy can bring to sore and weary bodies. Gradually I reduced my hours per week in clinical practice and invested more time in academic teaching and research. When my peers enquired, I glossed over these changes in my work by explaining that I loved academic life and I found research challenging and fun. These explanations of the joys of academe are true for me, however, it is also true that manual therapy work places strain on my hands, elbows, and shoulders, aggravating the rheumatoid changes in these joints.

I had never invested in establishing my own business, so I could not reduce my clinical workload by employing an associate practitioner. I was a sole trader who sub-contracted to other practitioners. In reducing my clinical hours to move into academe, I reduced my income from clinical practice. Later, when a change in Australian tax laws meant I could not offset practice income against academic wages, I found myself running my clinical practice at a financial loss. I could not afford to keep a financially unviable business going, and I found the physical costs of manual therapy work too high to consider returning to full-time clinical practice. Again, I count myself fortunate because when I explained this difficulty to my academic head of department, he suggested that I consult for the university, and he offered a financial arrangement that ensured that both the university and I got paid. This solution allowed me to keep an open window into clinical practice, and meant that I did not need to admit to my colleagues that I was really not physically able to practice much anymore.

My whole life I have been interested in exercise, not so much competitive sport as exercise for wellbeing and wholeness. Physicality and physical activity matter deeply to me, but somehow, in using exercise as therapy for myself, I was slow on the uptake. During my doctorate I conducted research into warm water exercise for people with arthritides, but it wasn't until after my own diagnosis, and almost a decade after my first symptoms, that I actually tried warm water exercise for myself. Why did I leave it so long? I wish I knew. All I can say is that sometimes illness blinds you to something right under your nose. I am sure that as clinicians we have seen this phenomenon, clients who overlook obvious or simple remedies for their woes, and seem astounded when we point them out. As a client myself, I was no different, unable to see what was right in front of me.

Also in my studies I had learned about Kate Lorig's work in patient education and self-management in arthritis (Lorig & Holman 1989; Lorig & Holman 2003; Lorig et al 1993; Lorig et al 1989). There is an established community of practice around this work, and a body of scientific evidence supporting its use. More, it doesn't seem to matter which form of arthritis clients have, or the stage of diagnosis, self-management offers some benefits to clients so long as they are ready to adopt recommended lifestyle changes (eg: healthy eating, moderate and paced exercise, stress reduction, improved sleeping habits). Despite knowing about self-management, I didn't take part in any self-management education for myself until some years after I had a formal diagnosis.

When I did decide that I should undertake some self-management training, I entered the training program thinking it was professional development, an opportunity to increase my work-related skills. As I moved through the 6 session program, I discovered that self-management was not only a well-researched intervention for people with arthritides, it was a system through which I could take care of myself.

My commitment to exercise and self-management has grown over several years with the positive reinforcement of successes. I am now confident that I can manage my arthritis well. I exercise everyday, using exercise to regulate my sleep, balance my mood, keep my joints mobile, and supporting muscles strong. As well as warm water exercise, I engage in regular walking, dancing, netball, and some swimming. I play netball in gloves, and I acknowledge that I will never be an elite athlete or dancer. I must exercise daily or I do not sleep well, and if I do not sleep well, then I risk a flare. These costs of arthritis on exercise, and the cost of regular and necessary exercise on my lifestyle and time, do not grieve me to the same extent as the changes to my manual therapy clinical practice, but they are still costs. This disease exacts its price.

No one feels this price more dearly than my family. It is my partner and my children who see

me shuffle around the house early on the mornings of a flare. They feel the effects of fatigue from the arthritis, when I fall into bed in the evenings rather than joining them for movies, games, and other entertainment. They see my deep frustration at not being able to make this disease go away. I love them, and they love me. Of all the ways I count myself fortunate, their love is the greatest.

I have, with time, some further study, and the support of some wonderful colleagues, been able to turn my research into exercise and my personal commitment to exercise into a refreshment of my academic and clinical careers. Now I am accredited as an exercise physiologist as well as an osteopath, recognised in both disciplines under the Australian health system. My present academic work includes educating students training to be allied health practitioners who intend to use exercise for clinical gains. Sometimes I open myself up to my classes in discussion of my own journey. I tell students my story, much as I have done in this case study, and let them ask me whatever they wish. I try to be open with them about the wrestles of being a clinician, knowing a lot, and yet feeling unable to help yourself.

These days my clinical practice, still undertaken as consultancy on behalf of a university, is mostly in clinical exercise, both individual and group exercise consultations. I practice little manual therapy now, although I recognise a place for passive care, I have come to find exercise a satisfying way to engage with clients and maintain my interest in physical wellbeing. I choose how much I exercise along with clients, and pace myself, demonstrating self-management of arthritis in my daily practice. Of course, it is somewhat self-serving to have reconfigured my clinical practice in this way, and I have an ongoing conversation with myself that includes calling my desires and motivations into check. I believe that clinical practice, regardless of the particular discipline, is about service, and to serve, clients' needs must be at the centre of clinical encounters. There is nothing wrong with shaping my clinical practice so that it is good for me as well as good for my clients, but I need to be sure that I serve my clients in my actions.

After some years of living with me with rheumatoid arthritis, my partner recently offered to relocate with me to a warmer climate. Although disease flares still occur, I experience less stiffness and pain in the heat. He supported me through an application for a job 1700 km north of our then home in southern Australia. This decision to move north also comes with cost, particularly leaving extended family and friends, but I am hopeful that the costs will be balanced out by the benefits. As a practitioner and as a client, my journey is not done, but I have walked some way on the path of healing myself.

MARK: THE IMPAIRED PRACTITIONER MALGRÉ LUI: TWO TALES OF SELF-CARE

For the title of this section, I have borrowed from Molière's comedy Le Médecin Malgré Lui (The Doctor Despite Himself) because many health practitioners experience ailments and impairments similar to those of their clients, but may not be so good at 'taking their own medicine'.

Professional impairment can manifest in multifarious (and nefarious) forms. The broadest description of impairment would be: when the actions and inactions of the practitioner serve some other purpose than the health, happiness, and welfare of the client. The 'serving some other purpose' of this overly general and sweeping definition is often difficult to determine. The seemingly helpful interventions the practitioner introduces may be based on sound theory and clinical practice, but if the professional doesn't have much time, has an overloaded schedule, and does not get the 'whole' story on the client's experiences, then the intervention prescribed may be useless or possibly even counterproductive. My position may sound harsh, but this scenario represents a common form of impairment. The action prescribed is, in part, in service of the practitioner's hefty schedule. Such impairment is almost unavoidable given the demands in the biomedical and psychosocial professions. I believe it would be safe to say that physicians completing their residencies are nearly all in an almost constant state of impairment. We should be kind to ourselves; this sort of impairment often comes with the territory.

As one moves through the spectrum of impairment, the consequences of substandard professional practice and potential damage to clients take on darker and darker tones. There may be impairment in learning in that the practitioner does not have the knowledge to deal with a client's concerns, but thinks they do and continues treatment as they see fit. Narcissistic

professionals may use clients for their own aggrandisement, manipulating them to become dependent on their services or exploiting them by requesting they recommend the professional to their friends. And then the darkest of all impairments is when the practitioner enters into a sexual relationship with his client. The 'his' here is intentional because even though women do exploit their clients in these sorts of ways, the overwhelming number of romantic/erotic/sexual boundary transgressors are men.

In this chapter, however, I want to focus on two different forms of impairment other than overwork, incompetence, personality pathology, and sexual exploitation. My concern here is when a reasonably sane and competent practitioner becomes impaired either through a relatively acute deterioration in mental health or because of some (in the first case below, apparent) physical ailment. Before I launch into the stories of my physical illness and psychological impairment as a graduate student and a psychologist, I need to lay some background as to how I view the human condition. I guess I could say, as a first maxim, that none of us get out of life unscathed. We are all damaged goods. Humans can be glorious, magnanimous, heroic, even almost super-human, but we all have frailties, and somewhere along the line many of us will crack in some fashion.

I also find the academic and quotidian use of the words 'mind and body' to be a false dichotomy and a vulgar (in the original Latin sense of the word) misrepresentation of how we are built. This Cartesian division of thinking substance (mind) and extended substance (body, the physical world) holds sway over how many of us think about ourselves and is probably one of the root sources as to why we view psychological disorders as different from other medical conditions. Philosophically, I guess I would have to say I am a monistic materialist and a reductionist, and that 'minds' are functions of nervous systems interacting with the world. One consequence of splitting mind and body is that we regard them as different, and when something goes wrong with either one, we treat them differently.

Most all readers of this book would have little trouble seeing a doctor for a respiratory infection or a broken bone, but when it comes to mental disturbances, help-seeking behaviours may not eventuate as they would with a busted thumb. Psychological problems are somehow more personal, intimate, and even shameful than something one can point to and say, 'There's the nasty little microbe causing you difficulties. Here are some antibiotics.' Microbes are unwelcomed 'others' that are hurting us. Mental disturbance feel more like 'us', like there is something wrong with our core beings. They indicate that we are constitutionally weak, and that weakness, if possible, should be hidden (by a process called compensation). In the rugged individualism of many societies, there is often a cultural pressure to work things out on one's own when it comes to mental and behavioural issues. This self-sufficient individualism is also a contributor to the stigma attached to seeking help from the psychological professions. Even psychologists are not immune to cultural influences and stigma. I know many psychologists who think that if they needed to go into therapy that it would be embarrassing and shameful, and ascribe to a secular corollary to the biblical admonition found in Luke 4:23, 'Psychologist, heal thyself'.

First tale: impairing somatization

My first story is about a young psychology graduate student during the time of his first major clinical psychology internship and the completion of his master's thesis. It is a tale about the inseparability of minds and bodies, but it starts first with the body. That student was, of course, me. I was thrown in the deep end for my clinical internship; it was on a locked psychiatric ward of a US Veterans Administration Hospital shortly after the end of the war in Vietnam. I only half-believed that my anxieties about my competence as a psychology intern (and my physical safety) might possibly have been sources of my physical ailments, but there were a lot of seriously damaged, unstable, and scary people on that ward (one of the reasons it was locked).

When I was completing my internship and thesis, I developed a chronic gastrointestinal problem. I would eat something, and within a few hours I would evacuate it. Food was sprinting through my body. At first, the problem was mildly disconcerting, but as I began to lose weight (I was slim to begin with), I became seriously anxious. On the locked ward I would often have to excuse myself because of an urgent need. My gut problem was starting to impair my work. I can't recall how

many medical tests and samples were taken, but I was poked and prodded (often in vulnerable and indecorous positions), irradiated and X-rayed repeatedly over a couple of months. Nothing. My frustrated physician finally said, 'Do you think you are experiencing a lot of stress?' I responded, 'Yes, my gut problem is scaring the crap out of me' (pun intended). He then asked me about other stressors in my life, and I told him that I was completing my master's thesis, but I didn't think I was that stressed out about it. I also told him about my internship situation. He suggested that I have some psychotherapy. I didn't really think my problem was in my head or that it was closely connected to the internship, but I went anyway.

My psychologist was a young woman, and we had a great time in psychotherapy. I learned some important and sobering stuff about myself. My anxieties about the locked ward were diminishing as I got used to the patients and the routines, but my guts were not getting much better. Maybe I wasn't going deep enough in therapy. The turning point came after I handed the first full draft of my thesis to my supervisor. He had helped me immensely with the design and the analyses, but he had not seen much of my writing. A few days after handing in the thesis, he called me into his office and said, 'Your thesis is very well written. I don't see how you really have much more work to do on it.' The next day my gut problem disappeared. Mind and body are one. Even though my problem did not manifest in psychological ways with anxiety (probably through ego-defence mechanisms such as denial and repression), the stress became expressed through somatic channels. My anxieties about my internship were conscious; my anxieties about my supervisor's evaluation of me, of me possibly disappointing him (I admired, adored, was in awe, and had a huge crush on him), and my competency to do and write up research were largely unconscious. The problem was both in my head and in my guts. My supervisor and I labelled my condition as 'somatic thesis disorder'. I have been a staunch monist ever since.

My thesis disorder is now an amusing tale I occasionally tell my students when we are discussing the trials and tribulations of graduate school. I was doing all the right things. I was seeing a physician, getting tested in all sorts of ways, and I was in psychotherapy. But all this self-care was still failing. Luckily, my cure was delivered through chance and circumstance and the words of my supervisor. Try as I might, the psychologist in me could not heal me because the source of the problem was unconscious and inaccessible. Maybe several more months of therapy would have done the trick, but I have never seen a treatment work as fast as the words 'well-done' from my supervisor. His words worked because of the phenomena of transference, idealisation, the internalisation of the love object, and of course, love itself. But it would take another chapter to explain those processes.

Second tale: impairment and maladaptive self-care

Now, I would like to tell a tale that to this day still seems paradoxical, but understandably so. Before I launch into the tale, however, I need to write about depression. In clinical psychology circles it has been called 'the common cold of mental health'. I both like and dislike that appellation. In one way it normalises the condition and may help people look upon depression with sympathetic eyes because it is so common. In the US, major depressive disorder affects approximately 16% of adults at least once in their lifetimes (Gartlehner et al 2007). In another way, however, this 'common cold' analogy trivialises depression, and it is anything but trivial.

As one becomes depressed there are changes in thoughts, feelings, and behaviours, and the level of previous overall functioning decreases. From the *Diagnostic and Statistical Manual of Mental Disorders* (DSM; American Psychiatric Association 2000) a diagnosis of major depressive disorder is made if a person meets the following criteria: for at least a 2-week period, the person has experienced depressed mood or loss of interest or pleasure in many activities. Also, within that time period, the person reports at least four of the following symptoms: (a) significant changes in weight (up or down); (b) significant changes in appetite (increase or decrease); (c) significant changes in sleep (insomnia, hypersomnia, early awakening and trouble returning to sleep); (d) indecisiveness, (feelings of worthlessness or emptiness); (e) fatigue or low energy levels; (f) agitation or lethargy; (g) concentration difficulties; and (h) thoughts of death or suicidal ideation.

Many years after my somatic thesis disorder, over a period of a couple months, I began to lose interest in food; I was losing weight. I had difficulty

sleeping, and I was ineffective in my work. I was beginning to feel worthless, but also agitated. I was working on a book and not getting anywhere. I would stare at the manuscript on the screen for an hour or so, obsessing over a sentence only to throw my hands up and go lie on the couch. I was ticking off most of the diagnostic criteria for depression. I could compensate for short periods of time, such as going into work and teaching, but then I would drive home and fall in a heap. These symptoms were all the more confusing because I should have been entering a happy period of my life. A year-long trans-Pacific romance was going to come to an end soon with my partner from the USA coming to Australia to live with me.

I know depression well. My mother had many bouts of depression from her 30s until her death. A good deal of my overachieving is probably connected with her depression. I was the son of a depressed mother using his achievements to distract her from her unhappiness ('See, Mom, look what I did! Please be happy'). The flawed logic is, 'When you are depressed Mom, you move away from me and all of us. How can I get you back? Maybe if I do something grand you will come back and love us again.' It actually worked sometimes, and thus, my achieving was reinforced. It is often children's lot to feel responsible for parental happiness. It's an impossible and doomed job, but we take it on anyway.

I could not get over the paradox of feeling sad and worthless at the happiest time of my life. I figured it would pass, and I would have a couple of good days here and there, but my sleep was becoming more and more disturbed. So I started some self-care with some self-medication; Benedryl™ (an antihistamine that causes drowsiness) is a wonderful thing. Then I discovered doxylamine (an even better antihistamine). I thought, 'I'll just get on these drugs until my partner arrives, and then all will be right with the world'. But it didn't stop there; I added ethanol into the mix. Pretty soon I was popping pills and drinking over a bottle of wine a night with no more than two alcohol-free days in a row. I knew it was all wrong. The psychologist in me knew it was all wrong, but I still continued. My deeply flawed self-care regimen had gone pear-shaped. Psychologist, heal thyself. Yeah, right.

One night, in the lachrymose stage of ethanol consumption, I started making a connection that might explain my sadness. I realised that my partner was arriving in Australia within a couple days of the 10th anniversary of my mother's death. I am my mother's son, and she still visits me often in dreams. When she died, I was partnerless, and even though she never said anything, I know she was worried sick about me finding love and happiness (my two sisters were, and still are, both happily married). She died without me accomplishing something that probably would have worked better, in terms of her happiness, than any of my other accomplishments. I was in grief for her (the 10th is a big anniversary), in grief that she never got to see her son with a loving partner, in grief that she died without me making her happy in the end, and in grief over all my failures at saving her. I am such a mama's boy, still intimately tied to her 16 years after her death.

That night I said to myself, 'OK, Mark, you have the Big D. Now do something about it.' The next day I was on a plane to visit my best psychologist friend in Canberra. I told him the whole sad tale, and he immediately called up his physician (I also knew him and his family well). We had a long chat, and I began taking anti-depressants. When I got home, I started psychotherapy to go through, not just what had recently happened, but also to do some archeological digging into my past. It helped.

I think this tale illustrates that even a well-trained professional in psychology can be blind to his own psychopathology, can languish in denial, and can choose maladaptive self-care tactics that actually exacerbate his condition. My story reminds me of one of my doctoral students. He was an Olympic hopeful in rowing, but he worked so hard to get on the Olympic squad that he overtrained and incurred a serious injury. He didn't make the team. He then did his PhD on over-training at my university. He knew everything about over-training, its signs, its symptoms, how to avoid it. He was jam-packed with knowledge. He believed he was now prepared to train properly for the next Olympics. So he had another go, but he succumbed to the intense pressures of Olympic-level rowing to train more and more. Even when he was starting to see signs of over-training, he would not stop or drop back because the coaches and other athletes would start to look at him funny, as though he didn't really have the gear to be an Olympian. Like the last time, he overtrained, became injured, and didn't make the team. Even knowledgeable experts, who should know better, fall into traps of irrational thinking and maladaptive behaviour.

Self-care through another's care

The last words the Buddha spoke to his monks were, 'Work hard to gain your own salvation. Do your best.' The Buddha knew that we are all flawed; he knew that we all struggle. He brought himself to enlightenment, but the rest of us mortals probably can't see our way clear to solving many of our troubles. We need help, and that help may come in the form of a thesis supervisor, a psychotherapist, a guru, a teacher, or a wise friend who may assist us in gaining some measure of our own salvation. Many of the readers of this book are in the helping professions. They help people exercise; they help people heal. Their service to others, in many cases, brings about some small (or even large) changes that increase health, happiness, and wellbeing. But helpers sometimes need help to get through difficult times, or to remove blind spots that they cannot see because they are, in a word, blind.

I really like the Buddha's last three words, 'Do your best.' Those words speak of a deep compassion and say to me, 'We are all imperfect; we are all flawed. All of us struggle with some major or minor demons, but there is hope. Keep trying; keep having a go at figuring things out. You may not reach enlightenment, but if you do your best you will be moving in the right direction.' I would add, 'and find someone to help you along the way.'

HELEN

I have been a front line paramedic for 13 years. Prior to that I was a physical education, health, and science teacher. The major subjects studied in my physical education degree were sports medicine, exercise physiology, biomechanics (kinesiology), and health.

Being a front line paramedic means that you are exposed not only to traumatic incidents and sometimes multiple casualty incidents, but also to long and gruelling hours of shift work. The average paramedic either works a 4 × 4 roster which includes 2 × 10-hour day shifts, followed by 2 × 14-hour night shifts, with the possibility of overtime and no fixed meal breaks during each shift. The 4 × 4 roster is followed by 4 days off. The other common type of shift is day shift followed by on-call at night. While on-call you have to take the ambulance home with you and cannot be more than 30 seconds from your vehicle during the on-call period. You must be contactable at all times and can be called out to any type of incident at any time during the 5 to 7 continuous periods of day shift and on-call. I have worked both types of shifts, the 4 × 4 roster at Kings Cross in Sydney and the on-call roster in remote New South Wales. Kings Cross was a busy area and it was nothing to work 16 hours straight and complete 14 jobs in the 16 hours and then have to drive an hour to get home. In remote country areas, it was not unusual to work as a single response paramedic with 10 hours of driving each shift.

After a 4 × 4 roster or 5 days of on-call, you are exhausted, sleep deprived, mentally fatigued, hungry and dehydrated. The longest period I have worked during a 24-hour period is 20 hours straight. I had a 4-hour break and then had to go back to work. I survived on caffeine to stay awake during the day and often skipped meals due to work commitments. Sleep was elusive when I finally got a break as the caffeine and adrenaline were still affecting me. I often consumed two straight whiskies to sleep after each shift. If I woke up or could not get to sleep, I had another one. I was desperate to sleep and suffered significant sleep disturbance. Many of my nights were filled with vivid dreams of jobs I had attended or I spent hours awake, reflecting over my time at work.

A few of the types of cases that I have been exposed to include: cardiac arrests (too numerous to count); traumatic injuries (multiple organ injury, traumatic amputations, traumatic brain injuries, multiple casualties, gun-shot wounds, stabbings, motor vehicle collisions); deaths (due to medical or trauma causes, death of a child); responding as the paramedic to a person known to me; sieges; assaults; sexual assaults; child sexual assault; murders (including child murder); responding as a paramedic to the murder of a person known to me; suicides; fires and horrendous burns injuries; drownings; and births. (I have delivered two babies. It was nice to be part of a happy occasion; they were good jobs.)

I believe that I was continuously fatigued and sleep deprived for a period of 10 years. I was underweight, according to the body mass index scale. I was also suffering from post traumatic stress disorder for a significant part of that 10-year period. The job turned me into a different person.

I was sceptical, detached, intolerant and not able to maintain a long-term personal relationship with a partner. The person I really loved at that time said to me 'you are always out helping others and you are never here when I need you'. The relationship ended. I could not see the impact the job was having on me. I did not talk about my feelings with anyone. Counselling or emotional support was not readily available to paramedics and no one wanted it anyway as it was seen as weak. Moreover, mental health issues were entered onto your personnel file and no one wanted that recorded.

I learned an amazing thing about continuous exposure to traumatic incidents — it is cumulative and the images stay with you and remain locked away in your memory. Vivid details of jobs come back to you and you remember them with surprising accuracy, many years after the event. You also relive the sensory experience. The senses of vision, touch, sound and smell collide. When you have to not only see an event, but to also hear it, feel it and smell it, it becomes a 'sensory overload' situation. You also relive the experience of fear, which is associated with some jobs. This is the phenomenon that eventually wears you down.

Fortunately, I had acquired valuable knowledge during my university studies. I knew how to stay physically fit. I maintained a continuous exercise regime which included weight training, riding an exercise bike and some walking. On-call prevented me from exercising away from home and shift work prevented participation in team sports. Exercise was an individual activity in a confined space. The time away from work was spent predominately on my own. The sports psychology I had studied helped me stay focused and motivated. I believe that this was the only thing that saved me from physical injury at work. I never suffered a back or musculoskeletal injury due to the weight training. If I had, I am sure it would have impacted on all aspects of my health.

Good nutrition was important to me. When I got a chance to eat properly, the meals were always nutritious and well balanced. I ate lean meats, low GI carbohydrates and lots of fresh fruit and vegetables. I rarely ate take-away foods or 'junk' foods. The knowledge in diet and nutrition I had gained during my physical education degree was invaluable.

To maintain some degree of good mental health, I had to actively seek positive and rewarding experiences. For every one bad thing that I experienced, I actively sought 10 good experiences. I ardently looked for beauty and joy in all aspects of life. This was difficult to maintain at times.

Others were not as lucky — many of my colleagues suffered from depression, hypertension, hypercholesterolemia, gastrointestinal disorders, myocardial infarction, back injury, musculoskeletal injury and obesity or weight-related problems. In one 12-month period, four of my colleagues attempted suicide and three were successful. Many went through relationship break downs and divorce. Paramedics have twice the divorce rate as the average population.

Since becoming involved in paramedic education, I have developed a stream of subjects in the area of 'practitioner health'. Three subjects have been included into the curriculum of a university-based paramedic degree. The units of study focus on physical fitness and health, diet and nutrition and the mental health of the paramedic throughout the lifespan. I see this as the most positive thing to come from my experiences as a paramedic. I have had a chance to give back to the profession and if the knowledge imparted by these units of study improves or maintains the health of just one paramedic, then my experiences have all been worthwhile.

DENNIS: TAKING CARE

What does it mean to take care of yourself, especially when much of your professional life involves taking care of others? I am not referring to getting enough sleep, eating regular, nutritious meals or keeping fit, although these are key ingredients of a healthy lifestyle. Rather, I am referring to the care that it takes to ensure that your professional life has an enduring sense of purpose and meaning.

I would like to weave together several personal experiences into a story about taking care in professional life. The first has to do with my first experience of using crutches, after suffering a knee injury playing Canadian football.

The crutches feel like an external object, an instrument separate from my body. Normal, taken-for-granted daily activities such as showering, getting dressed, travelling to and from classes are now awkward, cumbersome and annoying. I eagerly and gratefully accept the assistance of others. My flatmate carries my books, and people go out of their way to hold doors open for me.

However, I am gradually 'incorporating' the crutches. That is, they are becoming an extension of me. I buy a backpack. I am becoming more mobile, and more independent. I rely less now on other people, and I'm even starting to resent unsolicited assistance.

I am approaching yet another closed door. I stop before it, just to the right of the handle. I use my left hand to grab the handle and swing the door open wide enough to get the left crutch and hip planted in the door before the door swings shut. I pivot on the left crutch and swing my right leg through the door. I'm in. No problem.

I recall gaining more confidence with the use of crutches and feeling quite pleased about my ability to manage my day-to-day affairs.

I didn't think much more of this incident until some years later. I was asked on relatively short notice to cover a colleague's exercise-to-music class, which I was happy to do. I had taught at this leisure centre once before, but I always found it refreshing to work with a different group of people in new surroundings.

As I strode past the reception desk I could see the swimming pool ahead of me and the exercise studio just beyond it. Walking past the pool I happened to notice out of the corner of my eye a woman in distress. On the stairs leading to the pool deck, there she was: hands clawing the handrail for dear life as her legs dragged limply behind her. I immediately ran to her aid, and as I reached down to support her, I was met with a gruff: 'Leave me alone; I can do this myself!' I backed off and watched as the woman literally dragged herself along the pool deck and into the pool, where she proceeded to swim like a champion.

I found out later that the woman was an avid swimmer, despite a car accident that left her without the use of her legs. She always left her wheelchair in the change room and crawled to and from the pool. This was part of her daily routine.

As teachers, instructors or therapists, we clearly have a duty of care to ensure the safety and wellbeing of students and clients. Sometimes, though, we might be unwittingly paternalistic. That is, in our zeal to help, we can sometimes take away a person's capacity for self-care. Looking back, I recall my self-satisfaction at becoming more adept with crutches, and now I could better understand the resentment the woman must have felt by having to deal with well-meaning people who try to help too much. If I had I known better, I would have left the woman in her capable hands. Since I didn't, I should have offered, rather than imposed my assistance, so as to give her a choice in the matter.

The next experience relates to teaching a beginning weight training class.

There is a group of four girls huddled together at the back, waiting for the class to begin. They are the only girls in the class of 20. There is the characteristic male banter and swagger, but the girls try to be as inconspicuous as possible.

I begin the class using a (male) anatomy chart to illustrate the major muscle groups and basic weight training exercises for each. Just as I begin talking about the bench press as a core exercise for the development of the pectorals, one female student exclaims: 'We can't do that exercise; we don't have those muscles!' I reassure her that girls do, indeed, have these muscles, and I promise to bring in a female version of the anatomy chart to prove it.

The first 'prac' session with the girls, who insisted on working together, involved learning to perform squats. This is an 'old school' weight training class; no sleek, shiny machines, just free weights and pulleys. One by one, each girl practiced the technique by using only the bar, but when the time came to progress, they were apprehensive about putting on additional weights. I try to encourage the girls by saying that they are yet to realise how strong they are.

The student who thought that girls lacked the muscles to do weight training, now stands in the squat rack facing the bar. She steps under the bar, aligns her feet and hips, adjusts her hand grip, and looks in the mirror. She hesitantly bends her knees to perform the first repetition, which is then followed by several clean repetitions and a final shaky, tortuous one. She drops the bar on to the rack pins, steps out, then jumps up and yells: 'I did it!'

This was met by excited cheers and hugs from the other girls. The boys turn to stare, bemused by all the commotion. The female student turns to me and says: 'I really didn't think I could do that — thanks!'

I recall from this incident a quiet sense of satisfaction. I put it down to not only witnessing the transformation of a previously apprehensive girl into one with an expanded sense of her capabilities and power, but, yes, that I had something to do with it. To use what is now a cliché, I felt that I had made a difference. It was then and there that I thought: it is a 'break-through' moment like this for a student that makes teaching worthwhile.

There have been other experiences such as these. A corporate client was defensive when I was too prescriptive with an employee fitness program proposal; but he responded favourably when I provided informative program options which gave him the responsibility to decide what's best for the organisation. The moment after handing me a research paper on authenticity and personal values, a student confessed that he was attending university only to satisfy his parent's desires, but now was quitting university in order to pursue his dream of being a stand-up comedian.

The idea of participant self-care has found its way into my teaching philosophy, which I communicate to students as follows:

> It is my educational philosophy that I cannot 'teach' you anything. We are entering into a learning relationship that will require engagement and collaboration. I seek to provide opportunities, resources and support; but I insist that, ultimately, the students are responsible for their learning.

I have recently become a head of school. With it has come a steep learning curve, especially in the area of financial management. Yet, another significant part of the position is staff performance and development. The challenge here is to provide opportunities and support so that researchers, teachers, and support staff maintain productive and fulfilling careers.

This I am attempting to do in part by promoting a shift from 'compliance' culture to a 'collegial' one, where discipline or program groups provide the peer support and leadership to self-manage research and teaching/learning against standards of best practice. Professional development may also mean supporting a staff member's ambition to pursue a higher degree, or encouraging those with the potential to 'step up' to a leadership position, or providing a new opportunity to rekindle a staff member's passion and commitment. It is still early days, but I find myself relying on the notions of 'self-care', of 'break-through' moments as a guide for my efforts.

The promotion of self-care and the facilitation of 'break-through' moments give me a sense of purpose and fulfilment in my work. I have to take care that I don't get swept up in the daily detail of management. I have to pay attention to it, for my sake as well as that of staff members. The extent to which I can achieve this becomes my measure of a healthy professional life.

CLOSING REMARKS

It is not really possible to conclude this chapter. Each of us is on a journey. Along the way, we have discovered, unearthed, and sometimes tripped over ways to take care of ourselves. In the process of being human we learn more about being practitioners, and in the process of being practitioners we learn more about being human. Our journeys continue.

DISCUSSION Questions

1 Regardless of your age and experience, you are a practitioner on a journey. How do you care for yourself in your work?

2 Consider some of the ways that caring for your clients might conflict with caring for yourself. For example, you are tired and need to sleep, but your client is only available for early morning appointments. How might you foresee and manage some of these conflicting needs?

3 It is not always possible for practitioners to foresee how they will need to care for themselves. What other checks and balances do you adopt in your work to identify when your existing self-care approaches are inadequate or need to be modified?

REFERENCES

American Psychiatric Association (2000) *Diagnostic and Statistical Manual of Mental Disorders* (4th ed, text revision). Washington, DC: American Psychiatric Association

Arnett FC, Edworthy SM, Bloch DA, et al (1988) The American Rheumatism Association 1987 revised criteria for the classification of rheumatoid arthritis. *Arthritis & Rheumatism*, 31:315–24

Gartlehner G, Hansen RA, Thieda P, et al (2007, January). *Comparative Effectiveness of Second-Generation Antidepressants in the Pharmacologic Treatment of Adult Depression.* Rockville, MD: Agency for Healthcare Research and Quality. AHRQ Publication No. 07-EHC007-EF

Lorig K, Holman H (1989) Long-term outcomes of an arthritis self-management study: Effects of reinforcement efforts. *Social Science and Medicine*, 29:221–4

Lorig K, Holman H (2003) Self-management education: history, definition, outcomes, and mechanisms. *Annals of Behavioral Medicine*, 26:1–7

Lorig K, Mazonson P, Holman H (1993) Evidence suggesting that health education for self-management in patients with chronic arthritis has sustained health benefits while reducing health care costs. *Arthritis & Rheumatism*, 36:439–46

Lorig K, Seleznick M, Lubek D, et al (1989) The beneficial outcomes of the arthritis self-management course are not adequately explained by behavior change. *Arthritis & Rheumatism*, 32:91–5

Chapter 11

Case studies in exercise for the management of weight

Gina Mendoza, Dan van der Westhuizen and Steve Selig

INTRODUCTION

Obesity, generally defined as an excessive accumulation of body fat in proportion to lean body mass, is a key health problem of our time. Overweight and obesity is a worldwide or global epidemic that affects all genders, races, ages and socioeconomic groups (World Health Organization [WHO] 1998; Ross & Janssen 2007). Obesity is strongly associated with affluence — waistlines increase somewhat proportionally to gross domestic product, and wealthy nations, well able to feed themselves and fund high quality healthcare systems, find themselves with new problems — the disease burdens of being overweight or obese. Overweight and obesity are growing problems in developing nations too, and are more common than infectious diseases and malnutrition (Brown et al 2006).

Obesity alone (excluding overweight) accounts for 2–7% of total direct healthcare costs in developed countries (WHO 1998). The annual cost of weight reduction treatment in the USA is estimated to exceed US$117 billion (Stein & Colditz 2004), which does not include the psychosocial costs of obesity (eg: depression, lowered self-esteem and eating disorders) (Robbins et al 2009). The total estimated, financial cost to Australia of overweight and obesity rose from $3.767 billion in 2005 to $8.283 billion in 2008 (Access Economics 2008).

Obesity is regarded as a leading risk factor for chronic health conditions and premature mortality, which negatively impacts quality of life

(QoL) (Ross & Janssen 2007). A constellation of comorbidities are associated with obesity, including type 2 diabetes, dyslipidaemia, hypertension, arthritis, gallbladder disease, kidney disease, liver malfunction, musculoskeletal disorders, sleep disturbances and increased risk of cancer, stroke and coronary heart disease (Brown et al 2006; Thompson et al 2010).

The Centers for Disease Control and Prevention ranks obesity as second to cigarette smoking as the second leading cause of preventable death in the USA, which may overtake cigarette smoking as the leading cause in the next 10 years (Ehrman et al 2009; WHO 1998; McArdle et al 2009). Non-smoking, overweight but not obese men and women aged between mid-thirties to mid-forties die 3 years earlier compared to their normal-weight peers (Peeters et al 2003; McArdle et al 2009). Obese people can expect a 7-year shorter lifespan than their normal weight counterparts (Peeters et al 2003; Ehrman et al 2009).

In contrast to the health penalties of overweight and obesity, weight loss by as little as 3% has shown beneficial improvements in chronic disease risk factors (Donnely et al 2009). A modest reduction of 10% in body fat within 4–6 months is associated with a reduction in visceral and abdominal fat of 35% and 25% and leads to several health-related benefits including decreases in fasting glucose, insulin, blood pressure, mortality, social–psychological complications, C-reactive protein, triglycerides, low density lipoprotein (LDL) and total cholesterol (Haslem et al 2006; Ehrman et al 2009; Ross & Janssen 2007). These benefits are sustained through regular physical activity and maintenance of healthy body weight (Thompson et al 2004; Donnely et al 2009).

Willmore et al (2008) estimated that the average person, older than 25 years of age, gains 0.45–0.90kg fat mass, and simultaneously loses 0.25kg of muscle mass and bone each year, due to physical inactivity. These changes equate to a net gain of 0.7–1.4kg fat mass per year, which will result in 20–40kg fat gain over 30 years (ie: by age 55). Being overweight may be a double-edged sword. Being overweight makes it more difficult to be active, and physical inactivity amplifies expected age-related fat mass gain (Brown et al 2006; Voorrips et al 1992).

Exercise is a powerful intervention for managing body weight and maintaining weight within a healthy range (recognising that being underweight has serious health implications too), but there are considerable challenges for practitioners working with clients in weight reduction, weight management, and lean body mass increase. In the following four case studies we raise some concerns, and prompt thought, but do not resolve all the problems neatly. Anyone who has ever struggled to control their weight will tell you that it is not so simple as 'do x, achieve y'. For example, a weight management program is successful if body weight is maintained long-term, which depends on consistent, self-monitored, exercise supported by emotional coping skills (Brown et al 2006). Weight maintenance (ie: prevention of further weight gain) seems to protect against an increase in chronic disease risk factors (Donnely et al 2009), therefore, obese and overweight clients are best encouraged to improve their fitness through regular physical activity, rather than focusing on weight loss as the primary endpoint.

Considering the increasing prevalence of obesity worldwide, and the importance of exercise in weight control, clinical exercise practitioners' interactions with overweight and obese clients can be expected to grow. This chapter includes four case studies of clients who wish to use exercise for weight control; three case studies of overweight or obese clients, and one case study of a rugby player struggling to gain muscle mass, while minimising body fat increase.

CASE STUDY 1: BODY SHAPE, POSTURE, AND BODY IMAGE

Subjective

Judy, a 38-year-old full-time mother is referred for evaluation because she is having difficulty losing weight. She leads a fairly active and busy lifestyle in caring for two children aged 4 and 7 years. Judy wants to have another baby, and due to experiencing difficulty falling pregnant, she has been advised by her general practitioner (GP) to lose weight. For the past 2 months Judy has consistently stuck to a healthy, calorie-controlled diet, and is becoming frustrated that she has not lost any weight. Judy suffers from intermittent lower back pain which she believes to be weight related. Several months ago she was diagnosed with endometriosis and polycystic ovary syndrome (PCOS). Most evenings she and her family take an evening walk with the dog which lasts approximately 30 minutes. Judy feels self-conscious and physically restricted by her large, apple-shaped belly, and says she hates this area of her body.

Objective

Postural examination reveals an anterior pelvic tilt with the appearance of an exaggerated lumbar lordosis, a forward head position placing stress on the upper cervical and thoracic regions of the spine, and slightly raised shoulders with the appearance of breathing high in the chest. Alignment of knees and ankles: no problems noted. Judy's stride is shortened due to restricted hip flexion. Normal stride length is about 70–82cm, with normal step length being between 35–41cm. Judy's step length was measured at only 20cm with stride length being approximately 40cm. Associated with this, Judy walks flatly on her feet with observable movement into plantar-flexion during push-off phase of gait; her gait appears as a 'shuffling' motion (Magee 2008). Slump test and straight leg raise are negative. Standing balance test reveals that Judy can balance for greater than 30 seconds on either leg independently. Judy's measurements are: height 165cm; weight 142kg; waist 130cm; hips 142cm; waist/hips ratio: 0.9; BMI 52.1; blood pressure 128/80mmHg. Lower body strength was measured using sit-to-stand test with a score of 9 seconds. Upper body strength was measured using biceps curls with dumbbell free-weights:

one repetition maximum (1RM) lift capacity is 10kg for both right and left arms. Judy's aerobic fitness, calculated using a predictive step test, was estimated as average for a female of her age at 32 ml.kg^{-1}.min^{-1}.

Assessment

The overall picture for Judy is of a woman who is in quite good health, relatively fit and active. The most outstanding problem was noted through observation of her posture and movement. Postural examination revealed Judy's pelvis to be in anterior pelvic tilt probably due to the excess weight on her abdomen. When asked if she understood how to engage her core postural muscles, Judy did not understood. Observation of Judy's functional movement indicated very little awareness about her core abdominal region. Judy expressed that she hated this area of her body. Functional movement analysis also revealed that she was somewhat disengaged from her core abdominal region; so much so, that her breathing appeared to be occurring as far away from her abdomen as possible.

Plan

Primarily, to assist Judy in developing an awareness and appreciation for her abdominal region. The approach will be focused on Judy understanding how to engage the core abdominals, and the positive health outcomes from this. Additionally, time will be spent learning to implement postural awareness to her daily activities through some techniques adapted from the Alexander Technique. Ultimately, the plan will be for Judy to be able to apply both core and postural techniques to any daily activity she undertakes. The proposed outcome from this plan will be for Judy to learn to move freely and with a new appreciation for her body as an integral and important part of her, rather than something that she particularly separately hates. By learning how to engage her core Judy will in an overall sense, be effortlessly drawing her abdomen back towards her spine, thus allowing it to return to neutral spine and away from lumbar lordosis. She will also be learning to use her breath deeply in a nourishing way, rather than 'chest-breathing' as she appears to have been doing. As Judy already leads a very busy lifestyle the approach will be more about maximising what she is already doing instead of adding to her full schedule. Firstly, by adding core exercise as a way of

going about her daily activities, Judy will be subtly increasing her metabolic cost, albeit minimally, but the benefits from this will assist her adaptation to movement efficiency. Some simple whole-body resistance type exercises will be given to Judy to practice on a daily basis. These will be designed to target the chest, waist and hips. They will be more concerned with bringing about changes in body composition than being specifically for weight loss. Her evening walks will take on additional fitness components. To encourage weight loss, there will now be a need to add eg walking at a speed so that Judy becomes breathless but can still talk. There has been no health indication that Judy cannot exercise to her maximum heart rate for short periods of time, however, the approach is intended to work towards gradually making this a goal. The main focus in the beginning will be for Judy to increase her perceptual motor skills awareness, which will assist her in learning to enjoy the way she feels about her entire body/self in human movement.

Outcomes

Judy embraced her exercise plan by religiously adhering to her 3-month program. Although weight loss was the primary reason for Judy being referred to an exercise physiologist, weight loss achieved was relatively minimal. The major change which occurred with Judy over this period was in her body composition. At the start of the program she had a waist measurement of 130cm and on completion of the 3-month program it was 121.5cm. Despite having a significant change in her body composition, Judy had only lost a total of 6kg in total body weight.

Discussion

There may have been a variety of reasons that will have contributed to Judy finding it difficult to shed unwanted kilos at a faster rate. This could have been in part due to the fact that Judy was already leading a fairly active lifestyle and following a healthy diet prior to the program. The exercise program which was added to her normal daily routine was not extreme by any means. Each day Judy practiced a short routine of whole-body exercises specifically designed to target the chest, waist and hips. Judy's daily walk became a workout in itself. This is where she learned to increase her heart rate by building on the intensity, speed and duration of this activity. This had always been a family activity, so when the walk became more of a workout, the rest of the family joined in making it fun for them all, and making it easier for Judy to stay motivated to exercise purposefully. Most importantly, the way in which Judy began to use her body brought about a most remarkable change in her movement carriage. It was this key factor which acted to empower her, because she grew to enjoy how she felt about herself, through exercise.

The abdominal region is the area of the body that houses the majority of metabolic and postural distress in overweight and obese people. Alongside obesity, there are often associated fertility issues in females, gastrointestinal problems, low back pain, PCOS, diabetes and other weight related metabolic disorders. During the initial stages Judy was learning how to engage her core abdominal musculature and how to integrate this with postural awareness. Judy remarked on how different she felt when practicing this activity. She also commented that she had 'never experienced this kind of feeling before'. Judy learned to breathe deeply, imagining that her breath was reaching as far down as her pubic bone. All the while she did this, her attention was on her core remaining engaged, thus her spine was being supported by her deep postural muscles. She felt the expansion of her ribcage as it moved in and out like a concertina. She allowed the tension to release from her hips and learned to comfortably maintain a neutral spine position. This was all a new experience for Judy.

After a month her back pain vanished, and realising the benefits from this, Judy enthusiastically applied this technique as often as she could remember throughout her regular daily activities. She had previously believed that to stand up straight the shoulders should be pulled back. Her new training had taught her that she should allow the shoulders to simply 'fall apart' effortlessly. In doing this, as she walked with chest open, Judy learned to enjoy the feeling of the breeze moving under her chin and onto her lengthened neck. When she increased the intensity of her walking, the goal was for her not to lose the feeling of core engagement and postural lengthening achieved through relaxation.

The key message from this case study is that there are many women like Judy who have difficulty losing weight due to a variety of factors, medical and/or lifestyle related. These women simply do not feel good about the way they look and they will often feel self-conscious about their body shape. Media advertising everywhere promotes the hyper-sexualised, perfect-figured young female wearing skin-hugging skimpy clothing. Overweight and obese women do not fit the above model. It can be difficult to feel good about the way you look in a culture that promotes an image of women which is in stark contrast to what you actually look like. In turn, movement and exercise can become a very self-conscious making activity for the overweight/obese. If one does not feel good about the way they look, or how it feels to move, then why would they feel inspired to exercise?

It could therefore be very short-sighted for a practitioner to believe that the only focus for an overweight client should be weight loss. For a clinical exercise practitioner to merely prescribe a strict exercise routine for their obese client, along with explanation about, for example, the benefits of increasing muscle mass for weight loss, could be equally lacking insight. It is not that this method will not work, but the feeling of punishment that may be associated with it, is unnecessary. The main issue for an overweight woman such as Judy is for her to learn how to feel good about herself through exercise by increasing her awareness about the way in which she uses her body. A positive outcome of this case study was that Judy proved to herself that she could actually lose weight. The more significant outcome was her change in body composition, and how this altered the way she felt about the way she looked. With some simple, yet quite specific instructions, Judy was able to increase her perceptual motor skills in movement through a heightened sense of body awareness.

What followed next was the easy part. Caring for the client is about caring for the whole individual. Caring for an overweight or obese woman will always contain emotional and self-confidence issues. An obese woman is not just a body, and designing her exercise program involves focusing her mind, training her body and lifting her spirits. The final message from this case study is that the body is the easy part. Once Judy had learned to enjoy how she felt about herself, through exercise, she wanted to do it, so the main battle was over.

Summary of key lessons

- Weight loss and obesity often involve matters of emotion and self-confidence.
- An exercise program can be holistic, encompassing focusing the mind, training the body, and lifting the spirits.
- An understanding about core control, postural awareness and breathing should be used in tandem with an exercise routine and applied to regular daily activities so that this becomes a way of being.
- Exercise for empowerment: guide the client toward growing to enjoy the positive way in which they can learn to feel about themselves, through exercise.

DISCUSSION Questions

1 Your client doesn't want a 'warm and fuzzy' style practitioner. She wants to get on with it and get straight down to the business of losing weight as fast as possible. Describe your approach to working with this client. Would you adopt the same approach as the clinical exercise practitioner who worked with Judy?

2 Your client doesn't believe in core exercise. She has been told by another practitioner that core exercises are 'a complete waste of time because if you are exercising you will be using your core anyway'. How would you respond to this assertion?

3 A fellow practitioner criticises your method. He claims that your client must perform at least three intensive 30–40 minute resistance training workouts per week, plus at least 30–60 minutes walking each day to be on an effective weight-loss exercise program. Your colleague says that any less than this and you are not doing your client justice. How would you respond to this assertion?

4 If clients do not feel good about the way they look, or how it feels to move, what might happen to their motivation to exercise?

CASE STUDY 2: A SPORT WHERE 'SIZE MATTERS'

Subjective

CJ, a 22-year-old university student and keen rugby union player, had unsuccessfully been trying to gain some muscle mass over the last 2 years in an attempt to improve his rugby performance and reduce risk of injuries. He had started several exercise routines during this time, but never continued the program for an extended period of time. He had been told by a friend that in order to gain muscle mass he needs to begin a resistance training program and ensure that he is in a positive energy balance (ie: consuming more calories than he is expending). Given this advice, CJ decided that his lack of results in the past may have been as a result of an insufficient energy intake and ineffective resistance training program.

At the start of December 2007, prior to commencement of the 2008 rugby season, CJ made a commitment to himself that he was going to persist with a resistance training program and make an effort to eat more. Upon discussion with his friend, CJ informed him that he is really busy with his university studies during the academic year, and doesn't really have the time to perform more than two resistance training sessions per week. His friend fully understood CJ's position, and was in fact an advocate of infrequent resistance training sessions (training each body part once per week) so as to avoid over-training. The friend provided CJ with a 2-day per week resistance training program, and recommended that he train his entire upper body in the first session of the week, and his lower body in the second session. In addition, the friend had CJ performing a total of only five sets per muscle group per week by doing only 'muscle isolation' exercises such as pec deck for chest and knee extensions for quadriceps. He explained to CJ that performing muscle isolation exercises such as pec deck and knee extensions are superior to compound movements like the bench press and squat, since he will get a better 'pump' and really feel his muscles become engorged with blood, particularly if he works within the 10–20 repetition range. Furthermore, he recommended that CJ avoid all forms of aerobic training while trying to gain muscle mass since there is some evidence that it may interfere with the recovery process and prevent the hypertrophy of fast twitch muscle fibres. CJ's friend then designed him a dietary plan which would hopefully assist him in gaining some lean body mass, and told CJ to weigh himself nude after using the toilet every Monday morning. Prior to commencement of CJ's new resistance training program, his friend also took CJ's girth measurements (upper arm, mid thigh, chest, and waist circumference); numerical values which he claimed would enable CJ to monitor his progress on a weekly basis. CJ reported that his waist was 90cm at initial testing.

Two weeks down the track, CJ is confused since he has gained 2.5kg, but his upper arm, chest, and mid thigh girth measurements remained unchanged. However, his waist circumference had expanded out to 94cm, an increase of 4cm. He is bitterly disappointed that his girth measurements have not increased despite complete commitment to the training and eating plans prepared for him by his friend. He consults his friend on the issue, and expresses concern that he believes his

weight gain to present has been entirely fat. After asking CJ a few questions regarding his training and dietary habits, it is of the friend's opinion that CJ's disappointing results thus far are as a result of an insufficient energy intake and being over-trained. The friend is particularly concerned that CJ has been taking all sets of all exercises to failure (the point at which the load can no longer be moved despite trying as hard as possible), blaming this strategy as the number one reason for being over-trained. Instead, he suggests that CJ stop all sets 2–3 repetitions short of failure as to ensure that he does not enter an over-trained state. Furthermore, he suggests that CJ further increase his energy intake by eating even more throughout the day.

Given this advice, CJ commits himself to avoid training to failure, but states that he simply can't eat anymore since he is already force feeding himself and literally feels sick after some meals because he is so full. He also questions the friend's advice to further increase his caloric intake since he has gained 4cm around his waist in 2 weeks, and really doesn't want his waist to expand any further. In response to this question, the friend claims that the increased waist circumference is normal while on a higher caloric intake, and is simply intestinal bulk from the larger food intake, rather than deposition of fat. He advises CJ that the easiest way for him to increase his energy intake will be to incorporate additional high energy liquids throughout the day since they don't bloat you as much. He recommends that CJ consume an additional 600ml of sports drink, and 500–600ml of flavoured milk throughout the day, stating that this will provide him with an additional 360kcal per day. He also informs CJ that adding the sports drink and flavoured milk to his daily diet will prove beneficial since they are predominantly simple carbohydrates, which have a profound stimulatory effect on the release of the body's most anabolic hormone, insulin. The friend explains to CJ that insulin aids muscle growth by facilitating the uptake of carbohydrates and amino acids into the muscle cell. Given this advice from his friend, CJ once again feels more optimistic at achieving his goal of an increase in lean body mass.

CJ continued his new modified resistance training program and diet for another 3 weeks before he eventually lost motivation as a result of lacklustre results. By now, after 5 weeks of training and following the higher calorie diet he hadn't made any noticeable gains in his muscle girth measurements. However, despite the lack of any noticeable muscle size gains, he has gained a total of 6kg in body weight, and now weighed 97kg. Although he achieved his goal of increasing his body weight, he believes that the vast majority of the additional mass was fat, and was particularly concerned that his waist circumference had increased to 98cm, an increase of 8cm in 5 weeks. Given these disappointing results, CJ speculated that his training program may in fact be ineffective, and opts to seek a second opinion. CJ has just started a Bachelor of Science degree at one of the local tertiary institutions, and from what he has learned thus far he believes that the training principles he has been following may be flawed. He decides to seek the opinion of one of his lecturers whom is a clinical exercise practitioner.

Objective

Upon discussion with the clinical exercise practitioner, CJ learns that several of the training principles which his friend promotes and that he has been following are completely illogical. CJ asks the clinical exercise practitioner to design him a new resistance training program. The exercise practitioner assists CJ, and also recommends that he should consult a dietitian regarding a suitable and effective dietary plan. The clinical exercise practitioner, who is also a trained anthropometrist, conducted some measurements on CJ. He is 186cm tall and weighs 97kg, with a BMI of 28. In addition, based on the sum of seven skin-fold measurements, CJ's body fat percentage is 16%. He also confirms that CJ's waist circumference (around the belly button) is in fact 98cm, which according to CJ is an increase of 8cm in 5 weeks.

During his initial consultation with the dietitian, CJ gives her a quick briefing on his dietary history, as well as the undesirable fat he has gained over the last 5 weeks. He informs her that he would like to gain some lean body mass, but first wants to get rid of the excess fat that he has gained. The dietitian then informs CJ that in order to achieve both of those goals they will have to determine the proper energy intake for him given his goals. She believes that the most accurate method of doing this will be for him to complete a-3 day diet record in which he uses

an electronic food scale to weigh and record all the foods and beverages which he consumes over a 72 hour period. In addition, over the course of the 3 days she expects that CJ weigh himself nude every morning prior to breakfast and after voiding. CJ returns to the dietitian later on in the week with all the information which she expected from him, anxiously awaiting feedback from her. Based on the information provided, the dietitian estimates that CJ is currently consuming about 3000 calories per day, and is in energy balance since his weight only changed by 0.1kg over the course of the 3 days. Given this information, the dietitian then designs a dietary plan for CJ to follow which should assist him in achieving both goals.

Assessment

CJ's BMI of 28 classifies him as being overweight in relation to his height.

Plan

The dietitian knows that research has indicated that an additional 2800–3500 calories per week above maintenance intake should theoretically result in a lean mass gain of 454g (nearly 0.5kg) per week. Conversely, 2800–3500 calories per week below maintenance intake should assist a fat loss of 0.454g per week (in conjunction with an appropriate exercise program). Therefore, the dietitian advises CJ that if he were able to decrease his caloric intake by 500–700 calories per day, along with an appropriate exercise program, then he may well be able to lose 3–4kg of body fat in 6–8 weeks time. Once he has lost the excess fat, he would have to increase calories by 500–700 per day along with an appropriate resistance training program to encourage a lean body mass gain over a period of several weeks or months. Provided with this knowledge, the dietitian firstly devises a dietary plan to encourage fat loss. The dietary plan includes a few daily sample meal plans for CJ to follow, each of which provides roughly 2200 calories per day (800 calories below CJ's estimated daily maintenance intake). In addition, each of the daily sample meal plans provides roughly 190g of protein per day from complete protein sources (2g per kg), and focuses on complex carbohydrates rather than simple carbohydrates as the main carbohydrate source. The dietitian suggests that CJ should spread his meals over the day to combat low blood glucose levels, that is he should not stay longer than 3 hours without having something to eat. He may have three meals and two snacks (eg: one snack 3 hours after breakfast and 3 hours after lunch). The dietitian also encourages CJ to eat plenty of fruits and vegetables, as well as making an effort to increase his dietary fibre intake. The dietitian tells CJ to visit her again once he has lost the excess fat, so that she can design a lean mass gain dietary plan for him to follow. This diet will provide roughly 3800 calories per day (800 calories above maintenance energy intake), and have a strong emphasis on ensuring that he consumes sufficient protein (2g per kg), as well as complex carbohydrates.

The clinical exercise practitioner plays an important role in enabling CJ to reach both of his goals. Firstly, he designs a program which successfully assists CJ in losing 4kg (he now weighs 93kg) in 8 weeks time, while following the dietitian's dietary recommendations. After taking skin-fold measurements, it is confirmed that CJ has decreased his fat percentage by 2.3%, and now possesses a fat percentage of 13.7%. The clinical exercise practitioner mentioned to CJ, that as a rugby backline player who has to be quick, he should not carry excessive body weight (eg: >12% fat) as he needs to move his total body mass swiftly and horizontally through space on the rugby field and an additional load might impair his performance. Thus it seems that CJ's fat percentage is slightly too high. Following this 8-week fat-loss plan, the clinical exercise practitioner designs CJ a new exercise plan aimed at increasing lean body mass. After following this routine, along with the lean mass gain dietary plan, CJ increases his weight to 100kg in 11 weeks time, a weight gain of 7kg. After taking skin-fold measurements, it is determined that CJ's fat percentage only increased by 0.5% (CJ's fat percentage is now 14.2%), thereby proving that the vast majority of his weight gain is in fact lean body mass. Generally, CJ is delighted about the results he has achieved over the last few months, and now realises that there is no reason why anyone shouldn't be able to gain some lean body mass provided they follow an effective exercise and dietary plan. Though he has not achieved the 12% body fat as suggested by the exercise physiologist he realises that he needs to adhere to his exercise and nutrition plan in order to get closer to his goal of 12% body fat.

Discussion

BMI may not always give one an accurate indication of whether an individual is overweight or not, particularly in the case of relatively short muscular people as it is not distinguishing between bone, muscle and fat. The large increase in waist circumference (and most likely associated fat) experienced by CJ while following his friend's exercise program and higher calorie diet may well be as a result of excess calories. Reported ranges of relative body fat values for male rugby players are between 6–16% (Wilmore et al 2008).

Although a positive energy balance is necessary to assist a lean body mass gain, an excess surplus will result in unnecessary body fat increases. The friend made no attempt to determine the proper energy intake for CJ to follow before designing a higher calorie diet. This may well have lead to CJ consuming more calories than actually required to build lean body mass. Furthermore, the fact that CJ obtained a relatively large percentage of his total energy intake from simple carbohydrates (from the sports drinks and flavoured milk) may have compounded the problem. Simple carbohydrates digest very quickly, causing a rapid increase in blood sugar levels, thereby stimulating the release of insulin. Insulin then helps to lower blood glucose levels by facilitating the uptake of blood glucose and other nutrients into muscle and fat cells. Therefore, although insulin may assist muscle mass gains, this hormone may also encourage the deposition of additional body fat. In order to maximise the muscle building benefits of insulin, most simple carbohydrates should be consumed within 30–60 minutes after a resistance training session. At this time, the body will hesitate to store the excess blood glucose as fat since the muscle cells are greatly fatigued and in search of nutrients, consequently resulting in the vast majority of excess blood glucose being stored and used by muscle cells for anabolic purposes. Hence, the dietitian recommends that CJ focus predominantly on complex carbohydrates. In addition, the training program designed for CJ by his friend appeared to lack intensity and included no aerobic training, thereby also possibly contributing to CJ's fat gain during this time.

Summary of key lessons

- Before designing a diet aimed at increasing lean body mass, the proper energy intake for that individual should be determined in order to minimise the likelihood of excess fat gains as a result of excess calories.

- Complex carbohydrates are the preferred form of carbohydrates. Medium and low GI foods should make up 60–65% of the total energy intake as intense training depletes glycogen stores. However, simple carbohydrates may actually assist lean body mass gains and speed up recovery if consumed within 30–60 minutes after a strenuous training session.

- Athletes who participate in sports requiring high levels of aerobic conditioning are ill-advised to completely avoid aerobic training in the fear that it may compromise their muscle building ability. The benefits of aerobic training far outweigh the slightly negative impact on muscle hypertrophy.

- Lean body mass gains should be slow, ideally no more than 1kg per week as to minimise the likelihood of an unwanted excess increase in fat mass.

- Although monitoring waist circumference can give one an indication of changes in fat percentage, caution should be taken when using this as the sole source of information to determine body composition changes. An increase in waist circumference is normal while following higher calorie diets due to increased intestinal bulk. For this reason, other measurements, such as skin-folds, should be used.

- An additional 700–1000kcal (2900–4200 KJ) per day is required for gains of 0.05–1.0kg muscle mass per week.

DISCUSSION Questions

1 Why do you think CJ was initially unsuccessful in achieving his weight management goals after following his friend's advice?

2 Considering the initial diet and exercise plan CJ followed resulted in a fat mass gain, how would you suggest that CJ's friend alter the advice he offers his peers if they wish to increase muscle mass and reduce fat mass?

3 Many clients have well-meaning but misinformed friends. How might you counter the flawed advice they receive?

CASE STUDY 3: MIDDLE-AGE SPREAD

Subjective

BK, a 34-year-old businessman, is referred by his GP to a clinical exercise practitioner because he struggles to take control of his 'creeping obesity' and his health in general. His doctor is concerned that his obesity may contribute to comorbidities (eg: diabetes, heart disease, stroke, hypertension, kidney disease, cancer). BK is also concerned that he may also succumb to heart disease at a relatively young age, just like his biological mother who passed away due to sudden death at the age of 56 years. His father was diagnosed with lung cancer at the age of 58 years. BK has no siblings.

Apart from playing one nine-hole round of golf fortnightly, using a golf cart, BK leads a sedentary lifestyle. He states that he struggles to complete a brisk, continuous walk of 20 minutes without taking a brief rest. However, he has experienced no previous history of chest pain or dyspnea during physical exertion. BK consumes three beers daily after work, while watching his favourite TV programs for 5 hours before bed time. His dietary habits consist of at least five fast food meals per week and he ingests fish, fruit, salads and vegetables no more than once per week. He mentions that long hours at work (10–12 hours daily) makes it difficult for the family to do proper cooking. BK also revealed that he has experienced repeated cycles of weight loss–weight regain throughout his life with little long-term success at keeping the weight off. BK mentioned that his mates frequently teased him about his weight issues during his childhood and that he did not enjoy sport participation and exercise as he was not very good at it. Due to this he struggled to make friends, was very lonely and admits that he has a lack of self-confidence. He also believes that these circumstances contributed to his depression and that eating helps to comfort him, offers him security and companionship.

He quit smoking (20 cigarettes per day) 7 months ago. His spouse indicated that she would like him to start a regular exercise program. His GP prescribed some medications (Xenical and Reductal) to assist with his treatment.

Objective

The report from his GP indicates that BK's fasting serum glucose, total cholesterol, high-density cholesterol, low-density cholesterol and triglycerides are respectively 5.9, 5.8 (223.9 mg/dl), 0.83 (32.05mg/dl), 3.31 (128 mg/dl) and 1.45 (128 mg/dl) mmol.L^{-1}.

During the first consultation with BK a pre-participation health screening was administered, that included the following categories: medical history; risk factor assessment and stratification; prescription medication use; current physical activity level; and establishing whether physician consent is necessary. A physical activity readiness questionnaire (PAR-Q) and a health status questionnaire were also included. This information provided more clarity about any obesity-related comorbidities of BK. Due to his moderate obesity BK was asked if he has a history of diabetes, thyroid dysfunction or impaired blood glucose. BK was also asked if his parents, siblings, aunts or uncles have been overweight or obese to deduce if genetics may have contributed to his obesity. BK's response to both questions was negative.

Consequently there seems to be no propensity toward genetic obesity in BK's case.

BK's posture shows an android body type. His body composition measurements were: height 174cm; body weight 107kg; BMI 35.4kg.m^{-2} and waist circumference 118cm. His blood pressure during rest is 128/84mmHg and 218/110mmHg during activity at 85% of his heart rate reserve. An aerobic fitness level of 28 ml.kg.min^{-1} was determined by means of a sub-maximal YMCA cycle ergometer test. A 3-day dietary record of BK indicated that he consumes approximately 3750 kcal/day. His dietary fat intake accounts for 38% of total energy intake and 65% of his carbohydrate intake is refined sugar.

The second consultation with BK focused on: goal setting; beliefs; behaviour modification; exercise-specific self-efficacy measures; benefits and barriers to exercise (eg: time management and past experiences to exercise); and eating habits (reflected in 3-day dietary record).

Discussion

Orlistat (Xenical) as a gastrointestinal lipase inhibitor which decreases about one-third of fat absorption in the small intestine and Reductal that helps to promote satiety and decreases appetite is part of BK's prescribed medication from his physician. Fortunately BK does not have any comorbidities, which allows him to engage in a safe exercise program. However, obesity-related comorbidities can become a severe risk for people with a BMI ≥ 35. BK's BMI of 35.4kg.m^{-2} is moderately obese (class II) and many of his measurements are close to abnormal, which can potentially contribute to comorbidities in the near future, if he is not taking control of it. Unfortunately BK has a family history of heart disease and his mother succumbed to sudden death before 65 years of age. Family history is an important non-modifiable risk factor for heart disease.

According to the transtheoretical model (Robbins et al 2009), BK is in the preparation phase as he is doing some exercise (golf), though realises that it is insufficient and he needs some assistance to resolve his exercise barriers and with designing his personalised program. Fortunately his spouse is very supportive of his intention to engage in exercise. This social support for exercise from his spouse should have a positive influence on

BK's exercise participation. His chronic tiredness may be related to poor eating habits and poor fitness. BK's indirect VO_{2max} of 28ml.kg.min^{-1} is below the 20th percentile for his age and gender, which is indicative of his sedentary lifestyle (and is associated with an increased risk of death from all causes).

Exercise for BK should be enjoyable to ensure adherence as he states that he does not enjoy exercise much, though he is prepared to give it a go. BK has a low level of exercise self-efficacy (ie: task-specific self-confidence). BK's past experience with sports and physical activity, most likely due to his weight issues and lack of skills, contributed to his lack of confidence and not enjoying participation in physical activities.

The 3-day dietary record reveals that BK's total daily caloric intake is too high considering his sedentary lifestyle, with a disproportionate amount of total energy intake coming from fat and refined sugars. It appears that a large part of his poor eating habits are probably linked to emotional eating, including depression and lack of confidence that trigger eating for comfort.

Ongoing plan

It is important to identify the factors that cause BK to deposit excess body fat and try to control those contributors. BK is willing and able to safely participate in a regular exercise program, as it seems that he does not possess any comorbidities.

The overall aim is to promote physiologic changes which could reduce potential risk of disease and improve BK's health status. BK is discouraged to exercise and diet for the sole purpose of trying to achieve some predetermined weight. Improved health and QoL should be the focus of treatment. BK is encouraged to initially follow the 'health at every size' (HAES) paradigm for the first 2 weeks of his intervention (Brown et al 2006). This will provide him with some opportunity to gradually start introducing regular physical activity as part of his busy daily routine. This approach implies that the overweight and/or obese person wants to eat healthy food and be active and that once diet restrictions and barriers to activity have been removed, the individual will develop healthier eating and activity patterns that lead to a genetically determined healthy body weight. In this respect adherence, consistency and enjoyment, rather than mode or intensity

of exercise, are the goals of exercise for weight control.

Consequently, BK trained the first 2 weeks only three times per week to allow his body to adapt to exercise and to avoid musculoskeletal injuries, before the frequency was upgraded to five times per week. BK decided to reduce his daily television watching during the week by 2 hours and replace it with exercise time. Four key factors — motivation, self-responsibility, self-motivation and expectation — are important for successful intervention. BK shows self-responsibility by his willingness to exercise, which will make it easier to accomplish his exercise goals. Goals that are specific, measurable, achievable, realistic, sustainable, self-determined and time-oriented should be followed. For example, a modest reduction in caloric intake of 400kcal/day (two beers contain 218 kcal and two slices buttered bread contain 200kcal) and an increase in physical activity of 300kcal/day (eg: 4–5km brisk walk) should result in a deficit of 3500kcal or 0.45kg loss in adipose tissue per week.

BK's medium-term goal is to shed 11kg over 4–6 months, which will calculate to a body weight of 96kg and a BMI of 31.7kg.m^{-2}. This implies a 10% weight loss which is associated with several health-related benefits. BK's long-term goal is to shed 22kg over 12 months. This will result in a body weight of 85kg and a BMI of 28.1kg.m^{-2} (overweight, but not obese). This weight reduction should also reduce his waist girth and decrease his risk of comorbidities.

The fact that BK is self-motivated and willing to alter his current, unhealthy lifestyle by adopting more healthy eating habits and regular physical activity as part of his lifestyle can assist in contributing to a higher QoL. The last mentioned reason should motivate him to adhere to his exercise intervention. However, BK has to be educated that success with body fat loss does not occur overnight and a healthy, sensible approach should be followed. For example, if fat loss does not always meet a client's expectations, one can become discouraged and quit the intervention. A decreased rate of fat loss (plateaus) may have a similar effect. Verbal encouragement and the teaching of positive self-talk can play an important role in this regard.

BK decided to choose walking as his exercise mode to improve his aerobic fitness, as increased walking fitness will also enhance his personal golf performance. Due to BK's low fitness level, he can begin with five walking sessions per week (frequency) of 15 minutes (duration) brisk walking per day. A gradual, progressive increase of 5 minutes walking duration per session can be added each following week. This could result in 60 minutes of walking by week 9; if BK's body adapted well to the walking and no injuries restricted his performance. The intensity is set at 50–80% of his heart rate reserve or a reported perceived exertion (RPE) reading of 12–4 on the Borg 6–20 scale (or 5–7 on the Omni 1–10 scale). Because heart rate is influenced by air temperature, medication, caffeine and psychological stress, the RPE scale method is preferred over percentage of heart rate reserve. Also, one does not want BK to become a 'pulse counter' who gets little pleasure from exercising. A critical factor in exercise for weight control is high-energy expenditure, thus, BK should try to burn 300–500kcal/day or 1000–2000kcal/week. Due to the fact that BK's aerobic fitness level is low, he should start at 1000kcal/week at an RPE reading of 12 on the Borg scale. Because heat dissipation is a problem in obese clients, BK is advised to walk during cool times of the day and he should drink at least one glass of water within the 30 minutes preceding each training session and approximately one glass of water for every 20 minutes of aerobic exercise.

In addition to the abovementioned walking sessions, two resistance training sessions per week of 30 minutes each, covering the major muscle groups by means of two sets of 10–15 repetitions per exercise, is incorporated. The intensity during resistance training should be at an RPE between 11–15 on the Borg 6–20 scale (or 4–7 on the Omni 1–10 scale). The rest period is 60–90 seconds between exercises. Emphasise correct technique and breathing during execution (ie: exhale during exertion and inhale during relaxation) to avoid the Valsalva manoeuvre and unnecessary strain on the blood pressure during activity. BK also commits to include lifestyle-based activities (eg: taking the stairs at work and a 20 minute walk during lunchtime each working day) that could further assist in burning calories. BK is encouraged to gradually increase total daily exercise (over and above that required during 'normal' living) to at least 75 minutes to effectively counteract further adiposity. Because high exercise-specific self-efficacy is associated with increased exercise participation, BK is verbally praised when he reported on successful execution of his exercise guidelines. He is also informed that there is no need to follow a vigorous intense exercise program to become an elite athlete and therefore he does not need to compare himself with athletes' performances. It is more important for him to adhere to the exercise in order to progress from the preparation stage to the action and eventually the maintenance stage in the transtheoretical model (Robbins et al 2009).

BK's high self-motivation should help him with his goal setting and he may need less external encouragement to adopt and adhere to his intervention. BK committed himself to a contract stating the following goals (during the upcoming 12 months): to drink only one, opposed to three, beers each evening; to gradually increase fibre intake to 38g per day by ingesting an average of two fruits, legumes and five vegetable servings daily; replacing all refined foods with wholegrain products (eg: brown rice, wholegrain pasta, cereals and bread); to eat no more than one fast food meal per week; and to execute two resistance and five aerobic training sessions during weekdays. BK's self-selected reward on achievement of his goal weight (85kg) is an overseas holiday for the family (extrinsic reward).

Outcomes

Eventually, BK achieved his medium-term goal of 96kg at the end of 14 weeks, 2 weeks earlier than anticipated. Unfortunately he sustained acute plantar fasciitis and on his GP's recommendation, decided not to proceed with his brisk walking as it aggravated his injury. BK was very frustrated and he did not discuss any alternative plan with the clinical exercise practitioner. At the time BK contacted the practitioner, BK had not exercised at all for 2 weeks, which resulted in an increase of 3kg weight during this time.

Summary of key lessons

- Self-responsibility to exercise, including willingness to commit to, and engage in, regular exercise training (because it is regarded as a high priority), is of paramount importance to reach the maintenance phase in the transtheoretical model.

- To achieve a healthy body weight, a healthy diet and regular exercise (sometimes accompanied by drug therapy) combined are more effective than dietary change or exercise training alone.

- The 'health at every size' (HAES) paradigm that incorporates adherence, consistency and enjoyment, rather than focussing on mode or intensity of exercise, may be helpful to motivate overweight or obese people to engage in physical activity.

- The RPE scale is very somewhat under-utilised in clinical exercise practice. Clients tend to enjoy exercise more when using this approach rather than pulse counting to reach a target heart rate.

- Regular exercise training that targets individual capacity is more important than trying to compete and compare oneself to high levels of performance of elite athletes.

DISCUSSION Questions

1 What alternative plans and recommendations would you (as clinical exercise practitioner) suggest to help BK accomplish his long-term weight-loss maintenance of 85kg?

2 Using the American College of Sports Medicine's risk stratification levels as your guide, do you consider that BK has a low, moderate, or high risk of adverse events during exercise? Refer to Chapters 3 and 6 for detail of the theoretical basis for exercise use in clients with cardiac and metabolic conditions.

3 Why is resistance training an important part of the recommended exercise regimen for BK?

CASE STUDY 4: WEIGHT GAIN AS A MARKER OF OTHER MATTERS

Subjective

SL is a 41-year-old female allied health assistant who works in a nursing home. Her job includes attending to the washing, feeding and toilet needs of dementia clients, as well as making beds, tidying rooms and general duties. Some of her work involves lifting clients or moving furniture. She always asks for help when performing these roles. She spends about 60% of her time doing office work (reception duties, phone calls, computer work). Overall she describes the physical intensity of her job as mainly light with occasional moderate levels of exertion, but her shift of 8 hours leaves her feeling very tired at the end of each day. She is involved in the social program in the nursing home too, organising social outings and in-house concerts and games. She loves her job and sees her role as helping her clients to live out the last years of their lives in happiness. But during the past 4 years SL has suffered the breakdown of the relationship with her partner of 14 years, and her mother, whom she was very close to, developed an aggressive form of breast cancer and died within 12 months of diagnosis.

During this 4-year period of stress, her weight ballooned from 57kg to 75kg. Six months ago, she decided that she would no longer eat breakfast, lunch or snacks and just eat one meal per day to try to get her weight under control. She finishes work at 6 p.m., and then often shops on the way home for food to cook for the evening meal. When she gets home, she has a glass of wine while watching TV or reading, and then she cooks for herself, cleans up and goes to bed exhausted but can not get to sleep easily. She often wakes at about 2 a.m. and can't get back to sleep until about 5 a.m.

Her GP arranged for a referral to a clinical exercise practitioner for advice on exercise and lifestyle. She told the exercise practitioner that she is rarely hungry during the day even though she is not eating, and then eats a large meal quickly at night and frequently retires to bed feeling full. She has recently been feeling cold, even when the weather is warm. During this most recent 6 months, her weight has increased by a further 8kg to 83kg and she is now extremely distressed and anxious about her weight, appearance and health. She has not enrolled in a weight loss program and is not planning to see a dietitian at this stage as she prefers to try an exercise approach for weight loss.

Objective

The clinical exercise practitioner has taken responsibility to work with SL and her GP to try to get her lifestyle, fitness and health back in order. The clinical exercise practitioner estimates that SL expends an average of 800kcal per day at work. This is about double that of an office worker and is clearly not responsible for her recent weight gain. However, apart from this occupational exercise, SL engages in almost no other exercise or physical activity.

During the past 18 months, she has been diagnosed with hypertension (155/105mmHg, treated with Atenolol), hyperlipidemia (total cholesterol of 6.6 mmol.l^{-1} and chol:HDL of 5.5, treated with Lipitor), depression (treated with Zoloft), and recently recorded a fasting blood glucose of 7.4 mmol.l^{-1}. This is being followed up with an oral glucose tolerance test (OGTT). SL is an ex-smoker with a 15 pack/year history of smoking; she finally quit after 33 years of smoking.

Pre-exercise physical examination

Height 160cm; weight 83kg; BMI 32.4; waist 94cm; hips 109cm; waist-hip ratio 0.86; blood pressure 138/88mmHg; resting heart rate 88bpm in rhythm.

Incremental exercise test

A symptom-limited incremental exercise test for the assessment of aerobic power (VO_{2peak}) was conducted using a STEP test (see Table 11.1). The STEP height was determined as 0.125 of SL's height and the STEP speed commenced at 12 ascents per minute and increased at a rate of 2 ascents per minute. A 12-lead ECG was used to monitor heart rate and rhythm and signs of ischaemia continuously, oxygen saturation in the blood ($HbO_2sat\%$) was monitored by pulse oximetry, blood pressure was recorded at 2 minute intervals, and 6–20 point scales were used to monitor self-perceived ratings of breathlessness and exertion (Borg 6–20 point scale). The criteria for stopping exercise tests are breathlessness, fatigue (failure to maintain the required stepping speed) or tests are stopped earlier in the event of adverse signs or symptoms.

The test was terminated at 8 minutes of exercise and the reason for stopping was severe breathlessness (18/20) associated with mild arterial desaturation. SL had not exercised at this intensity for some years, and her breathlessness was unexpected. VO_{2peak} was estimated to be 24.6 ml.kg^{-1}.min^{-1}, which needs improvement compared to SL's age peers. Her blood pressure, heart rate and heart rhythm responses to the STEP test were normal, and there was no electrocardiographic evidence of myocardial ischaemia.

Lung function testing

Following the discovery of severe breathlessness and mild desaturation in the STEP test, it was decided to test lung function at rest and during a subsequent exercise test on a different day (see Table 11.2).

Functional tests

A 6-minute walk test (6MWT) was conducted on a different day, and SL completed 440 metres without the level of breathlessness that she experienced in the STEP test. She also completed some lifting, carrying and placing tasks and demonstrated safe techniques and capacities that suggest that she is not limited in her job requirements with respect to these.

Table 11.1 Results of incremental step test

Time	Step speed	VO_2ml.kg^{-1}.min^{-1}	HbO$_2$sat%	Heart rate	BP (mmHg)	ECG	Breathing rating (6–20 points)	Exertion rating (6–20 points)
Pre-exercise	–	4.1	95%	88	138/88	Sinus rhythm, no ischaemia	–	–
2 min	14	13.3	95%	122	142/85	As above	6	6
4 min	18	16.1	94%	129	155/88	As above	11	8
6 min	22	19.0	94%	140	158/83	As above	15	13
8 min	26	21.8	92%	149	168/91	As above	16	15
8 min	30	24.6	92%	160	188/101	As above	18	16
Recovery 3 min	–	–	96%	112	122/76	As above	–	–

Table 11.2 Results of lung function tests

Stage	FVC	%pred	FEV$_1$	%pred	FEV$_1$/FVC	Peak capacity	Comment
Pre-exercise	3.6	88%	1.9	68%	53%	MVV = 51 l.min^{-1}	FVC test indicates obstructive disease
Peak exercise						VE$_{peak}$ = 53 l.min^{-1}	SL stopped exercise due to breathlessness
Pre- vs peak	Breathing reserve = 2 l.min^{-1}						Breathing reserve is very low

Assessment

The clinical exercise practitioner followed up the first exercise test with a subsequent test that included resting and exercise spirometry to further investigate the breathlessness (see above). These latter tests were consistent with SL's symptoms in the STEP test and so the clinical exercise practitioner referred SL back to her GP for further investigation and treatment of her obstructive lung patterns. Chest radiographs revealed panacinar emphysema of the lower lobes of both lungs.

There was no evidence of lung carcinoma. The GP prescribed both reliever and preventer medications for obstructive lung disease, and advised SL to attend the clinic whenever symptoms worsened or she caught a respiratory tract infection as antibiotics may be needed to treat infections. The clinical exercise practitioner also advised the GP of her recent rapid weight gain and so the GP ordered a thyroid function test that indicated that her thyroid function was borderline low, but no treatment was indicated or commenced at this time.

The clinical exercise practitioner supported SL to develop a lifestyle plan that focused on a core program of moderate-intensity aerobic exercise combined with short bursts of high-intensity resistance exercise. Healthy nutrients and eating patterns, and attention to her stress levels were also emphasised. The exercise plan needed to challenge SL to cope with some exercise-induced dyspnoea and SL was counselled to 'enjoy' this as it will help to clear her lungs, but not to the extent that her breathing made exercise too difficult for her as this will almost certainly lead to discontinuation in the short to medium term.

Plan

Barriers to exercise intervention

- SL remains extremely distressed and anxious about her weight, appearance and health. She is suffering from depression and this is de-motivating for exercise and physical activity. SL lacks self-confidence and self-efficacy in relation to any physical task, including exercise.
- Her weight is now at the point of becoming a barrier for high intensities and volumes of exercise and some modes of exercise, and may cause or exacerbate musculoskeletal injuries.
- SL continues to work long shifts, but there are no big demands placed on her time outside of work.
- Emphysema causing breathlessness and mild arterial desaturation at relatively high intensities of exercise, but she exhibits a normal response to exercise at low and moderate intensities.
- Lack of recent regular elective exercise, with almost all current participation being confined to vocational physical activity that will continue to be encouraged.

Immediate goals of exercise and lifestyle intervention

- To improve self-confidence and self-efficacy in relation to exercise and physical activity.
- To relieve stress, anxiety and the symptoms of depression.
- To stimulate SL's resting, exercise and recovery metabolic rates using a properly designed program of moderate-intensity aerobic exercise combined with short bursts of high-intensity resistance exercise. To educate and counsel SL about this.

- To stabilise SL's weight and to counsel her that exercise will cause slow, permanent, rather than rapid, temporary weight loss. SL will also need to be counselled and reassured that weight gain is normal early in an exercise program for someone who has not engaged in exercise recently.
- To break the cycle of anorexia during the day followed by a single large meal at night that is contributing to SL's metabolic problems.
- To improve glucose and lipid metabolism.
- To reduce blood pressure, resting and upon exertion, and to improve self-reported ratings of breathlessness and exertion.

Immediate exercise strategies

- SL will be advised that exercise is possibly even more effective if the total volume is distributed among several periods that 'break up sedentary behaviour' and stimulate metabolism.
- SL will be counselled that exercise, including brief high-intensity exercise, can help to break the stress cycle. The QoL questionnaire to be completed prior to starting the exercise program.
- The clinical exercise practitioner will accompany SL on at least one aerobic and one resistance exercise training session per week for the first 2 months.
- Commence with 30 minutes daily of easy to moderate constant aerobic exercise (eg: walking; indoor and outdoor cycling; swimming; aquatic exercise). Aerobic exercise intensity should be undertaken on most if not all days in the week and be in the range of 9–13 on the 6–20 point scale of breathlessness: very slightly breathless to somewhat breathless. RPE should also be limited to a similar range.
- Two to three sessions (20 min) weekly of moderate-intensity resistance training, flexibility exercises and stretching. Self-reported ratings of breathlessness and exertion in the range of 11–15 points, and recovery periods dropping these to 9 points before commencing the next effort. During the early sessions and also whenever intensity is increased, blood pressure will be measured by brachial artery sphygmomanometry while SL is undertaking an exercise such as leg press or leg extension to check safety; intensity will be modified if necessary to keep blood pressure below 210/110mmHg.

- SL will not be weighed during the early weeks, and advised not to weigh herself at home. Instead, SL should focus on how her clothes fit, and how she feels.
- The clinical exercise practitioner should stress to SL that any signs or symptoms such as severe breathlessness, dizziness or chest or other pain should be reported to the AEP and SL's GP. However, occasional mild symptoms should not preclude SL from doing low to moderate-intensity exercise.

Long-term goals of exercise intervention

- At 6 months, SL has achieved self-efficacy and has adopted her exercise and lifestyle plan for the long term. SL has come to realise that health and fitness are associated with increased metabolism at rest, during exercise and during recovery from exertion.
- SL's symptoms of anxiety and depression are alleviated and she associates these with fitness and healthy lifestyle.
- SL has reduced her self-reported ratings of breathlessness and exertion for a given level of exercise (both aerobic and resistance) by at least 2 points (= one whole category).
- SL has lost at least 10kg of weight and reduced her clothing size by at least one size.
- SL has reduced the risk of further cardiac events by reducing weight, blood pressure, heart rate and cholesterol (total cholesterol, LDL, triglycerides).
- Blood pressure, lipid and glucose metabolism are all improved, and these improvements are clinically significant (eg: reduced need for medications).

Long-term exercise strategies

- Exercise comprising aerobic and resistance training is maintained at a minimum of 60 minutes per day, and includes at least two exercise episodes per day.
- Now that exercise-induced breathlessness is not as severe, SL will engage in bursts of high-intensity resistance training ($15 \leq RPE \leq 17$) in order that the gains with this intensity of training are available to SL. Each week, SL will be encouraged to undertake 2–3 sessions of resistance training of 10 exercises, 2–3 sets, 8–12 repetitions.

- SL will be encouraged to use her new health and fitness by joining active recreational activities and this should help her to recover her self-esteem and enjoyment of life.
- Add physical challenges to motivate SL (eg: Heart Foundation walks, fun runs, ocean swims, charity events).
- Other allied health professionals such as a dietitian and psychologist may be brought in if SL feels that she can benefit from this additional support.

Monitoring outcomes

- The clinical exercise practitioner, the GP and SL will work together to try to achieve long-term health goals. This will include 6-month check-ups for blood pressure, lipids and glucose metabolism and symptoms of depression and anxiety. Medications will be adjusted downwards by the GP if her health continues to improve.
- Follow-up exercise testing for VO_{2peak}, and a range of strength, endurance and joint flexibility will be conducted at 3–6 monthly intervals.
- Quality of life questionnaires to be completed every 3 months for comparison.

Outcomes

At 6 months, SL had made clinically significant improvements in all of her vital signs for metabolic syndrome (MetS), with modest falls in blood pressure, and fasted lipids and glucose. Her symptoms of depression gradually improved and at 6 months she was able to describe a 'healthy addiction' to exercise. She started to lose weight after about 2 months and had lost 12kg at 12 months.

Discussion

SL's health and fitness had deteriorated markedly during the past 4 years in response to her changed behaviours and mental state following the break-up of her long-term relationship and death of her mother. Prior to this time, she had been a relatively healthy individual, even given her 15 pack/year smoking habit that she had successfully broken. She also had never suffered previously from depression or anxiety disorders. The role of the clinical exercise practitioner was to support SL and her GP in reclaiming SL's mental and physical health, fitness and happiness. Exercise and healthy lifestyle were the cornerstone strategies of this.

SL underwent a symptom-limited STEP test for the assessment of aerobic power (VO_{2peak}), and this uncovered some unexpected severe breathlessness that led to further tests of resting and exercise spirometry, and finally a diagnosis of emphysema. While this was a nasty surprise for all involved, this early diagnosis was used to the advantage of SL to improve her lung function at rest and during exertion.

An evidence-based approach to increasing SL's metabolism was used, with a combination of moderate-intensity aerobic exercise combined with bursts of high-intensity resistance exercise. Volumes of exercise were increased as capacity improved.

Summary of key lessons

- It is important to counsel the client on the reasons for her rapid recent weight gain. The main issue seems to be a slowing of metabolism due partly to anorexia during the day that is not fully offset by her vocational activity. Her thyroid function was borderline low, but the decision was made to use lifestyle strategies at this stage to stimulate her daily metabolic output. She was counselled on the thermogenic value of many foods and this is juxtaposed to diets and weight gain. She was also counselled on the thermogenic and/or metabolic value of moderate and high-intensity exercise, as opposed to the low-intensity physical activity that best describes her work activity.

- It is important to counsel SL that weight may not be lost as quickly as she would like through this lifestyle plan, but that the weight gain may be 'permanent' if she embraces a new healthy, active lifestyle.

- Even in clients with chronic diseases (eg: emphysema), exercise has some effect to relieve stress and reduce the symptoms of depression.

- SL's metabolic signs of elevated blood pressure, lipids, and glucose, together with her increasing weight, should respond to a combination of aerobic and resistance training, but the clinical exercise practitioner will need to carefully design the program and monitor these signs during the early phase. Evidence supports the use of both aerobic and resistance modes of exercise for improving these metabolic signs.

- It is important to monitor blood pressure during resistance exercise early in the program, and this will be done by using brachial artery sphygmomanometry while SL is undertaking an exercise such as leg press or leg extension to check safety. An ECG is not needed during training because her exercise ECG was normal during the symptom-limited test (VO_{2peak}).

- Significant reductions in blood pressure can occur with exercise, independent of medications. It must be stressed that clients should remain on their prescribed medications (and dosages) while participating in structured exercise programs, until a prescribing practioner revises drug management.

DISCUSSION Questions

1 What are the physiological mechanisms for SL's weight gain over the past 4 years? How might you explain these mechanisms to clients who avoid food throughout the day, and then overeat at night?

2 Are there any associations between depression and weight gain? Describe your own experiences of the effects of exercise on mood.

3 What should the clinical exercise practitioner do if SL's symptoms of depression deteriorate further? How could the practitioner monitor mood during supervised exercise?

4 What was the rationale for the early monitoring of blood pressure during the training sessions?

5 Changes in body weight (both loss and gain) may be markers of underlying disease. Recommend methods for a clinical exercise practitioner to investigate whether weight change is purely due to shifts in energy-activity balance or associated with other conditions.

REFERENCES

Access Economics (2008) The growing costs of obesity in 2008: three years on. Online. Available: www.accesseconomics.com.au/publicationsreports/showreport.php?id=172

Brown SP, Miller WC, Eason JM (2006) *Exercise Physiology. Basis of Human Movement in Health and Disease*. New York: Lippincott Williams & Wilkins

Donnely JE, Blair SN, Jakicic JM, et al (2009) American College of Sports Medicine Position Stand. Appropriate physical activity intervention strategies for weight loss and prevention of weight regain for adults. *Medicine and Science in Sports & Exercise*, 41(2):459–71

Ehrman JK, Gordon PM, Visich PS, et al (2009) *Clinical Exercise Physiology*. Champaign, IL: Human Kinetics

Haslam D, Sattar N, Lean M (2006) ABC of obesity. Obesity — time to wake up. *British Medical Journal*, 333:640–2

Magee DJ (2008) *Orthopedic Physical Assessment* (5th ed). St Louis Missouri: Elsevier

McArdle WD, Katch FI, Katch VL (2009) *Sports and Exercise Nutrition* (3rd ed). Philadelphia: Lippincott Williams & Wilkins

Peeters A, Barendregt JJ, Willekens F, et al (2003) Obesity in adulthood and its consequences for life expectancy; a life-table analysis. *Annals of Internal Medicine*, 138 (1):24–32

Robbins G, Powers D, Burgess S (2009) *A Wellness Way of Life*. Boston: McGraw-Hill

Ross R, Janssen I (2007) Physical activity, fitness and obesity. In: Bouchard C, Blair, SN, Haskell WL (eds) *Physical Activity and Health*. Champaign, IL: Human Kinetics, pp 173–89

Stein CJ, Colditz GA (2004) The epidemic of obesity. *Journal of Clinical Endocrinology and Metabolism*, 89:2522–5

Thompson DL, Rakow J, Perdue SM (2004) Relationship between accumulated walking and body composition in middle-aged women. *Medicine and Science in Sports and Exercise*, 36:911–14

Thompson WR, Gordon NF, Pescatello LS (eds) (2010) *ACSM's Guidelines for Exercise Testing and Prescription* (8th ed). Baltimore, MD: Lippincott Williams & Wilkins

Voorrips LE, Meijers JHH, Sol P, et al (1992) History of body weight and physical activity of elderly women differing in current physical activity. *International Journal of Obesity*, 16:199–205

Wilmore JH, Costill DL, Kenney WL (2008) *Physiology of Sport and Exercise* (4th ed). Champaign, IL: Human Kinetics

World Health Organization (WHO) (1998) *Obesity: Preventing and Managing the Global Epidemic*. Report of a WHO consultation on obesity. Geneva: WHO

Chapter 12

Case studies in exercise as therapy for musculoskeletal conditions

Melainie Cameron and Cilas Wilders

INTRODUCTION

Exercise has been used as an intervention for musculoskeletal conditions for longer than we can recount. Chapter 2 covers the evidence supporting exercise as musculoskeletal therapy and describes the breadth of conditions for which this approach may be useful. The case studies in this chapter have been selected not simply as illustrations, but to further comprehension of the widespread usefulness of exercise in clients with musculoskeletal conditions. We have selected a client for whom a specific diagnosis cannot be reached, a client whose condition is more cosmetic than pathological, and a client whose musculoskeletal decline might be attributed as much to ageing as to longstanding disease. In these clients exercise remains useful and returns widespread benefits, but the selection and application of exercise is more complex than stretching tight muscles, strengthening weak muscles, or training clients in co-contracting stabilising muscles.

This chapter may appear a little thin; it should not be considered complete in isolation. Musculoskeletal conditions occur when people are engaged in the tasks of life, including daily work and sporting activity, therefore, musculoskeletal conditions are explored in other chapters too. In particular, readers are directed to Chapter 18, case study 3, for two accounts of discogenic pain (one cervical, one lumbar) in athletes, and Chapter 19, case studies 1, 2a, 2b, and 3, for reports of employees with non-specific low back pain,

traumatic fractures, and lumbar disc protrusion requiring surgery.

CASE STUDY 1: MUSCULOSKELETAL PAIN

Subjective

Helen, a 32-year-old woman working in journalism, presents complaining of a swollen and painful right elbow that has persisted unchanged for 3 weeks. She cannot identify any particular cause of the elbow pain. As well as pain, her elbow is very stiff first thing in the morning, gradually becoming more mobile about an hour after waking, but with the feeling of stiffness never completely abating during the day. Pain is disturbing her sleep, and she appears tired with darkened creases beneath her eyes.

Helen is right handed, and reports that she finds typing, writing, and driving, tasks important in her work, difficult due to pain and stiffness. Prior to this episode of joint pain, Helen would play netball on Tuesday nights during netball seasons, and nine holes of golf twice each week, once on Saturdays and once on Wednesday afternoons. Although she has not taken time off work or reported her condition to her employer, she has missed the past 2 weekly games with her local netball team and has not played golf at all since the elbow pain began.

She reports no current pain in other sites, but previous episodes of pain, swelling and redness in the small joints of both hands. None of these episodes lasted more than 10 days, and previous laboratory investigations for inflammatory arthritides were inconclusive.

Objective

Helen cradles her right elbow in her left hand. She moves cautiously, but through full range during active examination. Physical examination reveals redness and moderate swelling of the right elbow. All elbow movements are available but painful. Pain is reported at rest with the elbow in mid-range, and aggravated by all full range passive and active motions: extension and locking, full flexion, and end-range of supination and pronation. Helen reports tenderness to palpation through the muscles of the extensor compartment of the right forearm. Helen describes and rates pain using the short-form McGill pain questionnaire: sensory pain 12/33, affective pain 4/12, total pain 16/45, visual analogue scale 63/100, present pain index 3 (distressing). Grip strength registered using a handheld dynamometer is 8Kpa lower on the right than left. Helen's oral temperature is 36.7 degrees centigrade.

Assessment

Helen has arthritis (non-specific joint inflammation) of her right elbow. The cause of the inflammation is unclear, but is probably not septic as demonstrated by her normal body temperature. At this time her presentation does not fit the diagnostic criteria for any particular arthritic disease. Helen is adopting pain behaviours that if prolonged, regardless of the specific diagnosis, may worsen her prognosis. In particular, Helen is at risk of physical deconditioning due to inactivity.

Plan

Helen is advised to keep a watching brief on symptoms, and to return for further investigations of arthritides if symptoms persist for 6 weeks or longer, or escalate to include pain, swelling, and redness of multiple joints, joints on both sides of the body, or small joints of the hands. The negative sequelae of fear-avoidance behaviour are discussed with Helen and she is encouraged to resume some physical activities, practicing joint protection where possible.

Helen is keen to return to some exercise. The clinical exercise practitioner reassures Helen that despite lacking a clear cut diagnosis for her joint pain and inflammation, she can safely commence some forms of exercise. Goals for exercise intervention at this preliminary diagnostic stage are to: (a) prevent deconditioning and further loss of function due to inactivity; (b) maintain current fitness status, including aerobic capacity, muscle strength, and muscle endurance; (c) maintain joint ranges of motion; and (d) protect joint surfaces during exercise.

Helen selects walking as her preferred primary form of exercise, although the practitioner explains that cycling and water-based exercise are sensible alternatives to achieve the agreed exercise goals. Helen agrees to walk on a treadmill at the gym for 40 minutes on Tuesday evenings instead of playing netball. Fortunately the gym is part of the same centre as the netball club, and the treadmills are positioned so that Helen can watch her team play while she walks. She also agrees to walk around the golf course twice each week in order to fit walking into her usual schedule. Helen understands that walking is unlikely to aggravate her upper limb joint inflammation.

The clinical exercise practitioner demonstrates some range of motion exercises, flexing and extending the elbows, first with the hands supinated, and then with the hands pronated. The practitioner advises Helen to perform these exercises when she is in the shower and her elbow is feeling warm, and cautions her to flex and extend within her available range only, not to force or load the joints at the end ranges of motion. Helen is asked to perform these exercises daily as part of her normal shower routine. Further, the practitioner recommends that Helen not shower (and exercise) immediately upon waking, but delay her shower by 30–60 minutes so that some of the stiffness has abated before she attempts the exercises.

Outcome

Helen exercised as agreed for 3 weeks. During this time swelling, pain, and stiffness in her right elbow eased somewhat, and with this resolution of symptoms, she sought no further investigations for arthritides.

In the third week after this consultation Helen 'swung a few clubs' during her walk around the golf course. The following week, she resumed playing. Her first game performance was not good, but she enjoyed the activity, and her elbow felt 'no worse' after golf than it had beforehand. Another week later Helen resumed playing netball, initially playing in the goal keeper position for the first half of the game only.

Helen is aware that she may experience further episodes of joint pain, swelling, and stiffness, and that these episodes may be similar or more extensive than past episodes. Helen is confident that she can continue to remain physically active during these undiagnosed episodes of arthritis.

Discussion

Arthritis is a general term; it just means a joint is inflamed, which is obvious from inspection and examination of Helen. As explained in Chapters 2 and 10, strict diagnostic criteria are applied to arthritides (eg: Arnett et al 1988), and Helen's initial presentation does not meet these stringent requirements for a diagnostic label. Only when a client's symptoms satisfies these diagnostic criteria can the client be told that she (most arthritides affect more women than men) has a particular arthritic disease.

Because Helen has only one joint inflamed at the moment, the relevant disease classification using the International Classification of Disease version 10 (ICD-10) schema is *M13 other arthritis*, specifically *M13.1 monoarthritis not elsewhere classified* (WHO 2007). This classification, although it sounds a bit like a diagnostic label, may offer little comfort to Helen because it is a classification of exclusion, telling her more about what she doesn't have than what she does.

A wait and see approach is recommended; quite possibly Helen's presentation will advance to include other joints (polyarthritis), and last 6 weeks or more, meaning that her presentation would then satisfy criteria for classification *M06 other rheumatoid arthritis*, and if the blood tests were repeated and remained negative, the classification could be further refined to *M06.0 seronegative rheumatoid arthritis*. In contrast, further invasive investigation (eg: radiographs or other imaging, blood tests for rheumatoid factor, erythrocyte sedimentation rate, or HLA tissue type) at Helen's initial presentation adds little diagnostic value (Pincus et al 1994), and exposes Helen to the physical risks of testing as well as the emotional upheaval of prolonged diagnostic uncertainty. The extensive, time consuming, process of searching for a diagnosis does not serve clients well. Practitioners similarly can get hooked up on finding the precise diagnosis and leave the client hanging around doing nothing, deconditioning with every day of inactivity, and feeling helpless because their presentations don't meet stringent diagnostic criteria so no one can say (will say) exactly what is wrong.

It takes considerable interpersonal skill for a clinical exercise practitioner to work with a client like Helen. In particular, it is important that Helen does not feel dismissed. Helen is distressed about her joint pain and the immediate costs on her life. She is also quite likely to be afraid of an unknown diagnosis and concerned that she has some serious, perhaps life threatening, disease. She may catastrophise her symptoms and lack of a definitive diagnosis into something enormous and terrible. Clinical exercise practitioners need to tread carefully, simultaneously avoiding temptations to claim more diagnostic certainty than is genuine, request a flurry of useless (or possibly harmful) tests, or dismiss Helen's pain as less than real because it cannot be fully explained.

In Helen's case, exercise interventions can begin safely before a definitive diagnosis is made. Helen has arthritis, and although we don't know which type, she can begin exercising with some sensible precautions and a watching brief on her symptoms.

That said, once a diagnosis of an arthritic disease is confirmed (ie: classification criteria are satisfied), early referral to a rheumatologist for pharmaceutical intervention is wise. There is substantial evidence that joint surface damage (eg: erosions) are markedly reduced by early medical management (Dougados 2004; Egmose et al 1995; van der Heijde 1995).

Important features of the exercise intervention in this case are that it was designed to keep Helen in contact with her existing social networks and maintain her normal routines. People with undiagnosed musculoskeletal diseases are at risk of fear-avoidance behaviours; they become fearful of their pain, of provoking it, of worsening the unknown disease, and consequently avoid doing normal activities or socialising in usual ways. Fear-avoidance behaviour is potentially debilitating, both physically and socially, and along with catastrophising and depression, is a key marker (yellow flag) for chronicity in musculoskeletal disease (Pincus et al 1994; Pincus et al 2002). In this case exercise was used well to maintain some social engagement and empower Helen to return to her usual routines as soon as possible.

Summary of key lessons

- Diagnosis of musculoskeletal diseases, particularly arthritides, can be prolonged. Exercise and physical activity can be part of clinical management to maintain or improve physical function before a specific diagnosis is established.

- Fear-avoidance behaviour is possible in any painful condition aggravated by movement, particularly arthritides with stress-pain or end-range pain as part of the clinical presentation. Education, positive communication, helpful social support, and graduated physical activity are constructive methods for changing fear-avoidance behaviours.

- Distress is an important emotion associated with Helen's presentation. Helen describes her pain as distressing and scores moderately on the affective sub-scale of the short-form McGill pain questionnaire. Distress is often a product of feeling powerless. Physical activity, particularly graduated exercise to maintain daily functioning, is a key tool for building self-efficacy and reducing distress associated with powerlessness.

DISCUSSION Questions

1 How will you explain to Helen the preferred 'wait and see' approach? Consider how you might respond if Helen disagrees with this approach as the preferred course of action (eg: she wants extensive blood tests performed immediately).

2 What personal markers (symptoms and signs) would you identify for Helen as prompts for her to seek further investigation of her 'arthritis'?

CASE STUDY 2: MUSCULOSKELETAL STRUCTURAL DEFORMITY SCHEUERMANN'S THORACIC KYPHOSIS

Subjective

CJ is a 15-year-old girl, who was referred to a clinical exercise practitioner by an orthopaedic surgeon, with a diagnosis of Scheuermann's thoracic kyphosis. She complains of stiffness in her upper back. CJ has worsening back pain while sitting for long periods of time at school or at home, the pain is worst in the late afternoon. CJ also experiences difficulty in executing certain movements while participating in sport, although physical activity in itself gives relief.

CJ's poor posture is an embarrassment for her at school and she doesn't have a good self image, therefore she feels lonely and suffers from bad mood swings. CJ had seen a psychologist for a few sessions and was referred to a general practitioner (GP) for management of the kyphosis. The clinical exercise practitioner noted that although a surgical opinion was sought, both the surgeon and the GP have told CJ that surgical procedures are a last option to treat the problem. Furthermore, CJ does not have any other medical problems that would justify a surgical intervention. CJ's (and her mother's) biggest concern is her postural appearance. CJ has not received any previous treatment for the postural problem.

CJ's father is a heavy smoker and workaholic, while her mother stays at home suffering from emphysema. A full medical history reveals a family history of primary coronary and pulmonary risk factors including smoking, overweight, emphysema and hypertension as well as postural deformities and depression. Unfortunately no radiographs accompanied the reference.

Objective

Height 167cm, weight 53 kg, body fat 15.76%, waist 66cm, hips 81cm. Flexicurve (a malleable, metal ruler covered with plastic) was used to measure the thoracic kyphosis at 40° from T1–T12.

A New York Posture Test chart was used to screen CJ for possible postural abnormalities.

- Side views: neck: full range of motion with a slightly forward movement — no tenderness or pain with palpation (3), shoulders: rounded shoulders (3), chest: flattened (3), upper back: a significant kyphosis; pronounced with the forward bending test (1), lower back: appearance of a mild lordosis (1), abdomen: protruding abdomen (3), uneven hips: none (5), uneven shoulders: none (5), rib hump: none (5).
- Posterior views: neck and head: straight (5), shoulders: even shoulders (5), back plumbline: straight (5), hipline: straight (5), feet position: inwards slightly (3), arches: lower than normal (3).
- The clinical exercise practitioner used the YMCA cycle ergometer protocol (leg ergometer) to execute a sub-maximal graded exercise test (see Table 12.1).

Functional tests were also undertaken: sit and reach test = 20cm; YMCA sit up test 11 in 1 minute; curl-up 10/min; pull ups 3/min; push ups 5/min. CJ reported fatigue in her arms and breathing after completing these tests.

Assessment

CJ has a Scheuemann's thoracic kyphosis without evidence of underlying respiratory or neurological pathology. Although she is essentially healthy, the results of incremental exercise and functional tests indicate that CJ is sedentary. CJ believes that the kyphosis produces stiffness and some pain, as well as a physical deformity that causes embarrassment, all of which may compromise CJ's desire to participate in physical activity.

CJ is conscious (and critical) of her body, and seeks exercise intervention to improve her physical appearance. Further, CJ is in the middle of adolescence, a time when female participation in physical activity declines precipitously. CJ is at risk of reduced health due to sedentary behaviour and limited sport and exercise participation.

Plan

CJ is advised to exercise aerobically at 70% of her estimated maximal heart rate (ie: 220-age). She is also provided with a routine of stretches and strengthening exercises for the shoulder girdles and chest cage, and deep breathing exercises, to perform daily as part of her usual dressing and grooming routine. Exercise progressions will be added as CJ grows in strength, flexibility, and confidence in using her own body (exercise self-efficacy).

Table 12.1 Results of incremental cycle ergometry

Stage (3 min)	Heart rate (bpm)	Blood pressure (mmHg)	Reported perceived exertion (Borg scale)
Warm up	60	100/70	
Stage 1	105	120/70	2
Stage 2	156	148/70	5
Stage 3	190	188/70	7
3 min recovery	100	110/70	

Note: incremental cycle ergometry is important to determine CJ's aerobic capacity and identify possible respiratory restrictions (see chapter 4 for further explanation of hyperkyphosis and respiratory function).

Immediate exercise strategies

- Start with a 3–5 days a week of moderate continuous aerobic exercise for at least 30 minutes (eg: walking, indoor or outdoor cycling, swimming, aquatic exercise) maintaining heart rate between 130–160bpm. Include warm up and warm down for at least 5 minutes each time. The clinical exercise practitioner stressed to CJ that any signs or symptoms such as breathlessness, dizziness or chest pain during exercise should be reported immediately.
- Deep breathing exercises (ie: diaphragmatic breathing, see Figure 12.1) to help strengthen the intercostals muscles and the upper part of the abdominal muscles as well as the abdominal diaphragm.
- Static stretches for the shoulder adductors and abductors, internal and external rotators, pectoralis major and minor, starting with 20 second holds and two repetitions.
- Passive stretches for the chest cage and shoulder girdle: lie supine over a towel rolled and placed along the length of the thoracic spine, abduct both arms to 90 degrees, turn palms to ceiling, and breathe deeply filling the chest with each inspiration.
- Scapula repositioning exercises: contact and hold in retraction and depression. Commence with holds of 1–2 repetitions of 3–4, and eventually increasing to 10 repetitions of 10 seconds each.
- Prone back extension: lying prone raise the head, neck, and thoracic spine into extension. Commence with holds of 1–2 repetitions of 3–4s, and eventually increasing to 10 repetitions of 10 seconds each. Progress further by raising arms into elevation above the head (ie: 'Superman' position).

Long-term exercise strategies

- Increase duration of aerobic exercise sessions to more days of the week, with higher intensities (not more than 90% of MHR), including varying intensities of exercise, to particular focus to promote a healthy lifestyle.
- Involve CJ in more recreational physical activity that she sees as enjoyable.

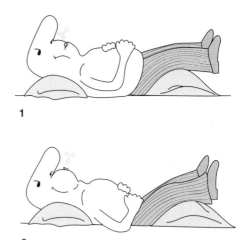

Figure 12.1 Diaphragmatic breathing

Notes. Step 1: Lie supine, rest one hand on the upper abdomen and one hand on the lower thorax over the distal end of the sternum, breathe in deeply, contracting the diaphragm and relaxing the muscles of the abdominal wall, feeling the abdomen push up into the lower hand.

Step 2: Breathe out slowly and fully, contracting the abdominal muscles and relaxing the diaphragm, feeling the abdomen sink below the lower hand.

Repeat up to five times. Rise slowly from the floor because deep breathing exercises can provoke light-headedness.

- Extend type of exercises to use all major muscle groups and all joints.

Progress

CJ exercised as agreed for 12 weeks. She met with the clinical exercise practitioner three times per week for supervised exercise. On the other days of the week she reported that she completed her home routine of breathing, stretching, and strengthening exercises. During supervised exercise sessions the clinical exercise practitioner taught CJ to measure her own heart rate during resting, training and recovery.

The first 4 weeks of supervised exercise were undertaken indoors in private (one-on-one) sessions with the clinical exercise practitioner. The only observer permitted in these sessions was CJ's mother. After 4 weeks of supervised exercise, the clinical exercise practitioner began varying the type of aerobic exercise, increasing the intensity of exercise, and adding some outdoor exercise. CJ was also encouraged to bring a teenage friend to these later exercise sessions if she wished. CJ brought a friend to three of the exercise sessions that included outdoor cycling.

Outcomes

Postural analysis, anthropometric and functional tests were repeated after 12 weeks of supervised exercise. The thoracic kyphosis was measured at 37° using the Flexicurve. CJ no longer stood with a protruding abdomen or rounded shoulders. Although the kyphosis persisted, CJ had altered her posture so that the kyphosis appeared less obvious. Functional test results (sit and reach, sit ups, curl ups, pull ups, push ups) were largely unchanged, except that CJ did not complain of fatigue during these tests.

Discussion

In this case the clinical exercise practitioner deliberately selected interventions that could be undertaken in the client's home without the need to join a gym or exercise in a public place. These recommendations are sensible given CJ's lack of self-confidence and poor body image which is likely to manifest while exercising within a fitness facility. CJ is also likely to have had negative experiences of trying to get involved in physical activity and exercise at school (eg: being selected last for a team game). Recently CJ has not been involved in any regular exercise; both a fear of pain while exercising, and some deconditioning due to CJ's sedentary lifestyle are to be expected. Further, CJ is a teenager: Teenagers are often reluctant to take advice from adults, therefore the risk that CJ might not adhere to exercise intervention is increased because of her age and stage of emotional maturity (see Chapter 7 for further discussion on working with adolescents).

Instability is an important problem to manage in many people with back complaints (eg: see Richardson et al 1999, 2004). Forces from the extremities are transmitted to the spine, and the abdominal muscles are recruited to stabilise the spine. In this case CJ did not display spinal instability, but the clinical exercise practitioner pre-empted this problem and taught CJ to identify and functionally isolate the muscles of her abdominal and her respiratory diaphragm. Being able to consciously distinguish between these muscles, and control contraction of each group independently, allows CJ to self-monitor exercise while progressing to more demanding exercises in which she might require increased respiratory exertion (eg: endurance running) or substantial spinal stability (eg: weight lifting).

CJ's problems associated with Scheuermann's thoracic kyphosis are not resolved by exercise alone. Further, most alterations in sagittal spinal curves do not appear to have a causal relationship to health problems (Christensen & Hartvigsen 2008). This condition is principally of cosmetic concern for CJ. It is unlikely to progress such that it leads to structural compromise of respiratory function. Rather, loss of respiratory exercise capacity is likely if CJ continued to be (or returned to being) sedentary, avoiding exercise and exercise environments. CJ's 'rehabilitation' is incomplete. She cannot expect that her kyphosis will go away. A wise practitioner will not make promises of postural change that are unlikely to be fulfilled, but will instead use exercise as a vehicle to improve and affirm CJ's body image and promote a physically active lifestyle for general health and wellbeing, particularly adolescent mood stability and restful sleep.

Summary of key lessons

- Perceived disability and the anticipation of pain contribute significantly to the loss of function even in the absence of underlying disease.

- Psychoemotional effects of cosmetic problems are particularly important during adolescence. Include the client in exercise goal setting and be in contact for support when needed.

- A rehabilitation program like this one takes some time, requiring the client to make a long-term commitment to achieve postural change.

DISCUSSION Questions

1 CJ is a young woman with concerns about her appearance. What words will you use to explain to her that her kyphosis is primarily a cosmetic problem rather than a structural one?

2 CJ believes that her kyphosis is causing her some pain, although a systematic analysis of the epidemiological literature suggests that a causal relationship between sagittal curves and spinal pain is unlikely (Christensen & Hartvigsen 2008). Discuss whether it is important for CJ to understand the cause of her spinal pain.

CASE STUDY 3: LONGSTANDING MUSCULOSKELETAL DISEASE

Subjective

Peggy, an 85-year-old woman, retired and living in her own home, presents as a participant in a community exercise class for people with arthritis offered at very low cost from her local church. Peggy reports that although she has widespread osteoarthritis, she experiences no major impairments. Instead, she has joined the exercise class in order to support the class leader, a 30-year-old woman healthcare practitioner who has volunteered her time to run the class as a show of solidarity for the church's community health and wellbeing project.

Because the arthritis exercise class is a group activity, individual consultations and assessments are not conducted. Rather, participants self-identify as people with arthritis, and complete a health screening risk assessment form prior to commencing the class. The class leader is an allied health practitioner, who ensures that the exercises undertaken in the class are low risk, as well as continuously monitoring the eight participants for signs of coping or distress.

Peggy reports some osteoarthritic pain, particularly in her knees, lower back and shoulders, but insists that she is not limited in doing the things she enjoys. Peggy says that she takes no regular medication. She uses 2 x 500mg paracetamol (acetaminophen) as required for pain, and admits that she can take up to eight a day when pain is severe. She also uses heated wheat bags and hot showers to manage her pain.

Peggy is married to Noel, an 87-year-old man who is an active member of the same church community. Peggy and Noel share a three bedroom unit in the same street as the church. They have four adult children, none of whom live at home. Peggy does not drive, but walks around her local community, both to church activities and to complete shopping and other tasks of daily living. She has never been particularly interested in exercise or sport. Involvement with church activities is her primary leisure.

Objective

Peggy walks with a steady gait. She wears flat shoes and loose, comfortable clothing. She participates fully in the class, which consists of a regular program of walking, then range of motion, balance, and core strengthening exercises, followed by stretching of large muscle groups. She appears to be able to complete all activities and complains of no pain during the class. She uses a chair for stability during some balance exercises, but does not appear particularly unstable or at risk of falling.

Assessment

Peggy has osteoarthritis with pain but little obvious impairment. She is engaged in exercise for leisure and social reasons rather than seeking health improvements.

Plan

Peggy is encouraged to participate as fully as she can in the exercise classes. 10 classes are offered at weekly intervals over the course of one school term. During the classes, participants are given the opportunity to ask questions about osteoarthritis and particular attention is given to explaining how exercise can benefit people with osteoarthritis in maintaining function for activities of daily living. Peggy and other participants are encouraged to repeat some of the low risk exercises (walking, range of motion) at home between classes. All participants are advised to cease any exercises that produce pain, and also, to ensure that other people are present at home when they are exercising in case they need assistance.

Outcome

Peggy participates in all classes and expresses enjoyment of them. She encourages the class leader, and commends her on her consideration, careful explanations, and care of 'us oldies'. As the term progresses, Peggy appears to move more easily, stretch a little further, and reach a little higher, but no measurements are taken, and Peggy reports no specific improvements in function. Rather, when asked to comment on the class and how it has affected her, Peggy reports that she has met some lovely new people, had an enjoyable time, and thinks the 'kind and enthusiastic young leader' is doing a 'wonderful job'.

On Sunday morning immediately following the end of the term of classes, Noel approaches the class leader privately and reports that Peggy no longer asks him to reach for items from the top shelves in their kitchen. The class leader replies that Peggy had not mentioned that she had trouble reaching high shelves or lifting things over her head. Noel says that although he is several inches shorter than Peggy, and the kitchen of their house is her domain, she has for the past 3 years, asked him to retrieve items stored up high. He has noticed that for the past 4 weeks, she has not asked him to do this task for her, and a few days ago he observed her successfully reaching for a high shelf herself.

Summary of key lessons

- Clients may be embarrassed to acknowledge loss of function, particularly if these impairments affect activities of daily living that are key to clients' self-perception and role. Embarrassment and reluctance to impart details may be amplified in a group or community setting.

- Social interaction may be an important driver for motivating people with little or no past experience of sport or exercise to become more physically active.

- Because regular activity is required for improvement or maintenance of function, exercises ideal for clients with longstanding disease will be safe to perform at home, easily remembered and repeated, require no specialised clothing or equipment, and be able to be broken into parts so that exercise sessions may be shortened or lengthened to adapt to clients' lifestyles.

DISCUSSION Question

In this case study Peggy engages in exercise to help the practitioner, and makes unexpected improvements in her shoulder range of motion. Because Noel observes and reports these improvements, it is possible that Peggy might not have noticed them in herself. If you were leading this exercise group, how might you encourage Peggy to identify her own exercise-related changes?

REFERENCES

Arnett FC, Edworthy SM, Bloch DA, et al (1988) The American Rheumatism Association 1987 revised criteria for the classification of rheumatoid arthritis. *Arthritis and Rheumatism*, 31:315–24

Christensen ST, Hartvigsen J (2008) Spinal curves and health: a systematic critical review of the epidemiological literature dealing with associations between sagittal spinal curves and health. *Journal of Manipulative and Physiological Therapeutics*, 31:690–714

Dougados M (2004) Monitoring arthritis progression and therapy. *Osteoarthritis and Cartilage*, 12 (Suppl A): S55–S60

Egmose C, Lund B, Borg G, et al (1995) Patients with rheumatoid arthritis benefit from early 2nd line therapy: 5 year follow-up of a prospective double blind placebo controlled study. *The Journal of Rheumatology*, 22: 2208–13

Pincus T, Brooks RH, Callahan LF (1994) Prediction of long-term mortality in patients with rheumatoid arthritis according to simple questionnaire and joint count measures. *Annals of Internal Medicine*, 120:26–34

Pincus T, Burton K, Vogel S, et al (2002) A systematic review of psychological factors as predictors of chronicity / disability in prospective cohorts of low back pain. *Spine*, 27:E109–E120

Richardson CA, Hodges PW, Hides JA (2004) *Therapeutic Exercise for Lumbopelvic Stabilisation: A Motor Control Approach for the Treatment and Prevention of Low Back Pain* (2nd ed). Edinburgh: Churchill Livingstone

Richardson CA, Jull G, Hodges PW, et al (1999) *Therapeutic Exercises for Spinal Segmental Stabilization in Low Back Pain*. Edinburgh: Churchill Livingstone

van der Heijde DM (1995) Joint erosions and patients with early rheumatoid arthritis. *British Journal of Rheumatology*, 34:74–8

World Health Organization (WHO) (2007) *International Statistical Classification of Diseases and Related Health Problems* (10th revision). Online. Available: www.who.int/classifications/icd/ICD-10_2nd_ed_volume2.pdf (accessed 20 August 2010)

Chapter 13

Case studies in exercise as therapy for cardiovascular conditions

Steve Selig, Dan van der Westhuizen, Suzanne Broadbent, Belinda Parmenter and Jacqui Raymond

INTRODUCTION

Exercise has been used as an intervention for some cardiovascular disease for several decades. Chapter 3 covers the evidence supporting exercise as cardiovascular therapy and describes the breadth of conditions for which this approach may be useful. The case studies in this chapter have been selected not simply as illustrations, but to further comprehension of the widespread usefulness of exercise in clients with cardiovascular conditions. We have selected clients with common conditions (older adults with coronary artery disease, type 2 diabetes, and peripheral artery disease) as well as clients with rarer but serious complaints. In these seriously ill clients exercise remains useful and returns widespread benefits, but the selection and application of exercise is particularly complex. These case studies offer examples of multidisciplinary care as clinical exercise practitioners interact with general practitioners (GPs), cardiologists and other allied health practitioners to serve clients. In case study 4 a change of voice is noticeable as clinical exercise practitioners describe working in a team with a client. Discussion is woven through these complicated case studies, and further investigation and study is prompted by the inclusion of discussion questions.

CASE STUDY 1: CORONARY ARTERY DISEASE

Subjective

TP, a 46-year-old senior male public servant, was overweight, hypertensive and suffered chest pain intermittently for 3 months. As pain worsened, his doctor diagnosed angina and recommended an angiogram, which showed a 75% block of his left descending coronary artery. A percutaneous coronary angioplasty (PTCA) was performed, and a stent implanted. After in-hospital Phase 1 cardiac rehabilitation (lifestyle advice and basic exercises for activities of daily living [ADL]), TP has been advised to undertake a regular exercise program and presents to a clinical exercise practitioner 6 weeks after being released from hospital. He has not participated in regular exercise since high school, and now only plays golf once a week. He is a non-smoker but does drink alcohol regularly (2 drinks per day). His father died from a heart attack aged 58, and his mother is hypertensive and overweight. TP currently takes aspirin (20mg), Lipitor (40mg), Dilatrend (40mg), and a sub-lingual oral nitrate when appropriate.

Objective
Medical history

A full medical history was taken, including: family history of chronic diseases; a history of signs and symptoms of cardiac disease; an exercise history; list of medications and a report from TP's cardiologist regarding the surgical procedures done. The clinical exercise practitioner noted that TP had not undergone a medically supervised incremental exercise test ('stress test') prior to or after the surgery.

Physical examination

Height 178cm; weight 107kg; body fat 33%; BMI 33.8; waist 116cm; hip 112cm; waist–hip ratio 1.04; resting blood pressure 142/92mmHg; resting heart rate 62bpm.

Recent fasting blood lipid test showed total cholesterol 5.8mmol/L, LDL 3mmol/L, HDL1.0mmol/L, triglycerides 1.8mmol/L. Fasting glucose test 6.8mmol/L.

Incremental exercise test

A medically supervised sub-maximal graded exercise test (GXT) on a treadmill (Modified Bruce protocol) with 12 lead ECG was conducted by the clinical exercise practitioner (see Table 13.1). The test was necessary to determine TP's aerobic fitness and to screen for any possible cardiac contraindications to exercise.

The test was terminated in the first minute of Stage 3 due to high blood pressure (234/108mmHg). Up-sloping ST-segment depression of 1.5mm was noticed in leads V4, V5 and V6 during the final stage of the test. Three ectopic heart beats (PVC) were also noted in the final stage.

Table 13.1 Results of sub-maximal graded exercise test on a treadmill (modified Bruce protocol)

Stage (3 min)	HR (bpm)	BP (mmHg)	RPE (Old Borg scale, 6–20)
Warm up	83	156/92	9
Stage 1	94	178/92	11
Stage 2	98	200/100	13
Stage 3	100	234/108	14
Recovery	90	192/92	9

VO_{2peak} was estimated from the GXT results using the ACSM metabolic equation (Thompson et al 2010):

$$VO_2 = ([S \times 0.1] + [S \times G \times 1.8]) + 3.5$$

Where S = treadmill speed in m.min^{-1} and G = grade (% incline) in decimal form (i.e. 10% = 0.1)

TP's estimated VO_{2peak} was 22.17 mL.kg^{-1}.min^{-1}, which was 'poor' for his age group.

Functional tests

These tests were conducted 15 minutes after the conclusion of the GXT to assess TP's muscle strength and endurance, and flexibility. Resting heart rate and blood pressure were taken prior to the functional tests (HR 85bpm; BP 146/90mmHg).

Hand grip strength left, 35kg; right, 40kg. Sit and reach test +5cm; YMCA sit up test 22 in 1 minute. 5RM leg press, pin-loaded machine 50kg. (5RM refers to the maximal load that can be lifted for 5, but not more than 5, repetitions.) No chest pain or symptoms of angina were recorded during these tests. TP reported fatigue in the legs and tightness in the lower back after the testing.

Assessment

As a result of the ST-segment depression during the GXT, and hypertension at low workloads, TP was referred back to his cardiologist for further tests. The ECG findings could indicate new atherosclerotic stenosis and ischaemia, or failure of the stent. The clinical exercise practitioner recommended that exercise workloads be currently set below the onset of ST-segment depression. Functional exercise test results show average hand grip strength; poor hamstring and lower back flexibility; poor abdominal strength; average leg strength.

Plan

TP was advised to exercise at a low to moderate intensity (9–12 Borg scale, HR to 98bpm) for at least 30 minutes daily, in line with ACSM and Heart Foundation guidelines (Thompson et al 2010; National Heart Foundation of Australia and the Cardiac Society of Australia and New Zealand 2008). Exercise intensities could be formalised after advice from TP's cardiologist. TP was also advised to consult his doctor about his high blood glucose, as his test suggests glucose intolerance or possible type 2 diabetes.

Barriers to exercise intervention
- Lack of previous regular exercise, and lack of knowledge about duration and intensities of exercise sessions.
- Recurring ischaemia and hypertension at moderate workloads.
- Anxiety and mild depression about his medical condition and management.
- Exercise intensities reliant on medical advice.
- Lack of time due to work commitments.
- Lack of self-confidence about doing regular exercise after a cardiac event.
- Possible fatigue and breathlessness during exercise.

Immediate goals of exercise intervention
- To maintain a basic level of cardiovascular fitness within symptom limits.
- To reduce or maintain blood glucose and cholesterol.
- To reduce body mass and body fat.
- To reduce resting and exercising blood pressure and RPE and heart rate.
- To reduce patient anxiety regarding his medical condition.

Immediate exercise strategies
- At least 30 minutes daily of easy to moderate constant aerobic exercise (eg: walking, indoor or outdoor cycling, swimming, aquatic exercise); HR 88–98bpm, RPE 9–13. Exercise sessions should be supervised by a clinical exercise practitioner for the first 6–12 weeks of the exercise program (standard Phase 2 cardiac rehabilitation exercise guidelines, for 12 weeks duration). HR and BP should be recorded at rest and during exercise and recovery.
- The clinical exercise practitioner should stress to TP that any signs or symptoms such as severe breathlessness, dizziness or chest pain should be reported to the clinical exercise practitioner and TP's GP. However, occasional mild symptoms should not preclude TP from doing low to moderate-intensity exercise.
- Two to three sessions (20 min) weekly of moderate-intensity resistance training, flexibility exercises and stretching. Can be included with aerobic exercise session. Can be home or gym-based. 10–12 reps, 2 sets, RPE 9–12. Sessions should initially be supervised by a clinical exercise practitioner.

- For sessions not monitored by a clinical exercise practitioner, TP takes his HR from radial pulse to monitor. TP to monitor his BP at home before and after exercise using a small electric BP cuff with digital readout.
- Encourage TP to walk to work, climb stairs instead of using the lift, be more active in the workplace.
- Encourage TP to reduce anxiety and depression by joining a cardiac rehab exercise group, involving family in his weekend exercise activities, discussing his fears with his GP or other health professionals.
- Quality of life questionnaire to be completed prior to starting the exercise program.

Long-term goals of exercise intervention
- Long-term goals relate to 3–12 months post-Phase 2 cardiac rehabilitation.
- Reduce risk of further cardiac events by reducing weight, blood pressure and heart rate, and cholesterol (total cholesterol, LDL, triglycerides).
- Reduce blood glucose and risk of type 2 diabetes.
- Reduce weight; reduce % body fat and increase lean muscle mass.
- Increase TP's exercise endurance — oxygen consumption (VO_2) and endurance, muscle capillary density and activity of oxidative enzymes.

Long-term exercise strategies
- Increase duration of aerobic exercise session to 60 minutes plus daily, including varying intensities of exercise. High-intensity exercise >90% maximum HR (RPE >16) should be avoided although intermittent higher-intensity exercise to 85% maximum HR (RPE 15) may be tolerated.
- Increase length of resistance training session to 30 minutes, three times per week.
- Involve client in more recreational physical activity that he sees as enjoyable.
- Add physical challenges to motivate the client (eg: Heart Foundation walks, fun runs, ocean swim, charity events).
- Maintain regular cardiac checks (eg: GXT every 6 or 12 months) in accordance with the cardiologist's advice.

Monitoring outcomes

- Follow up maximal or sub-maximal GXT after 12 weeks of exercise program (typical Phase 2 cardiac rehabilitation exercise program and follow-up).
- Client monitors his own resting, training and recovery heart rates.
- Weekly monitoring resting blood pressure.
- Fasting cholesterol and glucose tests repeated after 12 weeks.
- Quality of life questionnaire to be completed after 12 weeks for comparison with pre-program questionnaire.
- Anthropometric and functional tests repeated after 12 weeks.

Progress and outcomes

TP underwent a supervised maximal GXT with his cardiologist, with the ST-segment depression and high blood pressures occurring again during stage 3 of the treadmill test. Further tests showed that the original stent had failed, and it was replaced. Furthermore, a 50% blockage of the left circumflex artery had developed so a second stent was inserted. TP was also prescribed an ACE-inhibitor for his hypertension. TP began a Phase 2 cardiac rehabilitation exercise program, exercising with a group 3 days per week (indoor cycling and resistance exercises), and walking for 30 minutes on alternate days. He played nine holes of golf, and went for a long easy walk (60–120 minutes) with his family on most weekends. TP was also referred to a dietitian to discuss nutritional strategies to reduce weight, cholesterol and glucose.

After 8 weeks of rehabilitation exercise TP's outcome measures were:

- weight 100kg; body fat 29%; BMI 31.5; waist 109cm; hip 108cm; waist–hip ratio 1.01; resting blood pressure 130/86mmHg; resting heart rate 60bpm
- functional tests: hand grip strength, left, 38kg; right, 41kg. Sit and reach test +11cm; YMCA sit up test 28 in 1 minute. 5RM leg press 60kg
- fasting cholesterol: total cholesterol 5.0mmol/L, LDL 2.3mmol/L, HDL 1.6mmol/L, triglycerides 1.0mmol/L. Fasting glucose test 6.0mmol/L.

The 12 week follow-up maximal GXT is recommended to monitor cardiac function. After 12 weeks of exercise and another GXT TP had no further problems with his stents and was referred for annual GXT with is cardiologist. It is recommended that TP continue with his exercise and dietary plan, and that these be monitored regularly. TP may need further treatment for high blood glucose.

Summary of key lessons

- It is important to monitor cardiac function using ECG and exercise responses during the rehabilitation process. The onset of signs and symptoms could indicate the need for further surgical procedures or changes in patient medication. Referring cardiologists or doctors should be advised of any signs of deteriorating cardiac function, angina, breathlessness or adverse changes in blood pressure during exercise.

- Significant reductions in blood pressure can occur with exercise, independent of patient medications. It must be stressed that patients should remain on their prescribed medication dosage while participating in structured exercise programs, until such time as their doctor decides to reduce or change the medication.

- TP was taking a beta-blocker medication, which is commonly prescribed to lower heart rate and cardiac output, and to help reduce blood pressure. As TP's heart rate remains low during exercise, it is advisable to set exercise intensities using either the Borg scale for rate of perceived exertion, or by using METs corresponding to the RPE rather than using a target heart rate (% of age-predicted maximum heart rate).

- It was suggested that TP follow a more healthy diet (possibly with a dietitian's aid) to lower cholesterol and glucose, as well as body fat. Dietary changes as well as regular exercise will lower the risk of a further cardiac event.

- During the initial 8 weeks of the Phase 2 program, TP made significant improvements in weight, body fat, blood pressure, fasting cholesterol and glucose levels, lower back flexibility and strength. Because he was initially very unfit, we would expect him to improve relatively quickly during the first few months of exercise, and then to plateau. Clients should be advised to expect this common adaptation, and that their program may be modified to increase the stimulus to maintain further health and fitness gains. Intermittent higher-intensity exercise can be prescribed for stable Phase 2 cardiac patients but should be used in conjunction with low or moderate-intensity exercise bouts.

DISCUSSION Questions

1 Why is it important for regular incremental exercise tests to be conducted with diagnosed CAD patients, or those with a family history and high risk of CAD?

2 In TP's case, was there any significance in the fact that he had not done a graded exercise test (GXT) during the pre-surgery period when he was symptomatic for CAD?

3 Why did the clinical exercise practitioner decide to terminate the sub-maximal GXT? Why was TP recommended to undergo another GXT with his cardiologist?

4 What would be the recommended weekly energy expenditure for a client such as TP to maintain good health, maximise his weight loss and reduce cholesterol and blood glucose?

5 What are the benefits of using quality of life questionnaires with cardiac rehabilitation patients?

6 After 12 weeks of Phase 2 cardiac rehabilitation exercise, TP's cardiologist declares that he is haemodymically stable. Describe and justify the sorts of changes you would make to his exercise program after 12 weeks.

7 TP is taking a statin to control his cholesterol. What are some of the side-effects of this medication which may effect TP's exercise responses?

CASE STUDY 2: MODERATE AORTIC STENOSIS

Subjective

SL is a 57-year-old male who presented to his GP with a recent history of light headedness, two fainting episodes and some chest discomfort. His symptoms were associated with occasional episodes of physical activity during an otherwise sedentary existence, but light headedness occurred once whilst he was watching TV. Up until 12 months prior to these episodes, SL had been fit and very active in adventure sports and activities, had led many coastal and mountain bushwalks in Australia and New Zealand, and had been a member of mountaineering expeditions in Europe and North America. A change to his job and the break-up of his marriage led to depression, and he ceased regular exercise and gained 12kg in the previous 12 months. His blood pressure had previously been borderline high (average of 142/88mmHg for the preceding 3 years), but his lipids and fasting glucose were normal. He had never smoked and rarely drinks alcohol.

Objective

SL's GP measured his current blood pressure at 110/70mmHg, lower than previously, and noted a new ejection (early systolic) heart murmur. Given his previous active lifestyle that had recently been replaced by sedentary living and weight gain, the GP was concerned about the unexpected *fall* in blood pressure and the new murmur and referred SL for a stress echocardiograph. This test was conducted at a teaching hospital under cardiologist supervision 1 week after the GP appointment, using a treadmill and the Bruce protocol. At rest, a moderate aortic (bicuspid) valve stenosis was identified and the left ventricular:aortic pressure gradient was estimated to be 35mmHg using the modified Bernoulli's equation; the latter provided further clinical evidence that the level of stenosis was moderate.

There was no echocardiographic evidence of left ventricular hypertrophy. At peak exercise (2 minutes of stage 4 of the Bruce protocol), the ECG exhibited horizontal ST depression of up to 1.8mm in the anterior and lateral leads, accompanied by some chest discomfort and a plateau in systolic blood pressure. Immediately after exercise, the echocardiograph exhibited normal left ventricular wall motion and a mild aortic regurgitation that was not evident at rest. The left ventricular:aortic pressure gradient at peak exercise was calculated to have risen to 42mmHg.

Assessment

The cause of aortic stenosis in this case is unclear, but is most likely due to a congenital malformation of the aortic valve.

Progress

SL next underwent an angiogram to rule out atherosclerosis as the cause of his ischaemic signs and symptoms and the angiogram confirmed this. He was placed on a waiting list, estimated to be 9 months, for a percutaneous aortic valve replacement. (Anti-hypertensive medications were contraindicated because his blood pressure was unexpectedly low.) The client was advised that the best course of action whilst on the waiting list was conservative medical management and lifestyle interventions comprising exercise, nutrition, and treatments for his chronic anxiety and depression. Losing weight and gaining fitness were paramount to SL's recovery, rehabilitation and return to an active lifestyle following surgery. The client was referred to a clinical exercise practitioner for an appropriate exercise plan prior to surgery.

Plan

The clinical exercise practitioner obtained the results of all recent investigations and conducted a sub-ischaemic threshold exercise test on a motorised treadmill for the purposes of planning an appropriate program. The results of the exercise test are summarised in Table 13.2.

A second series of resistance exercise tests was conducted, using seven movement patterns involving all major joints. The client was asked to perform a 3RM test for each pattern; 3RM was considered safer than 1RM for this client. (3RM refers to the maximal load that can be lifted for 3, but not more than 3, repetitions; 1RM is a similar term identifying loads that be lifted just once.)

To eliminate an order effect, the same tests were repeated over the next few weeks using alternative sequences. An average of the results for three of the seven movement patterns is shown in Table 13.3.

The immediate goals were to assist the client to experience an active lifestyle again, albeit within the limits of his current condition, and to counsel him on both the safety and benefits of exercise. Emphases were focused on trying to achieve immediate improvements to his symptoms of anxiety and depression, and his self-efficacy with regard to exercise and physical activity. With regard to the latter, he was currently fearful of any form of exertion, and before and since his diagnosis, he followed a sedentary lifestyle. Counselling and motivational interviewing techniques were employed. He was reassured in plain language that there was no angiographic evidence of coronary atherosclerosis or left ventricular hypertrophy. Further, he was reassured that exercise and physical activity would not promote any progression of valvular, vascular or myocardial disease so long as he stays within the bounds of moderate-intensity training. The probable cause of his chest pain

Table 13.2 Results of sub-ischaemic threshold exercise test

Stage	Speed + grade %	VO$_2$(% peak)*	HR(% peak)	O$_2$sat%	BP	RPE	Comment
Rest (pre-exercise)	–	–	73 (43%)	99	133/83	–	BP higher than in GP clinic: anticipation of exercise test
Sub-maximal exercise	5 kph, 0%	17.5 (63%)	121 (72%)	99	155/82	11	Functional walking speed
Peak exercise	5 kph, 6%	27.7 (100%)	151 (90%)	98	156/75	16	Stopped when ST depression reached 1mm; not accompanied by chest pain; blood pressure plateau as for exercise test in hospital
1 min recovery	–	–	123 (74%)	98	152/79	–	Blood pressure remained at plateau
3 min recovery	–	–	110 (66%)	99	139/84	–	Heart rate slow to recover to pre-exercise level
10 min recovery	–	–	76 (46%)	99	110/70	–	Recovery to pre-exercise levels

Note: *Peak exercise for this test (below the peak intensity for the symptom-limited test conducted in the hospital clinic); RPE = Borg 6–20 point scale.

during exercise was explained to him in plain language and this served to reassure him further. It was helpful that this client had a long history of positive experiences of exercise and recreational activities, and he drew on those memories and understandings early in his program with the clinical exercise practitioner.

The main approach was for the clinical exercise practitioner to design a combined aerobic and resistance training program that did not produce signs or symptoms associated with his valvular disease. Blood pressures, heart rates, oxygen saturation (HbO$_2$sat%) and ratings of perceived exertion should all be monitored in the early sessions. This monitoring should be done during aerobic exercise and immediately following resistance exercises. The clinical exercise practitioner should estimate left ventricular systolic pressures by adding the expected left ventricular:aortic (= brachial artery) pressure gradient to brachial artery systolic pressures and ensure that peak exercise intensity does not generate left ventricular pressures above 220mmHg.

Exercise intensity and volume needed to commence at low levels, with gradual increases as SL gained both fitness and confidence. The clinical exercise practitioner needed to explain to SL that signs or symptoms may appear from time to time, and to report these as soon as possible to the clinical exercise practitioner and GP, but these should not preclude SL from continuing with the program, albeit with some modifications.

Intermediate goals were to prepare the client for surgery in approximately 9 months time, and to enhance SL's recovery from surgery, early

Table 13.3 Mean results for three of seven movement patterns

Stage*	HR(% peak)	BP	RPE	Comment
Rest (pre-exercise)	77 (46%)	138/81	–	BP higher than in GP clinic: anticipation of exercise test
Upper limb: bilateral elbow flexion/extension	159 (95%)	156/125	15	Upper limb exercises cause heart rate and blood pressure to rise higher, relative to similar intensities of exercise for lower limb and trunk
Lower limb: bilateral knee extension/flexion	144 (86%)	144/110	16	Make certain that the client does not hold breath during exercise
Trunk: sit-ups with disc weight across chest	145 (87%)	152/115	17	Breathe out on the way up; breathe in on the way down
10 min recovery	99 (59%)	110/70	–	Recovery to pre-exercise levels

Note: *Heart rate was permitted to return to within 10 b.min^{-1} of pre-exercise levels before commencing the next pattern; BP = blood pressure was measured within 30 seconds following each movement pattern. Inferences were then made about exercise blood pressures. It is recognised that it would have been preferred to measure blood pressure during the actual exercise phase, but the technology was not available for this; RPE = Borg 6–20 point scale.

rehabilitation and an ultimate return to an active lifestyle. Secondary goals include continuation of avoidance of symptoms, weight loss to reduce cardiovascular loads and improvements to SL's symptoms of anxiety and depression. Client goals need to gradually overtake practitioner goals in order to promote self-management and self-efficacy.

Monitoring of signs and symptoms should only be needed in the event that these have persisted. A careful progression from low intensity to moderate but not high intensity for both aerobic and resistance training should reduce the need for ongoing monitoring. However, it is advisable that the client continues to exercise at least once per week under the supervision of the clinical exercise practitioner in order that this can be checked.

In this case, long-term goals refer to those applying post-surgery and post-rehabilitation. Since SL does not have heart failure or coronary artery disease, SL is expected to make a full recovery following aortic valve replacement. The cause of SL's aortic stenosis was unlikely to be preventable. Therefore attention to risk factor modification for

secondary prevention or relapse of aortic stenosis is not an issue here. Rather, the focus should be on returning the client to his previously active lifestyle, and to use exercise and physical activity to improve his fitness, body composition and metabolic profile, quality of life (QoL) and anxiety and stress levels, and reduce the risk of a range of preventable conditions such as depression and cardiovascular and metabolic diseases.

Following discharge from hospital, SL will join a Phase 2 (out-patient) cardiac rehabilitation program mainly for the benefits of receiving advice and support as to which modes and intensities of exercise are appropriate during the healing and rehabilitation phases. Gradually upper body strength and flexibility exercises will be included.

Outcomes

SL recovered fully from the surgery and after 12 months of supervised exercise, he had returned to his previous active lifestyle of participation, but not leadership, in overnight bushwalks, mountaineering expeditions and other recreational pursuits. His symptoms of depression had resolved somewhat, but he needed to take care of himself in this area.

Discussion

Any exercise or physical activity that induces myocardial ischaemia or generates left ventricular systolic pressures above approximately 220mmHg is contraindicated. SL adopted a sedentary lifestyle since his life-changing events 12 months ago. This was reinforced by his recent diagnosis of moderate aortic stenosis, accompanied by a new fear of exercise and exertion. He was also confronted with the challenge of exercising at a higher weight than ever before.

Summary of key lessons

- *Severe* aortic stenosis is an *absolute* contraindication to exercise, whereas clients with moderate stenosis may participate in carefully supervised and monitored programs that do not provoke signs or symptoms of valvular disease.
- Clients with aortic stenosis should be monitored during aerobic exercises and immediately after resistance exercises to ensure that they do not become breathless, and that their left ventricular pressure does not exceed 220mmHg during systole.

DISCUSSION Questions

1 Why aortic regurgitation might appear at peak exercise in this case, but not be evident at rest?

2 What are the left ventricular:aortic pressure gradients for mild, moderate and severe aortic stenosis?

3 Can brachial artery sphygmomanometry be used to *measure* left ventricular pressure during exercise in this case?

4 Can brachial artery sphygmomanometry be used to *estimate* left ventricular pressure during exercise in this case?

5 Why is acute and severe breathlessness sometimes a problem for people with aortic stenosis when they exercise?

6 SL had extremely good outcomes from both the surgery and the exercise intervention. If SL had clinical evidence of left ventricular ejection hypertrophy at the time of the first series of investigations, then how might the outcomes and ongoing treatments have been different?

CASE STUDY 3: HYPERTROPHIC CARDIOMYOPATHY (HCM)

Subjective

JP, an 18-year-old male and talented young soccer player, who has been included in the Australian (u/19) National soccer team, struggles to improve on his current fitness level. The problem is that he experiences unexplained breathlessness after mild exertion, which he reckons hinders his ability to improve his fitness level. His coach believes that this symptom is all in the mind and due to inadequate physical conditioning and instructed JP to 'toughen up' and encouraged him to train even harder.

JP's BMI is 25.5kg.m^{-1} and he is not using any prescribed medication. JP's dad succumbed to sudden death at an age of 40 years when he played soccer for the local soccer club, while his uncle (JP's dad's brother) succumbed to sudden death during an athletic event at 17 years of age. JP's younger brother (16 years) is a keen cricket player who is asymptomatic. JP's mother was concerned about JP and makes an appointment with the clinical exercise practitioner to seek further advice.

Objective

A thorough questionnaire is important to screen the medical and family history of athletes and their relatives. Questions should comprise of the following: history of heart murmur, history of hypertension, history of unexplained shortness of breath, history of syncope during or after exercise, chest pain or discomfort during exercise, family history of cardiovascular disease or premature death before the age of 50, family history of significant disability secondary to a cardiac event or aetiology (eg: arrhythmias, hypertrophic cardiomyopathy [HCM], long QT syndrome, ventricular tachycardia, premature coronary artery disease, Marfan's syndrome).

During the assessment, JP's personal and family history is assessed for possible risk factors that could put him at high risk of sudden death. The family history revealed JP's uncle frequently experienced dizziness, sudden burst of palpitations and severe shortness of breath with exercise and competition. JP's uncle succumbed to unexpected sudden death, while collapsing during an 800m middle-distance race at school level, at an age of 17 years. According to JP's mother, her husband (JP's dad), who also succumbed to sudden death, did not complain of any abovementioned symptoms (indicated in the questionnaire), prior to his unexpected death.

A sub-maximal cycle ergometer test in conjunction with an exercise electrocardiograph (ECG) is conducted on JP to determine his aerobic fitness level and possible ECG abnormalities. JP's exercise ECG revealed ventricular arrhythmias, premature ventricular contractions (PVCs), in the form of a triplet and the clinical exercise practitioner decided to terminate the test. JP's exercise heart rate was 150bpm with an RPE rating of 15 on the 7–20 point Borg scale, prior to termination. The clinical exercise practitioner decided to liaise with JP's physician to be present during a maximal graded exercise test (GXT) to further explore JP's situation. During this GXT (in the presence of the physician), JP's test is terminated after he experienced near syncope, showed impaired systolic blood pressure response of > 10mm.HG^{-1} decrease from baseline blood pressure, despite an increase in work load, and an increased heart rate of 230bpm. JP's perceived exertion was an RPE scale reading of 19 (Borg scale) and 9 on the OMNI scale, prior to test termination.

The clinical exercise practitioner suggested that JP, as well as his brother, should undergo further clinical assessment with a sports cardiologist. The cardiologist used two-dimensional echocardiography to measure the thickness of JP and his brother's left ventricular wall and the size of their left ventricular cavities. His brother's left ventricular wall thickness and the size of his left ventricular cavity were within normal range, though JP's left ventricular wall thickness measured 15mm and his left ventricular cavity 42mm. In addition, the Doppler echocardiography also showed normal LV filling which did make it difficult for the cardiologist to differentiate, because it can be compatible with either hypertrophic cardiomyopathy (HCM) or 'athlete's heart'. The sports cardiologist also tested JP's dynamic left ventricular outflow by listening with the stethoscope to his left sternal border for murmurs (vibratory sound). A client with a significant obstruction usually presents a systolic ejection murmur. No murmur was detected by the cardiologist.

The cardiologist also asked JP to temporarily abstain from any exercise and soccer training in order to assess the dynamic changes occurring in his left ventricular wall thickness by means of high-quality echocardiography during a 3-month deconditioning period. This method can assist in distinguishing between pathologic (as in HCM) and physiologic (as in elite, conditioned athletes) left ventricular hypertrophy. JP was also asked to wear a Holter ECG for 48 hours to determine the presence of ECG abnormalities such as ventricular arrhythmias, sustained supraventricular arrhythmias or non-sustained supraventricular arrhythmias. JP showed a high level of exercise-specific self-efficacy toward walking as he believes with a 100% confidence that he is able to walk continuously for 40 minutes per session.

Assessment

In approximately 90% of clients with HCM, the ECG is abnormal. The ambulatory Holter ECG did show some PVCs at rest. Usually PVCs are harmless and often no treatment is required. The problem with the exercise ECG was that these PVCs did not disappear during physical exertion, but increased instead, which may be indicative of coronary artery disease or cardiomyopathy. In JP's case the sports cardiologist is concerned, because if JP has HCM, these PVCs can lead to more serious ventricular tachycardia or ventricular fibrillation, with life threatening consequences. The cardiologist concluded after the outcome of the GXT results that there is some reason to believe that JP may have some indication of possible HCM or heart disease.

JP's aerobic fitness (46 ml.kg.min^{-1}) was < below 50 ml.kg.min^{-1}. This finding was in line with asymptomatic clients with HCM who possess mild hypertrophy (between 13–16mm), which is usually associated with a lower aerobic fitness (< 50ml.kg.min^{-1}) versus higher aerobic fitness (> 50ml.kg.min^{-1} and often > 70ml.kg.min^{-1}) in elite well trained athletes.

The cardiologist mentioned to JP that due to the fact that some athletes (< 2%) with exercise-conditioned hearts, as well as some clients with HCM fall in the 'grey category' of those with left ventricular wall thickness of 13 to 16mm, it therefore creates diagnostic ambiguity. Differentiation between 'athlete's heart' and HCM can create economic, legal and ethical complications. For example, if the cardiologist concludes that the client's left ventricular (LV) hypertrophy is due to chronic exercise training, no economic losses/income from sport, due to unnecessary disqualification of the athlete from participation, would occur. In contrast, if the client is diagnosed with HCM, it would be in the best interest of the client's health to withdraw from all high-intensity competition sport as it may trigger possible sudden death.

In JP's case, he is one of the few people with HCM who possesses mild hypertrophy as reflected in his left ventricular wall thickness (15mm) that overlaps with the grey zone of 13–16mm, which could also be present in some elite athletes. However, his left ventricular cavity diameter that is less than 45mm is more typical of people with typical HCM.

Abnormalities in LV filling are present in 80% of HCM clients. Because the Doppler echocardiography also showed normal LV filling in JP's case, it was difficult for the cardiologist to differentiate, because it can be compatible with either HCM or 'athlete's heart'. The absence of a murmur in JP's case suggests that his condition was the non-obstructive form of HCM.

In JP's case no distinctive changes in left ventricular wall thickness has occurred due to the deconditioning phase of 3 months, which is indicative of HCM. In contrast, elite athletes showed a significant decrease in wall thickness of 2–5mm after three months of physical deconditioning. JP's three month deconditioning period, measured by means of high-quality echocardiography, showed no change in his ventricular wall thickness during this time period, which most likely indicates a pathologic enlarged left ventricle. The cardiologist concluded that this approach helped to distinguish between pathologic (as in HCM) and physiologic (as in elite, conditioned athletes) left ventricular hypertrophy. In an athlete's case, completion of a deconditioning phase usually leads to a significant decrease (2–5mm) in ventricular wall thickness. Considering all abovementioned findings, the cardiologist concluded that JP has HCM, albeit without specifically identifiable obstruction.

Plan

The 26th Bethesda Conference national consensus guidelines for athletic participation for selected cardiovascular abnormalities, recommend that athletes with HCM should not compete in vigorous, high-intensity activities or systematic isometric exercise (eg: heavy lifting) (Maron & Mitchell 1994). This recommendation is made regardless of medical treatment, absence of symptoms or implantation of a defibrillator. (Low-intensity sports such as rifling, golf, billiards and bowling are possible exceptions.) JP's cardiologist advises him to abstain from vigorous, physical activities and consider changing to a low-intensity sport. In addition, JP is prescribed beta-adrenergic blocking agents (ie: Metoprolol) to suppress PVCs during exertion and to prevent ventricular tachycardia and eventually ventricular flutter and fibrillation. The cardiologist also mentioned to JP that he would like to re-evaluate him at least twice a year, unless he experienced any symptoms which need further immediate medical follow up.

JP decided to take up ten-pin bowling as his future sport and expressed an interest in incorporating walking and light resistance training into his training. The clinical exercise practitioner designed the training programs (aerobic, bowling, and resistance) and discussed them with the cardiologist prior to implementation. The cardiologist was initially reluctant to allow JP to do resistance training, however, due to the fact that the medication controlled the PVCs (preventing ventricular tachycardia), he agreed to allow JP to commence resistance exercise.

It is also suggested that JP needs to follow a healthy diet in combination with regular walking at an RPE of 11–13 on the 7–20 point Borg scale or 2–5 on the 1–10 OMNI scale. JP committed himself to do two bowling sessions per week, in addition to three walking sessions of 40 minutes per session. Resistance training with light weights whilst focusing on slow, controlled movements is also part of his intervention. It consists of one set of 8–10 exercises (major muscle groups) with high repetitions (1 x 12–20 reps) at an RPE of 10–13 on the 7–20 point scale or 2–5 on the 1–10 point OMNI scale, twice per week (non-consecutive days). JP is instructed to avoid straining and to stop exercise, if warning symptoms such as dizziness, near syncope or syncope, unexplained breathlessness, chest discomfort or pain, palpitations or dysrhythmias, occur. He is taught the correct breathing technique (exhale during exertion, inhale during relaxation) to prevent Valsalva manoeuvre and only to increase the loads by 5% when he can comfortably execute 20 repetitions.

JP is wearing a medical bracelet as an important safety measure in the event of an emergency to provide first aiders with medical detail of his condition. Because it is stressful not only for JP, but also for the family, to adjust to a chronic disease such as HCM, a paediatric psychiatrist and accredited sports psychologist were also consulted to assist JP to lead and maintain a relatively normal life. For example, due to JP's competitive nature as a promising soccer player, it was a challenge to adapt to his lower-intensity exercise program.

Outcome

Fortunately, due to the fact that the cardiologist managed to diagnose JP with HCM, and the support of his medical team (cardiologist, clinical exercise practitioner, sports psychologist, dietitian), caring family and friends enabled him to adjust to a new lifestyle. JP expressed his gratitude being able to lead a relatively normal life despite his chronic disease, although he was initially very disappointed as he had visualised himself in the colours of the Socceroos — a dream that will no longer be realised.

Discussion

Sudden death during exercise is typically associated with two forms of heart disease; coronary atherosclerosis causing the acute heart attack (usually in those older than 40 years and the most common cause), and HCM (usually in those under 40 years and the second most common cause). Despite a preponderance in the young, HCM has the potential for clinical presentation during any phase of life (infancy to > 90 years of age). A practical concern is that HCM is a severe disease, and those with HCM are at high risk of sudden death, irrespective of whether they exercise or not. HCM is very hard to detect medically because many victims are asymptomatic until the fatal incident (sudden death). Also, the clinical differentiation of the exercise-conditioned enlarged heart of the athlete from the pathologic enlarged heart of those with actual hypertrophic cardiomyopathy is difficult to distinguish, even for those with specialist training.

Summary of key lessons

- Cardiomyopathies in the young (12–35 years of age) are the most frequent cause of unexpected, sudden, non-traumatic cardiac deaths (Liberthson 1996; Maron 2001; Noakes 2003).

- Hypertrophic cardiomyopathy is the most common cardiomyopathy (an estimated incidence of 0.2% in the general young population and at 36% the most prevalent cause of sudden death in young competitive athletes).

- Differentiation from the physiologic cardiac changes associated with chronic athletic conditioning (athlete's heart) and accurate evaluation of the morphologic cardiac abnormalities (left ventricular hypertrophy) form the basis of the diagnosis of hypertrophic cardiomyopathy.

- All children and young adults with HCM must be evaluated to define safe limits of physical activity and re-evaluated periodically to ensure the ongoing safety of participation, which would usually require referral to a cardiologist.

- Exercise ECG testing is not always a reliable measurement tool to detect the presence of HMC or predict risk of sudden death (Brukner & Khan 2007; Landry & Bernhardt 2003).

- Do not underestimate the value of a health risk questionnaire (with appropriate questions that also cover the medical history of close relatives) in the screening process of young athletes, especially if they show symptoms such as dyspnoea, dizziness, fainting, chest discomfort or pain during exertion, exercise intolerance or palpitations/dysrhythmias

- There are no therapies known that can cure HCM. Current therapies can only improve the symptoms and reduce the risk of HCM.

- Regular exercise may delay or prevent coronary atherosclerosis, but there is no evidence that exercise improves or aggravates HCM (Noakes 2003).

- Low-intensity physical activity may be allowed based on clients' clinical status, relative risk of arrhythmias and severe left ventricular dysfunction (eg: potential outflow obstruction from the left ventricle to the left atrium).

- Young competitive athletes with HCM should consider withdrawal from high-intensity sports/ exercise as high-intensity exercise may trigger sudden death. In the absence of specific obstruction, decisions to cease high-intensity training and competition are subject to much debate.

DISCUSSION Questions

1 List all the symptoms mentioned in this case example that may be associated with HCM. What other additional symptoms and clinical expressions may also be associated with HCM?

2 Do you think the clinical exercise practitioner decided wisely to terminate the sub-maximal exercise test?

3 What is the importance of listening to murmurs of the heart?

4 JP's intervention worked very well for 12 months and the cardiologist was satisfied with him adjusting so well to his new lifestyle. Unfortunately he experienced some palpitations and follow-up assessment showed ventricular tachycardia which worried his treating cardiologist. How might JP's exercise management be altered at this stage?

CASE STUDY 4: PERIPHERAL ARTERIAL DISEASE (PAD)

Subjective

James is a 62-year-old man with peripheral arterial disease (PAD), which he reports is beginning to limit his ability to walk to the shops, mow the lawn and walk the dog. His ankle-brachial index is 0.74 and he experiences intermittent claudication, usually with onset at 250–300m of flat ground walking. James was also diagnosed with type 2 diabetes 4 years ago. He takes his blood sugar readings regularly and his last fasting blood sugar level was 8.5mmol/L. There are no signs or symptoms of microvascular complications such as retinopathy, neuropathy or nephropathy. He also has mild hypertension and takes Ramipril and Metformin. James has been referred by his general practitioner (GP) for an exercise plan to target his functional limitations and to improve his health.

James works 4 days a week, 9 a.m. to 5 p.m., in an office job. He lives with his wife, who does not work and who is very supportive of her husband. He does not smoke, but consumes alcohol most days. James does not engage in regular exercise, mainly because he dislikes it and it causes too much discomfort in his legs and also leaves him a little breathless. He says that he is willing to give it a go though because the GP told him that it might make him feel better, but would prefer to undertake an unsupervised home-based program.

Objective

James weighs 110kg and is 179cm tall. He has a waist measure of 125cm, and his resting blood pressure is 142/82mmHg. A progressive clinical exercise test was initially performed to determine safe-training levels. During the test (see Table 13.4), James managed to begin stage 3, but stopped after 20 seconds due to ischaemic pain in the right leg (4/4 on claudication scale). Total exercise time

was 6 minutes 20 seconds. ECG and BP responses were normal. It took 3 minutes 15 seconds for his claudication pain to disappear completely. His calculated $VO_{2peak} \approx 20$ml/kg/min.

After recovery James completed a 6-minute walk test (6MWT) as a measure of functional performance; walked 440m in the 6 minutes and reached 3/4 on the claudication pain scale. His onset of claudication occurred at approximately 250m. Recovery to relief of pain took 2 minutes.

A series of 1RM tests for both upper and lower body muscle groups were also performed by James in order to determine training loads for resistance training.

Assessment

According to the Rutherford classification scheme for ischaemia (Rutherford et al 1997), James has moderate intermittent claudication. His ischaemic pain limits his walking distance and activities of daily living, James also has a range of other risk factors including obesity (BMI 34.3), in particular central adiposity (waist circumference >100), hypertension (mild hypertension with medication) and sedentariness (based on office job and lack of participation in regular exercise). The claudication pain experienced during walking would contribute to the risk factors. James' claudication pain will also be a barrier to exercise and his psychological response to the exercise training must be assessed and monitored closely in the initial stages in order to maintain adherence.

Plan

The aim of the exercise plan is to improve James' walking capacity and to target his risk factors. James will be encouraged to undertake an interval walking program to beyond onset of claudication pain beginning at 2–3 days per week, building to most days. He will also be encouraged to initially undertake a supervised progressive resistance

Table 13.4 Results of graded exercise test

| | | | | | Graded exercise test | | | | |
Stage	Time	Speed	Grade	HR	BP	ST	RPE	ECG	Claudication scale
Rest	0	0 km/h	0 %	79	142/82	–		N	0
1	3	2.7 km/h	0 %	93	146/80	–	9	N	0
2	6	4.0 km/h	2 %	102	152/80	-0.2	11	N	1–3
3	9	5.5 km/h	4 %	110		-0.5	15	N	4
4	12	6.7 km/h	6%						
5	15	8.0 km/h	8%						
6	18	8.8 km/h	10 %						
7	21	9.6 km/h	12 %						
Recovery									
1	1 min			106	156/76	–		N	2
2	2 min			100	150/76	–		N	1
3	3 min			92	144/78	–		N	1
4	4 min			88				N	0
5	5 min			84	144/78			N	0
6	6 min			84		–		N	0

training program 2–3 days per week, as well as some other form of aerobic exercise (other than walking), to help target his risk factors. Once he has had some improvement in his condition and is adhering to his exercise program, we will tailor a program for home based exercise. James will need to continue exercising on an ongoing basis so it will be important to discuss his barriers to exercise and options for support networks to help him with adherence. James will also be provided with educational materials on his condition, diet, foot care, and tips to avoid sedentary behaviours.

James presented with PAD and type 2 diabetes, which is not surprising because type 2 diabetes is a common comorbidity for PAD. Therefore, the exercise plan needed to account for both conditions, plus his risk factors, in order to meet the purpose of the referral. To begin with, we determined a series of short- and long-term goals in consultation with the client.

Short-term goals

- Increasing initial claudication distance on flat ground to 300m in 3 months.
- Reducing waist circumference to <115cm in 3 months.
- Completing three supervised sessions and one unsupervised walking session per week for the first 6–12 weeks.

Long-term goals

- To complete 500m 6MWT at the end of 6 months of training, while increasing the initial claudication distance during the test to 400m.
- Reducing waist circumference to <100cm in 6 months.
- Completing two supervised sessions and at least two unsupervised walking sessions per week by 6 months.

James' exercise plan included three main exercise strategies. First, to improve walking capacity, James participated in interval walking, starting with three times per week, but aiming to progress to 7 days per week. To improve walking capacity in those with PAD, provocation of claudication is recommended. However, the current research evidence suggests that walking to maximal pain is not necessarily better for improving walking distance than walking to tolerable pain levels. Therefore, interval walking commenced with James walking to pain onset, resting until pain subsided and then repeating the interval. This intensity was considered to be an appropriate starting point for someone who presented with a dislike for exercise and a history of sedentary behaviour. The intervals were repeated until 20 minutes of walking time had been accumulated. To progress the program, the total walking time accumulated was gradually increased to 40 minutes, and James also walked to beyond pain onset with each interval.

To target his risk factors, we included moderate-intensity aerobic exercise, 3 days per week. Exercise was commenced at 65% of age-predicted HRmax for 30 minutes, with the view to progressing to 70% HRmax for 50 minutes, 4 days per week. The key here though was the mode of exercise; the mode must be one that permits heart rate to be elevated sufficiently to ensure exercise is of the correct intensity, but not one that is limited by claudication pain. We used an elliptical machine to simulate pole-striding, Other options could be cycling, or arm cranking if cycling or pole-striding provoke claudication.

We also included a moderate to high intensity, progressive resistance training program to assist with improving walking capacity plus target risk factors and type 2 diabetes. Exercises included calf press, ankle dorsiflexion, thigh extension, leg press, leg curl, hip extension, hip flexion, hip abduction/adduction, chest press, seated row, and lat pull-down. Intensity was commenced at 8–10 repetitions at 60% 1RM, progressing to 8–10 repetitions at 80% 1RM.

Due to the walking program requiring exercise to pain and because of his history of low exercise levels and dislike for exercise, it was important to initially encourage James to attend supervised sessions so that we were able to assist with motivation and overcoming new barriers to exercise as they arose. Supervised sessions also allowed us to monitor subjective and objective responses to exercise, such as pain levels, rating of perceived exertion, heart rate and blood pressure, and educate James on self-monitoring these signs and symptoms. Once he was coping well with the program, meeting adherence goals and moving towards achieving his other short-term goals, we redesigned the program to increase the number of unsupervised sessions and allow more of his program to be completed at home. In particular, his entire walking program was able to be completed at home through education about, and self-monitoring of, claudication pain levels. Here, he was able to walk with his wife, who assisted with encouraging adherence.

Discussion

Two exercise tests were conducted as part of James' assessment. The symptom-limited clinical exercise test was used to assess his suitability for participation in an exercise program and to assess for thresholds in order to provide us with a safe yet effective exercise plan. Although we expected to provoke symptoms of intermittent claudication, we were also interested to find out whether his blood pressure and ECG response would be normal within his exercise limits. The data from this clinical exercise test provided us with information on walking speeds that led to maximal ischemic pain as well as heart rate and blood pressure responses that were safe in the event that non-walking exercise was included in our exercise plan. That is, based on James reaching a peak heart rate of 110bpm and his ECG and BP response being normal at this level, we know that we can have him exercising up to around 70% of his age-predicted heart rate maximum without undue risk. In addition to the exercise data, this test gave us an indication of the recovery time James would need while undertaking his interval training program.

We also wanted to include a functional walking test that allowed James to walk at a pace that better reflected what he might walk at in the community. The 6MWT was chosen because it has been shown to correlate better with physical activity during daily life, than treadmill measures in persons with PAD (McDermott et al 2008, 2009). The data from this test could also be used later to measure the effect of the exercise program.

Summary of key lessons

- Exercise assessments should be patient-specific, designed to gain information for a safe, yet effective, exercise program and to assist with evaluating the effectiveness of the exercise program.
- Clients with chronic, lifestyle-related diseases who attend for an exercise plan, typically present with more than one chronic disease plus risk factors. Type 2 diabetes, for example, is common in people with PAD, therefore, the exercise plan needs to account for comorbidities in addition to the primary presenting pathology.
- The patient approaches the exercise practitioner for advice and programming to help improve their condition and QoL. While it is important to address the patient's needs, it is also important that results are achieved, and sometimes this requires the patient to step outside their comfort zone.

DISCUSSION Questions

1 Why does James experience ischaemic symptoms during walking but not at rest?

2 Similarly, why do James' symptoms present during walking and not during upper body exercise?

3 An expected outcome of the walking exercise program is an increase in initial and absolute claudication times/distances. Discuss the physiological mechanism(s) which might explain these improvements in walking capacity.

4 What information about James' exercise program would you report back to the referring medical practitioner?

5 Explain James' fasting glucose test results. What are the risks during exercise for someone with elevated blood glucose levels?

6 James' clinical exercise program was developed by a team of allied health practitioners. What are the advantages and pitfalls of team-based care?

REFERENCES

Brukner P, Khan K (2007) *Clinical Sports Medicine* (3rd ed). Sydney: McGraw-Hill

Landry GL, Bernhardt DT (2003) *Essentials of Primary Care Sports Medicine*. Champaign, IL: Human Kinetics

Liberthson RR (1996) Sudden death from cardiac causes in children and young adults. *New England Journal of Medicine*, 334:1039–44

Maron BJ (2001) Sudden cardiac death due to hypertrophic cardiomyopathy in young athletes. In: Thompson PD (ed.) *Exercise & Sports Cardiology*, pp 189–209

Maron BJ, Mitchell JH (1994) 26th Bethesda Conference. Recommendations for determining eligibility for competition in athletes with cardiovascular abnormalities. *Journal of the American Cardiology*, 24:845–99

McDermott M, Ades P, Guralnik JM et al (2009) Treadmill exercise and resistance training in patients with peripheral arterial disease with and without intermittent claudication: a randomized controlled trial. *Journal of the American Medical Association*, 301(2):165–74

McDermott MM, Ades PA, Dyer A, et al (2008) Corridor-based functional performance measures correlate better with physical activity during daily life than treadmill measures in persons with peripheral arterial disease. *Journal of Vascular Surgery*, 48:1231–7

McGuigan MRM, Bronks R, Newton R, et al (2001) Resistance training in patients with peripheral arterial disease: Effects on myosin forms, fiber type distribution, and capillary supply to skeletal muscle. *J Gerontol Biol Sc*, 56A(7):B302–B310

National Heart Foundation of Australia and the Cardiac Society of Australia and New Zealand (2008) *Reducing risk in heart disease 2007* (updated 2008). Online. Available: www.heartfoundation.org.au/SiteCollectionDocuments/A%20RR%20RRIHD%202008Update%20Guideline%20pdf.pdf (accessed 31 August 2010)

Noakes TD (2003) *The lore of running* (4th ed). Champaign, IL: Human Kinetics

Rutherford RB, Baker JD, Ernst C, et al (1997) Recommended standards for reports dealing with lower extremity ischemia: revised version. *Journal of Vascular Surgery*, 26:517–38

Thompson WR, Gordon NF, Pescatello LS (eds) (2010) *ACSM's Guidelines for Exercise Testing and Prescription* (8th ed). Baltimore, MD: Lippincott Williams & Wilkins

Chapter 14

Case studies in exercise as therapy for respiratory conditions

Suzanne Broadbent, Gina Mendoza, Dan van der Westhuizen and Sarah-Johanna Moss

Exercise has been used as an intervention for respiratory disease for several decades. Chapter 4 covers the evidence supporting exercise as respiratory therapy and describes the breadth of conditions for which this approach may be useful. The case studies in this chapter have been selected not simply as illustrations, but to further comprehension of the widespread usefulness of exercise in clients with pulmonary diseases. We have selected clients with very common conditions (eg: exercise induced asthma) as well as clients with rarer but serious complaints (eg: occupational fibrosis). In these seriously ill clients exercise remains useful and returns widespread benefits, but the selection and application of exercise is particularly complex. Discussion is woven through these complicated case studies, and further investigation and study is prompted by the inclusion of discussion questions.

CASE STUDY 1: FIBROSIS (RESTRICTIVE LUNG DISEASE)

Subjective

EL, a 60-year-old ex-miner, has been referred to a clinical exercise physiologist for an exercise plan. EL emigrated to Australia from South Africa in 1980. He was diagnosed with silicon fibrosis 5 years ago, and suffers from dyspnea (shortness of breath), oxygen desaturation, fatigue and poor exercise tolerance. His doctor has recommended

EL to attempt some mild exercise as a means of improving quality of life (QoL), especially mobility for activities of daily living (ADLs). EL has difficulty with walking up a gradient or steps, and finds walking to the local corner shop an effort. He uses supplementary oxygen occasionally, and suffers from constant anxiety and depression. He has lost considerable weight in the last few years, and is underweight for his age and height. He would like to improve his muscle strength, and endurance.

Objective

A full medical history was taken, revealing the diagnosis of silicon fibrosis 5 years previously. EL had shown gradual onset of breathlessness, fatigue and repeated bouts of bronchitis over a 10-year period, exacerbated by a history of smoking since the age of 13. He had worked in the mining industry in South Africa and then in Western Australia for a total of 25 years, as a truck driver, sand-blaster of pipes and machinery, and with drilling and blasting equipment in an extremely dusty environment. In South Africa he had rarely used a dust respirator, although he adopted this safety practice once working in Australia. EL managed to stop smoking 4 years ago. X-rays revealed extensive fibrosis (pulmonary infiltrates) in both lungs. EL underwent a recent lung function test (see Table 14.1 and Figure 14.1).

Physical examination

Height 180cm, weight 64kg, body fat 12%, BMI 19.7, resting heart rate 76bpm, resting blood pressure 140/92mmHg.

Exercise history

EL had played rugby in his youth and also enjoyed playing tennis. By the age of 44 he rarely undertook any physical activity, weighed 94kg and was classified as overweight. He went fishing with friends, played golf once a fortnight and walked occasionally. The onset of dyspnea and fatigue in his 50s reduced his physical activity further and he was sedentary by the age of 60.

Psychosocial history

EL was asked to complete a QoL questionnaire and to also discuss his anxieties about his exercise capacity and feelings of breathlessness with ADL. His responses and exercise test results could be classified using the Baseline/Transitional Dyspnoea Index (The Australian Lung Foundation 2009; see www.pulmonaryrehab.com.au/index.asp?page= 21 for a comparison of QoL assessment tools in pulmonary rehabilitation).

Incremental exercise test

A medically supervised sub-maximal graded exercise test (GXT) on a cycle (Monark) with 12 lead ECG was conducted by the clinical exercise practitioner. EL cycled for 3 minutes with no load, and then the resistance was increased by 15W per minute until symptom-limited exhaustion. VO_2 was measured using a calibrated gas analyser (SensorMedics, Yorba Linda, CA). The test was necessary to determine EL's aerobic fitness and to screen for any possible cardiac abnormalities (See Table 14.2).

The test was terminated in the first minute of Stage 4 due to fatigue in legs and chest (rating of

Table 14.1 Results of lung function tests

Parameter	Measured	Predicted
Resting HbO_2sat%	97	98
FVC (L/min)	3.1	4.5
FEV1 (L/min)	2.6	3.5
FEV1/FVC (%)	83	80
$FEF_{25-75\%}$ (L/sec)	3.4	4.4
MVV (L/min)	50	90
Breathing frequency (b/min)	50	35

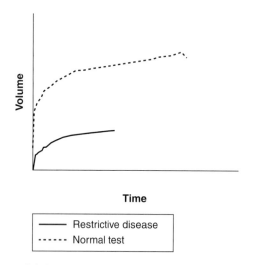

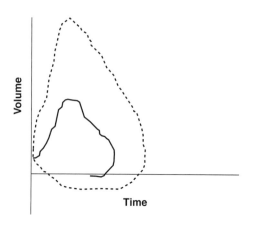

——	Restrictive disease
- - - -	Normal test

Figure 14.1 Flow volume loop

10, New Borg scale for chest; rating of 9 for legs). The ECG trace was normal. EL showed oxygen desaturation to 86%. Peak blood lactate was 12mMol.

6 minute walk test (6MWT)

The following day EL underwent a 6 minute walk test (6MWT) to assess his cardiorespiratory capacity during weight-bearing exercise. The test was timed on a treadmill, with ECG and pulse oximeter to monitor heart rate and oxygen saturation. Fatigue and breathlessness was assessed using a Modified Borg Dyspnoea Score. EL walked 283m and his oxygen saturation decreased to 90%. His dyspnoea score was 8. His peak heart rate was 118bpm.

Functional tests

These tests were conducted 15 minutes after the conclusion of the 6MWT to assess EL's muscle strength and endurance, and flexibility. Resting heart rate and blood pressure were taken prior to the functional tests (HR 85bpm, BP 146/90mmHg).

Hand grip strength: left 9kg, right 12kg. Sit-and-reach test: +5cm. YMCA Sit Up test: 10 in 1 minute. Sit-to-stand test: 15. No chest pain or symptoms of angina were recorded during these tests although EL became breathless during both the sit-to-stand and sit-up tests. EL reported fatigue in the legs and chest, and tightness in the lower back, after the functional testing.

Assessment

EL's test results are typical of a client with advanced restrictive lung disease (fibrosis). During the incremental cycle test, EL showed hypoxemia, low VO_2, high fatigue and high blood pressure at a relatively low workload of 60W. His 6MWT score was poor for his age group, and was combined with a high score on the dyspnoea chart. His exercise tolerance was classified as poor. Functional exercise test results show: poor hand grip strength; poor hamstring and lower back flexibility; poor abdominal strength; and a low sit-to-stand score indicating poor leg strength, compared to healthy men of the same age.

EL was advised to implement a combined aerobic exercise and strength and flexibility program that would improve his respiratory muscle strength, and overall muscle strength and endurance for ADL and increased wellbeing.

Although EL's condition is of occupational origin, his case is considered in this chapter rather than in Chapter 19, because he is seeking clinical care as a private client. Having migrated from South Africa 30 years ago, he is ineligible to claim workers' compensation from his former employer.

Plan

EL's exercise plan combined activities that would: (1) strengthen his respiratory muscles and improve his balance and proprioception; (2) improve his

Table 14.2 Incremental exercise test

Stage (1 min)	Work rate(W)	HR(bpm)	BP(mmHg)	RPE(0 – 10)	HbO$_2$sat%	VO2(L.min^{-1})
Warm up*	0	83	150/92	4	98	0.30
Stage 1	15	94	160/92	6	96	0.47
Stage 2	30	98	166/100	7	94	0.68
Stage 3	45	100	190/102	8	92	0.89
Stage 4	60	120	200/104	10	89	1.12
Recovery**	0	90	180/92	4	94	0.52

*Unloaded cycling for 3 min
**Recovery, 4 min

aerobic capacity by utilising intermittent exercise at a low to moderate intensity (5–6 New Borg RPE scale, HR to <100bpm) for 20–30 minutes daily; and (3) increase skeletal muscle strength and endurance through progressive resistance training (PRT) using therabands and light hand weights (home or clinic-based program).

- Qigong, tai chi or yoga, concentrating on breathing control and energy patterns; these activities also combine sequences of movements that strengthen muscles around the joints and improve range of motion, balance and proprioception. Concentration and relaxation is also enhanced with these activities.
- Intermittent walking, aqua exercise or indoor cycling; intervals of exercise alternating with intervals of rest. Total work can be increased from 15 minute per day to 30 minute per day as tolerated. Duration of exercise should be increased rather than intensity of exercise.
- PRT: upper and lower body strengthening; sit-to-stands; squats, step-up-and-downs; lunges; back, shoulder and arm exercises. Core abdominal strengthening can also be combined with deep breathing and diaphragm exercises.
- Stretching: muscle tightness can be caused by anxiety and depression, as well as physical inactivity. Stretching will improve range of motion and reduce the risk of exercise-induced muscle tightness.

Barriers to exercise intervention

- Lack of previous regular exercise, and lack of knowledge about duration and intensities of exercise sessions.
- Recurring breathlessness and hypoxia during low intensity exercise.
- Anxiety and depression about his medical condition and management.
- Lack of self-confidence about doing regular exercise unsupervised.

Immediate goals of exercise intervention

- To improve self-confidence related to exercise participation.
- To reduce anxiety and depression.
- To increase functional capacity associated with ADL.
- To improve muscle strength and endurance.

Immediate exercise strategies

- Initially 15–20 minutes daily of low to moderate (as tolerated) intermittent (interval) aerobic exercise. Indoor cycling or walking would be preferable to aquatic exercise to begin with; HR, BP and oxygen saturation should be monitored during exercise and recovery. HR between 88 and 100bpm, RPE 5–6. Exercise sessions should be supervised by a clinical exercise practitioner for the first 12 weeks of the exercise program.
- The clinical exercise practitioner should stress to EL that any severe signs or symptoms of hypoxia such as breathlessness, dizziness and desaturation <88% should be reported. However, occasional mild symptoms should not preclude EL from doing low to moderate intensity exercise. Length of exercise intervals and the exercise intensity can be adjusted depending on symptom limits.
- Initially 2–3 sessions (15–20 minutes) weekly of low to moderate intensity resistance training, flexibility exercises and stretching. Can be included with aerobic exercise session. Can be home or gym-based. 10–12 repetitions, two sets, RPE 5–7. Sessions should initially be supervised by a clinical exercise practitioner. If symptoms preclude a 20 minute session, then the exercises can be broken up into two sessions per day (eg: 10 minutes of lower body exercises in the morning, and 10 minutes of upper body exercises in the afternoon).
- Sessions of tai chi, qigong or yoga that use gentle exercises to improve flexibility, proprioception, lower limb strength and coordination, core stability; these types of exercises are very functional for ADL and also reduce stress and improve relaxation. Qigong improves breathing patterns through concentration on breathing as a means of conserving and utilising 'energy'.
- For sessions not monitored by an clinical exercise practitioner, EL may monitor his heart rate from his pulse oximeter. A pulse oximeter can be used with all home-based exercises to monitor oxygen saturation. EL should monitor his BP at home before and after exercise using a small electric BP cuff with digital readout. If EL can take more

control over monitoring his exercise responses, he may gain in self-confidence and reduce exercise-related anxiety.

- Encourage EL to be active as possible (eg: walking around the garden and to local shops); ADL; participation in family outings and activities as tolerated. An increase in self-confidence and reduction in anxiety associated with being active would improve EL's QoL.
- Encourage EL to reduce anxiety and depression by joining a rehabilitation exercise group specifically for chronic obstructive pulmonary disease (COPD) patients. He may also discuss his fears or concerns with his GP and other health professionals.
- Quality of life questionnaire (eg: Medical Outcomes Study 36-Item Health Survey, also known as the Short Form 36 or SF-36) to be completed prior to starting the exercise program, and at 12 weeks during the program.

Long-term goals of exercise intervention

- Improving respiratory muscle strength and endurance.
- Reduce dyspnoea.
- Increase EL's exercise endurance as measured by oxygen consumption (VO_2), muscle capillary density and activity of oxidative enzymes.
- Increase the duration of exercise sessions, hopefully to the stage where EL can participate in steady state exercise rather than intermittent training.
- Increase lean muscle mass and skeletal muscle strength for functional improvements.
- Maintain or improve QoL and reduce anxiety and depression.

Long-term exercise strategies

- Increase duration of aerobic exercise session to 30–40 minute plus daily, with an aim to increasing the intervals of exercise and reducing the intervals of rest between exercise bouts.
- Eventually increasing the intensity of exercise intervals, as tolerated by EL.
- Increase length of resistance training session to 30 minutes, three times per week.
- Involve client in more recreational physical activity that he sees as enjoyable, dependent upon symptom limits.

- Involvement of EL in community activity groups and group exercise rehabilitation exercise.
- Reduce reliance on supplemental oxygen.

Monitoring outcomes

- Client monitors his own oxygen saturation (use of pulse oximeter).
- Weekly monitoring resting blood pressure.
- Lung function tests to be repeated after 12 weeks.
- 6MWT to be repeated after 12 weeks.
- Quality of life questionnaire to be completed after 12 weeks for comparison with pre-program questionnaire.
- Anthropometric and functional tests repeated after 12 weeks and then at 24 weeks.

Outcomes

EL began his exercise program with three sessions of intermittent interval aerobic exercise per week. These sessions were supervised by a clinical exercise practitioner. EL chose to do the sessions in his home using a Repco indoor cycle. He cycled for 3-minute intervals with a 1-minute interval of rest. Oxygen saturation and heart rate were monitored using a pulse oximeter. Total session time was 20 minutes with a total exercise time of 16 minutes. Workload was set at 35–40W, with settings dependent upon the patient's symptoms. RPE for EL's legs usually varied between 5–7 for the first 3 weeks of training, with a dyspnoea scale score of 4 for breathlessness during the cycling intervals.

On alternate days EL did a home-based resistance training session using therabands, body weight and light free weights. These sessions were supervised by a clinical exercise practitioner to start with, but as EL became more confident, he did the sessions on his own. The resistance training was 20 minutes duration and consisted of half-squats, lunges, calf raises, seated and standing row (therabands), bicep curls (free weights), tricep kickbacks (free weights), deep breathing diaphragm exercises. EL started the training program with two sets of 8 repetitions, with a 2-minute rest in between sets. He was gradually able to reduce the rest time between sets, and after 4 weeks of training, had increased his number of reps to 10–12 depending upon his fatigue.

On Saturday EL joined in a rehabilitation exercise group that participated in a tai chi class specifically for chronic disease patients (cardiac, COPD and cancer), that was supervised by both a cardiac nurse and an clinical exercise practitioner. The class was run at a local hospital and concentrated on functional movement patterns, postural stability, core strengthening and some Feldenkrais breathing exercises (for both relaxation and breathing management). These sessions lasted for 30 minutes.

After 4 weeks of exercising, EL substituted one treadmill walking session for 15–20 minutes, in place of one cycling session, again at a very low intensity. He also walked on his own around a local park for 20–25 minutes on the weekend, with the proviso that he paused for a rest interval if he became severely breathless. He expressed an interest in doing some aquatic exercise during summer months. After 6 weeks of training, EL admitted that he did feel stronger and more able to cope with his disease, primarily the dyspnoea which had caused him a lot of anxiety. Although EL's lung function (FVC, FEV_1) had not really improved, his exercise tolerance had increased and he was able to gradually increase the total length of his exercise sessions. After 6 weeks of training, he increased the length of his exercise interval to 5 minutes, with a 1-minute interval of unloaded cycling as opposed to the previous no cycling rest interval.

After 8 weeks of training, EL had progressed to 30–40 minutes in total of 10 minute intervals of constant load or steady-state exercise, and was using both cycle and treadmill for alternating 10 minute sessions with a couple of minutes rest in between. These aerobic sessions were done three times a week, and on alternate days EL went for a 30 minute easy walk in a local park and reserve. EL continued with his resistance training sessions, making no change to length of sessions. He also continued with his tai chi class and occasionally substituted a gentle swim (breaststroke) and aqua walk session or a short game of lawn bowls with acquaintances he had met through his tai chi rehab class.

Lung function tests, and aerobic, strength and functional exercise tests were conducted after 12 weeks of training. Resting HR had decreased to 74bpm and BP to 138/84mmHg. Lung function parameters had not changed. EL had improved his 6MWT distance to 327m (15.6% improvement) with a peak dyspnoea scale score of 7, peak RPE of 5 and peak oxygen desaturation of 92%; hand grip strength: left 12kg, right 14kg; sit-and-reach test: +7cm; YMCA sit-up test: 14 in 1 minute; sit-to-stand test: 19.

Summary of key lessons

- Lung function *per se* will usually not substantially improve with exercise in patients with restrictive lung disease but respiratory muscles which aid in breathing may be strengthened and may increase in oxidative capacity, thus contributing to increased exercise tolerance.

- There is no optimal or generic exercise prescription for COPD and restrictive lung disease patients. Exercise intensity should be based upon clinical and exercise test data, with regard to symptom limits and to patient goals.

- Exercise intensity should generally be at least 50% of VO_{2max} for optimal improvements. Most COPD patients are de-conditioned but if they can initially exercise either intermittently or steady state at $\geq$50% VO_{2max} intensity, then their exercise adherence will be enhanced and their risk of injury or severe dyspnoea should be reduced. Oxygen consumption is correlated with levels of dyspnoea. For example, a Modified Borg Dyspnoea scale score of 2.5 or 'slight to moderate' breathlessness equates with 75% VO_{2peak}; a score of 5 or 'severe' equates with 50% VO_{2peak}.

- The use of the Modified Borg Dyspnoea scale to identify exercise intensities and limits is extremely useful, as the symptom limits for restrictive lung disease patients are defined by exertional dyspnoea. Both the normal Borg RPE and the dyspnoea scale can be used to self-monitor and quantify the amount of physical effort and breathlessness during exercise and ADL, and patients will also realise that some amount of exertional dyspnoea is normal and acceptable during physical activity.

- Anaerobic threshold (AT) may be used as a training intensity for patients who have mild COPD. AT is suitable for patients who have improved their cardiorespiratory fitness and are looking to increase their exercise stimulus for further gains. Minute ventilation (V_E) may be reduced by exercising for periods or intervals above AT, where some metabolic acidosis has occurred. As with a normal healthy population, V_E and lactate will decrease in COPD patients who train over AT, compared to those who train under AT. However, patients with severe restrictive lung disease or COPD may not achieve metabolic acidosis during incremental exercise, and these patients would be best advised to exercise below AT.

- Use of supplemental oxygen is recommended for patients, resting or exercising, whose oxygen saturation decreases to <88% whilst breathing room air (Australian Lung Foundation 2009; Thompson et al 2010).

DISCUSSION Questions

1 Why is it important for cardiac monitoring to be part of incremental testing in people with restrictive lung disease?

2 At what level of oxygen desaturation would you terminate a graded incremental test or an exercise session?

3 Suggest possible explanations for the lack of improvement in EL's lung function tests after 12 weeks of training.

4 Describe and justify the sorts of changes you could make to EL's exercise program, given the positive adaptations that have occurred after 12 weeks of training.

CASE STUDY 2: EMPHYSEMA

Subjective

Margaret, a 58-year-old office worker has been referred to you for an exercise plan. Margaret suffers from emphysema and is experiencing increasing difficulty with shortness of breath and associated lack of energy. Her doctor has advised her to take up mild exercise, such as walking. Margaret has found that any form of exercise tends to aggravate her breathing difficulties and for this reason she does not exercise. She used to smoke 40 cigarettes per day but gave up when she was diagnosed with emphysema 6 years ago. She maintains a slim figure and healthy appearance by sticking to an entirely organic and well-balanced diet. Margaret is irritated that her doctor says she is unfit because she believes that she cares for her body. However, Margaret expressed anxiety that her health is deteriorating due to her breathing problems, and is keen to find a solution for this.

Objective

Margaret's measurements are: height 154cm; weight 45kg; waist 68cm; hips 84cm; waist–hips ratio: 0.8; BMI 18.9; BP 110/70. Postural examination reveals pronounced kyphosis of the upper thoracic spine, forward head position and forward shoulders. Orthopaedic testing: tight pectoralis major clavicular and latissimus dorsi. Muscle testing: weakness in bilateral serratus anterior and latissimus dorsi. Thoracolumbar fascia test: tight/restricted ROM. Physical appearance of shallow breathing high in chest. Step length shortened with overall gait having very tight appearance. Straight leg raise: 50 degrees bilaterally (tight). Lower body strength measured using sit-to-stand test: unable to complete test due to breathing difficulties. Upper body strength measured using biceps curls with dumbbells free-weights: 1 repetition max 3.5kg weights capability bilaterally. Aerobic capacity (VO_{2peak}) of 17 ml.kg^{-1}.min^{-1} suggests an improvement when compared to age group normative data. Peak flow: 195L/min is low as predicted mean value for a healthy 56-year-old female is approximately 330–350L/min.

Assessment

Margaret presented as anxious about her current health dilemma. Whilst the underlying problem is emphysema, the stress this is causing her both mentally and physically appears to be the most globally debilitating health factor for her.

More, her pronounced kyphosis of the upper thoracic spine, forward head position, forward shoulders, tight chest muscles and weak upper back muscles, are all suggestive of an upper-cross syndrome (Magee 2008). These postural changes may also contribute to the development of thoracic outlet syndrome in which the neurovascular bundles supplying the upper limbs become compressed in the supraclavicular region. See Chapter 12 for a case study in which thoracic cage structure and posture potentially influence respiratory function.

Margaret has complained of lack of energy and her aerobic fitness level is comparatively poor. Margaret eats a very healthy diet which will assist her in building her energy levels once she commences a physical activity program. Being slim, Margaret has the energy efficiency advantage of not having to exercise with excess body weight.

Plan

There will be five main components to Margaret's exercise plan. The main barrier for her is the thought of exercise and her perception that it makes her feel unwell. For this reason, the word exercise will be eliminated. This terminology will be replaced by physical activities plan.

The first component will be focused on relaxation, stretching and breathing. The tension Margaret is carrying is expressed physically in both her posture and gait. To address this, relaxation techniques will be an important component of her overall individualised physical activity plan. For this, Margaret will learn concepts derived from the Alexander Technique of postural relaxation. Daily practice of this technique will assist her in releasing tightness and constriction in her upper-body region. The aim will be for Margaret to apply this concept to all her regular daily activities, for example, how she moves to sit in her work chair and how she stands up to get out of it, and especially when she walks, anywhere and everywhere. In this way Margaret's activity plan is more about a change in her physical lifestyle.

The second component will be stretching and breathing. Her tendency towards muscle tightness is consistent with her pattern of tension. Margaret would benefit from a daily stretching program and will be given ten daily stretches to do morning and night. They will be gentle stretches to be performed in a relaxed manner with structured counts for breathing in and out of the stretches.

The third component will be standing swings and breathing. Swinging the arms and spiralling the body on a transverse axis 'opens' the chest and enhances respiratory function by relaxing the thoracic region.

The fourth component will be deep water running in slow motion, to be done using a floatation belt. This activity will improve aerobic capacity and muscle strength/endurance using the resistance of the water. Stretching and relaxation exercises can also be performed.

The fifth component will be singing. This activity will be excellent for working the muscles in the thoracic region. The suggestion will be that Margaret sings every morning in the shower, expanding her rib cage and using deep breaths.

Discussion

Margaret related very well to advice that learning to relax was fundamental to her improving her overall health. In addition to her willingness to take on board all five suggested components of her activity plan, she also decided to take up yoga. Her yoga teacher has been very encouraging and Margaret is amazed at how much her flexibility levels have improved over a 3-month period. She said that she feels so much more confident in herself since she made these changes. Margaret knows that her lungs will never be what they once were, but she is very pleased at how much better her breathing feels since she began her gradual transition into exercise. The word exercise has now lost its fear and in fact Margaret proudly now talks about how she exercises at the pool. She has found that she can control her breathing whilst she performs her slow-motion deep water running. She worked out how to do this herself, by combining yoga breathing with her water activity. In addition, Margaret decided that she would take up singing lessons as her shower-singing improved her breathing and self-confidence.

Margaret's fear of exercise was real and very well founded. Having difficulty breathing properly can be frightening. Margaret had the good sense to know she needed to do something about her sedentary lifestyle, but she did not know how exercise could be the solution because exercise had been the very thing that had caused her to struggle to breathe.

The main message from Margaret's story, therefore, is that exercise does not always need to operate within the paradigm of 'faster, higher, stronger' for it to be beneficial. Margaret needed to become more active, and to release her thoracic region. It is quite likely that without it being the focus, Margaret will be increasing heart rate in the pool, during her singing and during yoga classes. The reward for Margaret from her lifestyle change is that she is no longer fearful of exercise. She has become proactive in choosing physical activities for herself which are both enjoyable and beneficial to her health.

Outcomes

Sit-bend test: successfully completed 11 seconds; straight leg raise: 70 degrees bilaterally; upper body strength: 5.5kg bilaterally. Aerobic fitness still needs improvement for a female of her age but has improved from 17 ml.kg^{-1}.min^{-1} to 20 ml.kg^{-1}.min^{-1}. Peak flow was 195L/min in pre-test and has improved to 270L/min.

Results show that although Margaret's cardiorespiratory capacity is impaired with emphysema, there has been significant improvement in exercise capacity and tolerance. Importantly, Margaret feels as though she is fitter, stronger and capable of gentle exercise without the fear of being unable to breathe.

Summary of key lessons

- Fear may be a barrier to exercise for people with chronic breathing difficulties. Fear about exercise and movement may impact on the level of tension held in their musculoskeletal system. This muscle tension/stress will most likely be linked to muscle weakness rather than strength. A focus on relaxation, posture and movement efficiency is of benefit to all, but vital to success for this specific population.

- When a client is sedentary due to illness, there are always fitness activity alternatives available for them: The priority is to get them moving and engaged in an activity. The key to keeping the client engaged and positive is usually to emphasise pleasure and participation (rather than power and performance).

- Practitioners are advised to help clients to build upon what they can do rather than attempt to make them learn to struggle through what they cannot do. Consider the age of the client when applying this concept. Young clients may be more adaptable to change than older clients. An older client may prefer to be validated for who they are rather than feeling as though they have been 'doing it all wrong' for a lifetime, and will now have to change.

DISCUSSION Question

A 55-year-old male client has emphysema, and his doctor has repeatedly tried to encourage this man to exercise. Exasperated that his patient refuses to exercise, the doctor has referred him to you for an exercise program. The referring medical practitioner is insistent that his patient must exercise to 70% of his maximum heart rate for a minimum of three 1-hour sessions per week, but the client is anxious about performing this exercise because he has difficulty breathing. Describe how you would handle this situation, including your communication with both the client and the medical practitioner.

CASE STUDY 3: EXERCISE INDUCED ASTHMA

Subjective

LM is a 55-year-old male, working as a school principal at a local high school. He is also a Masters athlete who intends to represent his state in cross country running. Since his secondary school years, LM participated in various sports including swimming, tennis and volleyball. He 'accidentally' got involved in cross country running to encourage his 16-year-old son during his training runs in preparation for middle distance athletic track events.

LM has complained lately of breathlessness, wheezing, coughing and chest tightness during and immediately after these high-intensity running sessions. LM experiences the abovementioned symptoms usually 3–8 minutes after starting intense running and they are most severe 5–10 minutes post-exercise, and it normally resolves 30 minutes to 60 minutes post-exercise. Initially LM thought that this breathlessness was just a lack of fitness, which reflected in his poor time trials. Despite the fact that he frequently partook in vigorous running sessions, he realised that he made no progress with his training. He believed that the abovementioned symptoms were not helping to improve his running performance and he experienced a lot of frustration. Consequently he decided to consult a clinical exercise practitioner for further advice.

Objective

A pre-test medical history questionnaire (see Carlin & Singh 2009 for suggestions) that emphasised the cardiorespiratory system and signs and/or symptoms related to asthma and EIA/EIB was conducted. For example: Does the client cough early morning, at night or after exercise? Does the client wheeze, cough or experience chest tightness when exposed to allergens or airborne pollutants or after exercise? Did the client experience an attack or recurrent attacks of wheezing? Did the client have a history of colds that 'go to his/her chest or take >2 weeks to resolve? Did appropriate asthma treatment alleviate the symptoms?

LM mentioned that besides the chest tightness, coughing, breathlessness and wheezing he experiences during and after a vigorous exercise bout, he occasionally experiences wheezing after exposure to grass and tree pollens when pollen counts are high in the late spring or early summer. LM was also questioned about his current medication use, his habitual physical activity participation and/or current active sporting participation. Considering his current habitual training it seems that despite LM's intensive training, his perceived and actual fitness levels were not equivalent.

First, the clinical exercise practitioner wants to ascertain if LM has asthma or another airway disease associated with increased airway responsiveness during or after exercise (eg: pneumonia, vocal cord dysfunction, chronic bronchitis, cystic fibrosis). He liaised with LM's physician and wrote a letter in relation to LM's complaints. LM's physician requested a pulmonary function test (spirometry testing) to confirm/disprove asthma. Besides confirming the diagnosis, the outcome of this measurement is also indicative of the severity of the airflow limitation, its reversibility and variability. LM's predicted baseline normal values for a male of his age (55 years) and height (185cm) were 4.14 L (FEV_1) and 5.41 L (FVC). LM is requested to execute a forced expiration, whilst measurements of forced vital capacity (FVC) and forced expiratory volume in 1 second (FEV_1) are obtained. His results regarding airflow limitation showed a reduction in FEV_1 to less than 80% of and a reduction in the FEV_1/FVC ratio to less than 65% of predicted normal value. LM also showed an increase in $FEV_1 > 12\%$ following administration of ventolin (salbutamol, a short-acting bronchodilator) compared to the pre-bronchodilator value, which suggests reversible airflow (or a positive degree of reversibility).

Second, the clinical exercise practitioner, with LM's permission and after informed detailed discussion, decided to conduct an 'exercise challenge' test in the laboratory and contacted a sports physician to attend. This decision was taken in view of the symptoms LM experienced during and after exercise (ie: breathlessness, wheezing, coughing and chest tightness). The clinical exercise practitioner was aware that although regular physical activity can be an important intervention for LM's health, it was also of paramount importance to cooperate with LM's sports physician in order to confirm or disprove EIA/EIB. Appropriate precautions must be taken for optimal exercise performance and to avoid a severe asthma attack that may result in suffocation and ultimately death.

LM was requested to avoid vigorous exercise for at least 12 hours prior to the running test, and to abstain from using any medication for a minimum of 24 hours prior to the test. The consumption of caffeinated foods and drinks (chocolate, coffee, tea, cola, Red Bull, etc) was not permitted within 6 hours prior to testing. LM underwent a single-stage, continuous test of 6–8 minutes duration, running at a high intensity (> 75–85% of HR max or 65–75% of VO_{2max}) in a laboratory on a treadmill. LM's forced expiratory volume (L) in 1 second was measured prior to exercise (3.22) and 3–9 minutes post exercise (2.57). The post-exercise results showed a decline of >15% in his forced expiratory volume in 1 second (FEV_1) compared to his pre-exercise values. During the test, LM was requested to

indicate his rating of perceived exertion on the 6–20 point Borg scale and his rating of breathlessness and/or dyspnea on the 1–4 point dyspnea scale. A pulse oximeter was used to ensure that the percentage saturation of the haemoglobin in LM's arterial blood (HbO_2sat%) did not fall below 90% during testing. Haemoglobin desaturation during a symptom-limited test may indicate the level at which a pulmonary client feels dyspneic. LM's exercise test was terminated at a rating of 17 and 3 on the Borg scale and dyspnea scale, respectively. At this stage he also experienced chest tightness, extreme breathlessness and wheezing, in association with an arterial blood saturation level of 89%.

The 'duration and severity' of EIA/EIB is determined by measuring the pre-exercise lung function values of FVC and FEV_1. The same lung function measurements are repeated immediately after and at frequent intervals of 5 minutes for 40 minutes after exercise. LM's values were: FVC (L): pre-exercise = 4.21; 15 minute post-exercise = 3.45; 30 minute post-exercise = 3.66; 60 minute post-exercise = 3.87 and FEV_1: pre-exercise = 3.22; 15 minute post-exercise = 2.67; 30 minute post-exercise = 2.88; 60 minute post-exercise = 3.05.

Another useful measurement is the mean flow rate between 25% and 75% of vital capacity (FEF_{25-75}) and the rate of flow at 50% of vital capacity (FEF_{50}) that require a 35% post-exercise reduction to confirm EIA/EIB.

Assessment

LM's symptoms of wheezing after exposure to grass and tree pollens in the late spring or early summer, in addition to his spirometry results, confirmed his asthma as mild intermittent. The decline of >15% in his FEV_1 is indicative of EIA. Healthy individuals should be able to exhale at least 80% of their FEV_1. LM's sports physician concluded that he has mild EIA/EIB and prescribed a reliever class of medication (eg: bronchodilator) which is the preferred treatment for clients with mild to moderate EIA/EIB. A fall in FEV_1 of 10–24% = mild, 25–39% = moderate, and $\geq 40\%$ = severe EIA.

LM's average FEF_{25-75} and FEF_{50} decreased >35% when his pre-exercise and post-exercise values were compared. These results were also helpful to confirm EIA/EIB. However, these measures have a high variability and can change from pre to post exercise and is therefore neither recommended nor accepted by sporting bodies. LM's final RPE of 17 (very hard) on the 6–20 Borg scale and his rating of 3 (moderately severe, very uncomfortable) on the dyspnea scale associated with symptoms of EIA/EIB and his below-normal low arterial blood saturation level of 89%, indicated that he has achieved his threshold level.

Plan

LM knows that if he avoids certain triggers (eg: air pollution, smoke, certain grass and tree pollens, and prolonged high intensity activity above 80–90% of HR max) he can minimise his asthma attacks. LM is taught how to monitor his airflow with a peak-flow meter twice a day and avoids exercise until the peak-flow reading returns to or exceeds 80% of his personal best peak-flow reading. LM also uses his prescribed pre-exercise short acting, bronchodilator medication (ie: ventolin [salbutamol] or bricanyl [terbutaline]), which involves one to two activations of inhaled beta-2 agonists bronchodilator spray 15 minutes prior to exercise and a second dose during exercise if breathing problems develop. If symptoms persist for longer than 20 minutes, despite repetitive inhalation of his beta-2 agonist, he should cease physical activity and seek medical treatment. In some cases exercise opens the airways of asthmatic runners and may reduce asthma symptoms, but many runners get worse with continued activity. LM's sports physician also prescribed inhaled beta-2 agonists that are permitted by the World Anti-doping Agency (WADA) and the International Olympic Committee (IOC) by means of an abbreviated Therapeutic Use Exemption which is required from the team physician (Brukner & Khan 2007; Landry & Bernhardt 2003). Because LM is a Master's athlete he may be subjected to sports drug testing, so the sports physician also provided written notification to the relevant medical authority by disclosing LM's medication use prior to competition, due to his diagnosed EIA.

LM's exercise plan is individualised and based on objective measurement of his exercise capabilities. General guidelines recommend that a client should start his/her initial cardiorespiratory program at an intensity level just below his/her anaerobic threshold (50–85% of max HRR), if his/her maximum level of exercise, as determined by measurement of oxygen consumption, is known. In LM's situation, it was suggested that he start at an intensity level below the level where he became noticeably dyspneic and thus he can exercise up to 15 and 2 on the Borg and dyspnea scales, respectively.

LM's goals are to exercise 3–5 times per week for 20–60 minutes duration and to progress by increasing intensity by 5% with each 1–3 sessions. When the recommended maximal level of intensity is attained, exercise duration can be increased by 5%. LM does a gentle and intermittent warm-up prior to training and competition to minimise or attenuate his EIB for up to 2 hours. The warm up consists of at least 10 minutes of moderate intensity jogging at approximately 60% heart rate max, followed by 5–7 sprints of 30 seconds at 100% effort with a 1.5 minute rest between sprints, followed by 20–30 minute of stretching. Following the warm-up, a slow increase in exercise intensity is necessary to allow minute ventilation to increase gradually.

Another example of a warm-up is a 2 minute interval of exercise followed by 2 minutes of rest for 6–8 minutes, with the exercise periods becoming progressively more intense. These two warm-up approaches reduce LM's episodes of EIA, as it takes advantage of the bronchospasm refractory period. After exercise sessions, LM cools down by easy walking until his heart rate decreases to within 20bpm of the pre-exercise heart rate. A sudden stop in exercise makes EIA/EIB more severe.

LM prefers to do cross training (cycling, tennis, swimming and aqua-jogging at least twice per week) rather than run outdoors, especially during cold weather or when pollen counts are high. Occasionally LM uses a surgical mask or scarf when running in cold conditions as it helps to maintain a warmer and moister air to prevent the asthmatic trigger. LM also includes frequent interval or intermittent activities such as short 'stop-and-go' bursts of running < 5 minutes each (eg: fartlek running, opposed to long intense, continuous exercise). LM is advised to avoid high-altitude mountain climbing and scuba diving because it exposes participants to dry, cold air which may trigger an acute EIB attack. LM is also advised to abstain from ingesting milk products within an hour or two before exercise and he is encouraged to drink plenty of water during endurance exercise, as it reduces the thickness of lung secretions which makes breathing easier.

Discussion

Although LM is aware that asthma cannot be cured, he realises that it can be controlled by establishing and following a lifelong management plan (monitoring airflow, avoiding allergic triggers, medication before exercise and modified exercise habits) as suggested by his sports physician and exercise practitioner. By following this comprehensive approach, LM improved not only his aerobic fitness, but also increased his exercise tolerance and asthma threshold. As a bonus for his dedicated perseverance and hard work, LM has been chosen to represent his State in the Inter-State Athletics Championships in the Master's age category.

Summary of key lessons

- More than 80% of children and 60% of adult asthmatics get EIA during or after exercise. However, those with EIA/EIB may have normal resting pulmonary function.

- Many asthmatics perform below par due to a lack of appropriate medical advice and medication, as they assume that a lack of fitness causes breathlessness (dyspnea). No two individuals with asthma are alike, thus interventions must be individualised.

- Asthma is estimated to affect >300 million people worldwide. Australia and New Zealand have the highest rates of asthma with incidence rates of approximately 11% amongst the general population and 20% in children.

- The prevalence of EIB in the Australian population is estimated to be 12% while 21% of the Australian Summer Olympics Games team reported asthma or EIB.

- Forced expiratory volume in 1 second (FEV_1) can increase with approximately 15–20% when unfit people achieve optimal, individual fitness levels.

- The beneficial effects of regular exercise on psychosocial development, cardiorespiratory function and improved work capacity makes it a vital aspect of disease management for the person with EIA.

- Australian athletes with asthma increased from 7% (1976) to 21% (2000) and asthmatic athletes have won gold medals at all but three Olympic Summer Games since 1956 (Brukner & Khan 2007). If asthma symptoms are well managed through appropriate prophylactic drugs, and non-pharmacologic treatment, EIB/EIA should not limit exercise performance in the elite athlete and the recreational athlete population.

- Exercise training does not cure asthma, but it can increase airway reserve and reduce the work of breathing during participation in exercise.

- EIB is the preferred term to describe post-exercise narrowing in the non-asthmatic population. EIA is used with specific reference to the asthmatic population.

DISCUSSION Questions

1 Your client is the child of a man who believes that swimming as a child cured his asthma and he wants you to endorse swimming as curative exercise for his son. Explain your responses and advice to both the father and the son.

2 Exercise < 2 minutes in duration is usually too brief to trigger EIB, but it is exercise > 10–12 minutes that is associated with a decreased incidence of EIB. Considering this disparity between comfortable and optimal exercise durations, what strategies might you adopt to encourage asthmatic clients to commence and progress with exercise?

CASE STUDY 4: CYSTIC FIBROSIS

Subjective

MV, a 16-year-old frail looking girl living with her foster mother, was diagnosed with cystic fibrosis (CF) at age 8 months. MV has done relatively well but had intermittent infections requiring antibiotics. She was underweight and with very little muscle strength. The GP suggested MV undertake a regular exercise program and referred her to a clinical exercise practitioner. MV has not participated in regular exercise previously. MV was on the following medication: asthavent, flexotide and seravent.

Objective

A risk assessment was performed that included a medical history incorporating any history of heart conditions, blood pressure abnormalities, medication use, exercise induced asthma, reparatory ailments, recent flu, blood circulatory abnormalities and diabetes mellitus. No other medical conditions except the CF were reported as well as a family history of an overweight direct family member. The only activity that MV participated in was swimming and trampoline. MV has not previously performed a functional capacity test to determine exercise intensity. No lung function tests were available.

The following measurements were determined during the physical examination: height 161.8cm, weight 45.6kg, body fat 11%, BMI 17.4kg/m^2, waist 69cm, hip 90cm, waist–hip ratio 0.76, blood pressure 112/64mmHg, resting heart rate 120bpm. Blood tests were not requested.

Lung function test: FVC = 72.5% of predicted, FEV_1 = 46.3% of predicted, FEF_{25-75} = 48.9% of predicted, FEV_1/FVC = 61%.

Incremental exercise test

A sub-maximal graded exercise test (GXT) on a Monark 843 bicycle ergometer (PWC_{170}) was conducted by the clinical exercise practitioner. The test was necessary to determine MV's aerobic fitness and response to exercise in order to compile an appropriate exercise program. The test was terminated at the end of Stage 1 due to breathlessness by the patient and the heart rate being near the target of 70% for age-predicted maximum heart rate (see Table 14.3).

$$VO_2 \; (mL.kg^{-1}.min^{-1}) = 1.8 \; (work \; rate)/(BM)$$
$$+ \; resting \; VO_2 \; (3.5 \; mL.kg^{-1}.min^{-1})$$
$$+ \; Unloaded \; cycling \; (3.5 \; mL.kg^{-1}.min^{-1})$$

where work rate = kg.m / min;

BM = body mass[kg])

MV's estimated VO_{2peak} peak was 12.94 mL.kg^{-1}.min^{-1} which is low for her age.

Functional tests

MV's muscle endurance and flexibility was assessed 10 minutes after the graded test. For the YMCA sit up test 15 in 1 minute was recorded. This is under the 10th percentile for her age group. The Canadian trunk forward flexion test was then performed, recording 21cm. This is at the 10th percentile for her age group.

Assessment

The tests performed on MV indicated that she is a low-body-weight-for-age girl with low percentage body fat. MV also has a low functional capacity for her age as well as low abdominal muscle endurance. Flexibility was also low. The spirometry test

Table 14.3 Results of sub-maximal graded exercise test

Stage (3 min)	HR (bpm)	BP (mmHg)	RPE (Borg scale, 1-10)
Rest	120	112/64	
Stage 1 (25 watt)	174	130/64	7
Recovery (1 min)	138	120/64	
Recovery (3 min)	126	116/62	
Recovery 5	120	110/64	

VO_{2peak} was estimated from the GXT results using the ACSM metabolic equation (Thompson et al 2010)

indicated moderate obstructive pulmonary disease as classified by the ACSM (Thompson et al 2010). The FEV_1 is between 30% and 79% of predicted and the FEV_1/FVC ratio is <70%.

The graded exercise test indicated that the heart rate increased rapidly with a low resistance and MV also perceived the cardiovascular test as 'very hard'. Breathlessness was reported by the patient during the graded test.

Due to the low functional capacity MV is advised to train at very low intensities (3–4 RPE scale) for 15 minutes, performing exercise with 3 minute intervals and 1 minute rest.

Barriers to exercise intervention
- Recurrent infections with the prescription of antibiotics.
- Lack of self-discipline and break down of family structure.
- Anxiety and mild depression about her medical condition and management.
- Exercise reliant on supervision by trained staff.
- Fear of training on her own.
- Reliant on her foster family and friends to go to supervised exercise sessions.
- Possible fatigue and breathlessness during exercise.

Immediate goals of exercise intervention
- To preserve the basic level of functional capacity while decreasing the breathlessness.
- To maintain muscle mass and prevent muscle wasting.

- To reduce exercise heart rate and RPE.
- To reduce patient anxiety with regard to exercise.
- To make the intervention enjoyable in order to enhance compliance.
- Present a structured exercise program built on mode, intensity, duration and frequency.

Immediate exercise strategies
- MV will perform her exercise program under the supervision of a clinical exercise practitioner. The first strategy will be to train the cardiorespiratory system by means of a bicycle ergometer. Cycling will be at a level of 25 watt for 3 minutes followed by 2 minutes of rest. This will be performed three times for a total of 15 minutes of exercise. Her heart rate should not exceed 170bpm. BP will be recorded in rest and during the final 3 minutes of cycling. Maximum heart rate will be recorded for each training session.
- Stretching of the hamstrings, hip flexors, pectoral and shoulder girdle muscles are each performed three times for 30 seconds.
- Three sets of inspiratory and expiratory muscle conditioning are performed with the Luft. The Luft setting is placed on 1. MV then inspires and expires 10 times through the device. Three sets are performed. The resistance is increased every week by increasing the setting with 0.5.
- Resistance training is finally performed for the biceps, triceps, abdominals, quadriceps,

hamstrings, erector spinae and calf muscles at two sets of 10 repetitions at a moderate resistance.
- Progression will take place at 10% increments every 2 weeks.
- Educate the patient about hydration during exercise. Fluids need to be taken every 20 minutes and not only when thirsty.
- Quality of life questionnaire to be completed prior to starting the exercise program.

Long-term goals of exercise intervention
- Long-term goals relate to 6–12 months since inception of the exercise program.
- Improve the lung function of MV in order to prevent breathlessness experienced during daily activities.
- Improve functional capacity to improve QoL.
- To increase body mass by preserving lean body mass.
- To control blood glucose and identify abnormal glucose concentrations early.
- To improve inspiratory and expiratory muscle function by training with the Luft daily.

Long-term exercise strategies
- Attend exercise sessions five times per week for 60 minutes.
- Perform aerobic exercise at an intensity of 70% of age predicted maximum heart rate (RPE = 5) at least three times per week for 30 minutes.
- Perform resistance training sessions three times per week for 30 minutes.
- Perform flexibility exercise at least two times per week stretching all the major joints for at least three sets of 30 seconds.

- Client to be involved in recreational physical activity that is enjoyable between once and twice per week.
- Perform regular progressive evaluations every 3 months.
- Report on hydration in general and during exercise.

Monitoring outcomes
- Repeat evaluation after 12 weeks of exercise program.
- Monitor training heart rate, blood pressure and breathlessness during training.
- Repeat lung function test after 12 weeks of training.
- Anthropometric and functional tests repeated after 12 weeks.
- Monitor blood glucose with every repeat evaluation.
- Monitor signs and symptoms of dehydration.
- Determine barriers to exercise during 12 week follow-up evaluation.
- Consult with medical practitioner on the outcome of medical tests that may influence the exercise program.

Outcomes
MV attended 10 supervised exercise sessions. Heart rate and blood pressure was measured during each training session. No repeat tests could be performed because she developed a respiratory infection (tuberculosis). She unfortunately did not return to her exercise program after the infection was cleared.

Summary of key lessons

- It is important to obtain the medical history and clinical information from the patient's general practitioner to be able to perform a comprehensive exercise test and exercise program prescription.

- When testing a patient with CF a lung function test should be performed. The outcome of the lung function test serves as an indicator for sub-maximal exercise testing by means of treadmill or bicycle.

- ECG, blood pressure and saturation should be measured as part of the incremental exercise test.

- Blood glucose should also be measured as pancreas function is influenced by CF.

- Due to regular infection of the lungs, exercise adherence is often difficult and irregular.

- CF patients often suffer from breathlessness. This should be monitored during each training session. In severe cases supplementary oxygen should be available.

- The medication used for CF patients may influence the exercise program. The patient should therefore be tested at the same time that exercise training would be performed to see the influence of the medication on the parameters measured during the incremental exercise test.

- Barriers to exercise should be determined especially in children who are reliant on parents to attend exercise programs. The advantages of exercise should therefore also be explained to the parents so that they can be part of the long-term goals that are set.

- Educate your patient about hydration in general and especially during exercise. CF patients become dehydrated easily and need to take fluids at regular intervals, not only when thirsty.

DISCUSSION Questions

1 Why is it important to measure blood glucose in MV, and what would you consider a normal glucose concentration? Refer to Chapter 16, case studies 1 and 2, for further discussion of glucose control.

2 What is the role of the clinical exercise practitioner in ensuring compliance with the exercise program?

3 What anticipatory counselling might you offer before the initiation of the exercise program?

4 In people with CF a postural kyphosis may be present. If this were the case with MV, how would you address this abnormality? Refer to Chapter 12, case study 2, for further discussion of thoracic kyphosis.

REFERENCES

Australian Lung Foundation (2009) *Pulmonary Toolkit*. Online. Available: www.pulmonaryrehab.com.au (accessed 22 July 2010)

Brukner P, Khan K (2007) *Clinical Sports Medicine* (3rd ed). Sydney: McGraw-Hill

Carlin BW, Singh A (2009) Asthma. In: Ehrman JK, Gordon, PM, Visich PS, et al (eds) *Clinical Exercise Physiology* (2nd ed). Champaign, IL: Human Kinetics, pp 391–401

Landry GL, Bernhardt DT (2003) *Essentials of Primary Care Sports Medicine*. Champaign, IL: Human Kinetics

Magee DJ (2008) *Orthopedic Physical Assessment* (5th ed). St Louis Missouri: Saunders Elsevier

Thompson WR, Gordon NF, Pescatello LS (eds) (2010) *ACSM's Guidelines for Exercise Testing and Prescription* (8th ed). Baltimore, MD: Lippincott Williams & Wilkins

Chapter 15

Case studies in exercise as therapy for neurological conditions

Marek Gorski and Cadeyrn J Gaskin

INTRODUCTION

The challenges of undertaking exercise therapy with clients who have neurological conditions are often as many and as varied as the impairments themselves. Motor impairments (eg: spasticity, tremors, ataxia) are often accompanied by a myriad of psychosocial issues. The case studies presented in this chapter touch on some of these issues. In case study 1, a clinical description of a case of exercise therapy for a young woman who experienced a subarachnoid haemorrhage is presented. In this case, the exercise therapist's role within a multidisciplinary team is highlighted. In case study 2, the emphasis shifts slightly from clinical aspects of exercise therapy to the motivation of a young man with cerebral palsy to perform exercise. Understanding clients' perspectives on exercise therapy and its meanings within the contexts of their lives can assist practitioners to design effective programs. In this case, the practicalities of assisting the young man to perform a weight training program are also discussed.

CASE STUDY 1: GEORGIA — LIFE CHANGES WITH A STROKE

Subjective

Georgia is a 28-year-old woman who suddenly collapses at home and is taken by an ambulance to an emergency department in a public hospital. She undergoes a computer-aided tomography (CT) scan and is diagnosed with a right subarachnoid

haemorrhage (SAH) due to a rupture of a right middle cerebral arterial aneurysm. Emergency craniotomy is preformed to drain a large volume of blood and to clip a right middle cerebral arterial bifurcation aneurysm. A bone flap on the right side of the scull is removed because of the swelling of the brain. There is no midline shift of the brain. A second CT scan shows secondary complications — right middle cerebral artery infarct.

Georgia has never been a smoker and has no previous history of any serious illness or hypertension. She is highly educated (higher degree in counselling) and has always been a supporter of the healthy lifestyle, with regular exercises and a healthy diet.

After 2 weeks in an acute hospital Georgia is transferred to a rehabilitation hospital for further treatment. On arrival, she is assessed by a multidisciplinary team including medical practitioners, a physiotherapist, an occupational therapist, a speech pathologist, a clinical exercise practitioner, a social worker and a neuropsychologist.

Objective

The initial findings are: dizziness, nausea, headaches, and absence of bone flap on the right side of the scull (Georgia has to wear a protective helmet at all times); decreased left visual field (hemianopia) and decreased left spatial perception (left side neglect); left hemiparesis including non-functional movement of the left upper limb (some adduction and elbow flexion); poor motor control of the left lower limb; decreased muscle strength of the left lower limb, particularly in the quadriceps, hamstrings, and gluteals (3/5 on the five point manual muscle strength testing scale); muscle weakness of the left shoulder girdle and risk of glenohumeral subluxation; increased muscle tone in left upper limb elbow flexors, particularly biceps brachii and brachialis; increased muscle tone and spasticity in left calf muscles, particularly gastrocnemius, soleus; left foot drop; and decreased sensation in the left upper and lower limbs. No speech or swallowing abnormalities are discovered.

Georgia is able to sit unsupported but she is unable to stand up independently and not able to walk.

Her exercise tolerance is very poor; she is able to tolerate about 30 minutes of seated exercise. Her resting blood pressure is 115/75mmHg, heart rate 78bpm.

Georgia refuses full psychology assessment. No cognitive abnormalities are discovered during the limited neuropsychology assessment.

Assessment

From the therapy point of view Georgia has to start physical therapy as soon as possible. The first 6 months are the most important in the recovery of a patient suffering from a cerebrovascular accident (CVA, 'stroke').

Multidisciplinary plan

Occupational therapy will provide a sling to support Georgia's left upper limb to prevent subluxation of the left shoulder. They also will be working with Georgia to improve her activities of daily living. Medical staff will provide necessary medications to manage her condition including headaches and nausea. They will also provide antithrombotic stockings to prevent deep vein thrombosis which is a very common complication for stroke patients. Psychologists and social workers will be providing an ongoing support for Georgia, her family, and also will monitor Georgia for signs of depression.

Due to a poor exercise tolerance, nausea, and dizziness, the team decides to limit the physical exercise program initially to physiotherapy only. Georgia's initial goals will be to improve strength and motor control of her left lower limb, transfers, standing balance, and function of the left upper limb. Georgia will start gait retraining and she also will be doing stretches to prevent contractions

and decrease spasticity of her left calf muscles. To work with Georgia, a physiotherapist will use motor relearning therapy as well as Bobath (neurodevelopmental) therapy. The emphasis will be on recovery and restoration of function rather than learning compensatory strategies.

Progress

After 4 weeks of physiotherapy treatment Georgia is referred to a clinical exercise practitioner for ongoing strengthening and cardiovascular fitness treatment. Georgia has made significant improvements. She now only occasionally suffers from nausea, dizziness and headaches. She is due to have a cranioplasty to insert a bone flap on the right side of her skull.

Her left visual field deficit and the left spatial perception have improved somewhat but are still significantly impaired. Tactile and kinaesthetic sensation in the left upper and lower limbs has improved.

Georgia's strength of the left lower limb has improved to 4/5. She is able to walk approximately 50m with minimal assistance. The motor control of the left lower limb is still poor.

A 10 metre walk test is conducted; Georgia takes 46 steps in 46.6 seconds to cover this distance. During this test Georgia requires close supervision, and her left knee is hyper-extended on every step. In a dynamic balance step test she takes 7 steps left leg and 6 steps right leg.

There is only minimal return of function in her dorsiflexors (2/5) and Georgia now wears an ankle foot orthosis (AFO) to prevent a foot drop. Spasticity in Georgia's left calf has decreased but is still significant, affecting her walking pattern, and together with the weakness of quadriceps (called 'quads lag') causing hyperextension of her left knee.

There is improvement in the muscular control of the left shoulder griddle but no significant changes in the function and muscle tone of the left upper limb. Georgia is now able to tolerate about 45 minutes of seated, standing, and walking exercises daily.

Georgia shows signs of depression. Although the function of her left lower limb has improved, she is very disappointed with the improvement in function of her left upper limb. She constantly seeks reassurance that she is going to recover completely. Although Georgia is a trained counsellor herself, she refuses to see a clinical psychologist or take antidepressant medication.

Ongoing multidisciplinary plan

Georgia will be discharged to the outpatients' clinic. Due to the increased level of depression, the team decides it would be beneficial for Georgia to live at home with her very supporting family and attend the clinic four times per week.

The medical staff will arrange as soon as possible the cranioplasty to insert a bone flap on the right side of Georgia's skull. That should have profound (if not quite immediate) affect on Georgia's mood because her physical appearance is very important to her.

Georgia's treatment will include physiotherapy, occupational therapy, and clinical exercise. Psychology will provide ongoing training and support for the other treating therapists to help the team to deal with Georgia's depression. A social worker will help to resolve any issues which may arise after discharge. Regular team treatment planning and review meetings will be organised every 2 weeks. Regular family meetings attended by all members of the treating team will be organised to inform Georgia's family on her progress. The emphases of interventions will be on recovery and restoration of function rather then learning compensatory strategies. Georgia is 28 years old and it is extremely important to restore function to her left side as much as possible.

Clinical exercise plan

Georgia will benefit from a cardiovascular exercise program. Severe cardiovascular deconditioning occurs as a result of immobility early after stroke. She now has sufficient strength in the left lower limb to be able to use equipment such as an exercise bike or stepper. The treadmill walking will be introduced to improve Georgia's ambulation as soon as her walking pattern improves. There is a risk of reinforcing unwanted movement patterns if treadmill exercise is started too early. The decision will be made jointly by a physiotherapist and a clinical exercise practitioner.

Georgia will start progressive resistance exercises to improve her strength, particularly the strength of her left limbs. Weakness is one of the major impairments after stroke. Exercises to strengthen her hip flexors and extensors, adductors and abductors, knee flexors and extensors, and ankle dorsiflexors and plantarflexors will be prescribed. Her strengthening program will include both open and closed chain exercises. She

will be doing exercises using the gym equipment as well as functional exercises. Strengthening exercises will not increase spasticity in her left calf.

Georgia will start left upper body exercises as soon as the strength and motor control of her shoulder muscles improves such that the risk of subluxation and damage to the glenohumeral joint is low. This decision will be made in consultation with a physiotherapist. Georgia will start with one easy exercise, such as using an upper body ergometer (Monark) with no resistance. She may have to have her hand strapped to a handle as she has very little activity in her hand. She also will need to exercise slowly to be able to turn off the muscle tone of her left elbow flexors. With time, she may progress to resisted exercises using equipment such as a functional trainer machine and weights.

To improve Georgia's spatial perception on her left side the following strategies will be used:
- Georgia will be advised to scan to her left side
- if unilateral exercises are performed she will start on her left side first
- when interacting with Georgia, the therapist will position themself on Georgia's left side.

Georgia will be doing balance exercises to improve her static and dynamic balance. She is at risk of falling and her balance has to improve to be able to walk independently.

Georgia will benefit from stretching exercises. Prolonged stretching will prevent contraction and also may decrease spasticity of her left calf muscles. She may also need to consider a Botulinum Toxin (Botox) injection to her left calf later on if the stretching has a limited effect.

Short-term exercise goals
- Improve Georgia's cardiovascular fitness so she can tolerate 60 minutes of exercises at the low/moderate intensity (estimated time to reach goal is 4 weeks: 4/52).
- Improve the strength of the left lower limb to 5/5 for major muscle groups, including resolution of quadriceps lag, and to 3/5 for ankle dorsiflexors (6/52).
- Improve dorsiflexion of the left ankle (2/52).
- Improve gait pattern to be able to start treadmill to improve walking endurance and speed (4/52).

- Improve balance for independent walking and enable safe negotiation of steps with rails (4/52).
- Start left upper limb exercises (4/52).

Outcome measures to be used
- Dynamic balance step test: consists of placing one foot forward on a 7.5cm high block and back on the floor in 15 seconds. The step test is commonly used to assess balance in persons with stroke.
- Timed up-and-go test: measures walking speed during several balance manoeuvres.
- Six-minute walk test (6MWT): to measure walking endurance.

Precautions
Unfortunately there is only limited data in the literature regarding intensity of exercises for subarachnoid haemorrhage survivors with clipped aneurysms. In general, recommendations are to avoid high intensity and heavy resistance exercises, which may cause significant increase in blood pressure (American College of Sports Medicine [ACSM] 2004; Gordon et al 2004; Williams et al 2007). There is also a one in five chance of the aneurysm recurring in people who survived SAH (Lindsay & Bone 2004).

Due to Georgia's condition, one repetition maximum strength and sub-maximal cardio-vascular fitness tests cannot be used. Exercise intensity will be restricted to 70% of the maximum predicted heart rate or 12–14 on Borg scale for rating perceived exertion (RPE). Heavy resistance exercises (4–6 on the 10-point RPE scale) and isometric exercises will not be included in Georgia's exercise program.

Outcomes
Georgia has been participating in the exercise program for 3 months now. She has improved in almost all problem areas. The strength of the main muscle groups in her left lower limb is now 4+ or 5/5. She can now walk independently, 6MWT = 285m. The spasticity in her left calf hasn't changed but with improved knee control she can walk slowly without hyper-extending her left knee. The strength of the dorsiflexors in her left ankle is now 3/5. She only uses AFO for long distance walking. Her dynamic balance has improved. Step test: 12 steps with left leg and 8 with right leg; timed up-and-go test 11.5 seconds. Her exercise tolerance

has improved. She is able to tolerate more than an hour of light to moderate intensity exercises.

Georgia's visual problems are slowly resolving and she is now well aware of her left spatial perception deficit.

Georgia's left upper limb has improved and Georgia is now able to use an arm ergometer with her left arm only. She still needs to have her hand strapped to the handle as there is only limited activity in her hand. Georgia is still unable to progress to more functional exercises with her left arm. The lack of return of function in her left arm is a concern for treating therapists and Georgia. She is reasonably pleased with her general progress but very depressed about recovery of her left arm.

Georgia still refuses to see a psychologist. She constantly needs reassurance about her progress and future recovery.

Recommendations
At this stage of Georgia's recovery the treating team will continue with an intensive treatment of her left arm to try to recover as much function as possible. Because there are no noticeable changes in the spasticity of Georgia's left calf muscles, the treating team has recommended a Botulinum Toxin (Botox) injection to her left gastrocnemius and soleus. She also will be working to improve her walking speed, walking pattern and motor control of her left leg. The more challenging balance exercises and high level skills, such as running and swimming, will be introduced to enable Georgia to participate in recreational activities. With time the issue of return to work will need to be addressed and Georgia will be discharged to a community based centre for ongoing rehabilitation.

Discussion
Georgia will keep improving as long as she has the motivation to attend therapy and exercise. It has been demonstrated that for stroke survivors the more they practice the more recovery can be achieved (National Stroke Foundation 2010). Because of Georgia's age (28) it is absolutely crucial to restore as much function as possible. With time she will make further improvements and new goals will be set. How much she recovers, nobody can tell. With the constant advances in medicine and continuing practice, she will keep improving. It is important that she sets achievable goals for herself but still see the big picture.

Summary of key lessons

- Stroke (CVA) is a cardiovascular condition with neurological consequences.

- It is often a very debilitating condition resulting in multiple physical, intellectual, and behavioural problems, which have to be addressed by a multidisciplinary team. All members of the team are equally important as they have different, unique skills and expertise to address specific aspects of the client's rehabilitation.

- The rehabilitation process should start as soon as possible to achieve the best outcomes for a client. The most return of function occurs in the first 6 months.

- Treatment goals should be achievable and set together with the client.

- Ongoing education should be provided for the client and his/her relatives.

- Post-stroke depression is very common.

DISCUSSION Questions

1 Consider how the exercise therapy provided for Georgia by the clinical exercise practitioner might differ from the exercise therapy provided by a physiotherapist and an occupational therapist. How do practitioners of these disciplines interact, and work together to offer care to a client?

2 Considering relevant risk factors, how could you design a safe exercise program for Georgia and still achieve significant improvements in her cardiovascular fitness and strength?

3 What adverse signs and symptoms are likely to appear as a result of exercise for this client? At what thresholds would you stop exercise?

4 Post-stroke depression is very common. What strategies would you use to motivate Georgia and manage her mood during and after exercise therapy?

CASE STUDY 2: EXERCISING FOR ROMANCE

Although therapeutic exercise is beneficial for people with cerebral palsy (Taylor et al 2007), many people who have this neurological condition lead sedentary lives (Gaskin & Morris 2008). Helping clients to develop and maintain motivation for exercise rehabilitation programs is often a difficult task. Superficial reasons for adhering to, or not engaging in, exercise rehabilitation programs can sometimes mask deep-seated motivations. Through gaining an understanding of these motivations, by carefully listening to their clients, clinicians are well-placed to help clients adhere to exercise rehabilitation programs.

This case is not typical of exercise rehabilitation. The 'client' (David) was 27 years old when he was part of a research project on physical activity in the lives of people with cerebral palsy. This research had a strong psychosocial bent, and incorporated over 4 hours of interviews with David about his life. The stories David told during these interviews were hugely informative about his life and his motivation to perform physical activity. These interviews occurred over a 10-week period, while David was participating in a weight training program. The description of the case that follows blends the practicalities of assisting David with an exercise program with interpretations of what motivated him to adhere to the program.

Cerebral palsy

Cerebral palsy is a neurological condition that affects between 1.2 and 3.0 of every 1000 live-born children in the developed world (Paneth, Hong & Korzeniewski 2006). The condition is 'not a single entity but covers neurological impairments characterised by abnormal control of movement or posture resulting from abnormalities in brain development or an acquired non-progressive cerebral lesion' (The Australian and New Zealand Perinatal Societies 1995: 85). Cerebral palsy is commonly described in terms of motor disorder and typography. Spasticity, in its purest form, is the most common type of motor disorder, and is evident in approximately 76% of all cases (Stanley et al 2000). Dyskinesia (occurring in its pure form in 6% of cases), ataxia (affecting 5% of cases in its purest form), and mixtures of all three motor disorders are also prevalent among cerebral palsy cases. Topographical classification refers to the limbs affected by cerebral palsy. Common distributions of impairment are hemiplegia (43%), diplegia (24%), quadriplegia (12%), and non-classical forms (21%; Stanley et al 2000). David's cerebral palsy was a moderately severe form of spasticity that mainly affected his lower limbs and, to a lesser extent, the left side of his body. Although he could walk independently at 10 years of age (250 consecutive steps was his reported best effort), this ability subsequently diminished due to severe pain in his lower back, which stemmed from tight hamstrings. At 12, David's hamstrings were surgically lengthened to alleviate the severe pain that he was experiencing. David used a motorised scooter for mobility, because he found walking extremely difficult and slow. He had minimal active movement in the hips, knees, and ankles, and he required the support of a walking stick in his left hand and assistance from a person on his right side to walk.

David's motivation

During the exercise program David's adherence was exemplary; he attended all exercise sessions except for one, when the battery in his scooter malfunctioned and could not be remedied quickly.

During the sessions he enthusiastically performed the prescribed exercises and regularly set new personal bests. The reasons why he was highly motivated to exercise became evident during the interviews.

As is often the case for people with cerebral palsy (Donovan 1995; Olkin 1995), David's condition not only affected his ability to perform physical tasks, but also his psychosocial functioning. Like many people who have cerebral palsy (Blotzer 1995), David found society to be judgmental and unaccommodating. His life had been characterised by an inability to demonstrate competence in several key settings (eg: education, physical, social) and by significant others in his life (eg: his father) emotionally abandoning him. This inability to show competence contributed to his development spiralling downwards into periods of depression, which included two suicidal gestures in his late teens and early 20s.

David, similar to many single people of his age, wished to have a romantic relationship. Like many men with cerebral palsy (Shuttleworth 2000), however, he struggled to attract potential partners. David had made numerous attempts throughout his adolescence and young adulthood to become connected with others, especially young women with whom he wished to form romantic relationships, but struggled to do so. Over time, his difficulties with finding love were prime motivators for him to be engaged in physical activity.

David's sexuality was intimately associated with his ability to walk. David felt that his limited ability to walk was the reason why attracting a romantic partner was so challenging for him. He attributed previous unsuccessful efforts to form romantic relationships to his walking ability and had fantasies of how his prospects would dramatically improve if he regained his ability to walk. Participating in the 10-week exercise program, then, was intrinsically linked to David's desire to walk again and to attract a romantic partner.

Exercise and cerebral palsy

To guide the prescription of exercise for David, we used guidelines from the American College of Sports Medicine (ACSM; Laskin 2003). These guidelines include advice on the prescription of aerobic, endurance, strength, and flexibility exercises for people with cerebral palsy. In regard to weight training, strength exercises can be performed using free weights or weight machines. With resistance set at a level that can be tolerated, the recommended program involves three sets of 8–12 repetitions of each exercise, performed 2 days per week. Laskin (2003) highlighted several special considerations for the practitioner to increase the effectiveness of exercise sessions for people with cerebral palsy. Because unwanted movement, caused by spasticity and/or athetosis, can make performing exercises difficult, the use of straps, wraps, or gloves can be useful to secure or stabilise specific body parts. In using these aids, however, care must be taken to avoid them being too tight, which may cause skin breakdown. Further, if these aids are causing pain or discomfort, spasticity may increase, which may result in a decrease in exercise performance. Certain exercises require a spotter to be present for safety reasons. For example, when using a treadmill, a spotter needs to be provided in case of a fall. Medications taken by some people with cerebral palsy to control epileptic seizures (eg: phenobarbital, phenytoin, carbamazepine) or spasticity (eg: benzodiazepines, baclofen) can confound the results of exercise testing and have an adverse effect on exercise performance (Laskin 2003). The anti-spasticity medications benzodiazepines and baclofen, for example, have sedation and weakness as common side-effects (Krach 2001). The use and dosage of such medications should be established during the physical screening of the person with cerebral palsy.

David's 10-week exercise program

Because the type of motor disorder and the extent to which cerebral palsy can affect a person's motor control can differ markedly between individuals, the prescription of exercise for people with this condition tends to be highly individualised. In designing the weight training program for David, we were cognisant of the spasticity and co-contraction of muscles in his lower limbs and the mild spasticity in his right upper body.

David trained 2 days per week (Tuesday and Thursday mornings), with each session being approximately 60 minutes long. Before the program started three daily workout plans were devised, with the intention of rotating these workouts, if David could perform all the exercises, or reducing the number of exercises to fit into two daily workout plans if David was unable to perform some of the exercises. Each workout contained three compound exercises for the chest (barbell bench press, seated cable press, or Smith machine bench press), back (lateral pull-down or prone barbell row), and legs (45° leg press or seated leg curl). The seated leg curl was the only isolation exercise, and was included because it was noted that David appeared to have weak hamstrings. When lying prone, David could not raise either foot off the floor by flexing the knee joint. The leg curl, in combination with the stretching of the quadriceps muscles, was prescribed in an attempt to improve his voluntary range of motion at this joint.

During the first three sessions, it was found that David could do all exercises, albeit with assistance and slight modifications. For the barbell bench press, a bench was placed under David's feet, because his feet did not come into contact with the floor due to the limited range of motion of his knee joints. This modification was not required for the Smith machine bench press, because the bench was long enough to fully support his legs. To give David extra stability, a weight belt, positioned mid thigh, was used to strap his legs to the bench. To ensure the strapping was comfortable, a weight belt with a broad back was chosen to disperse the pressure over a wider area, and the buckle was placed on the underside of the bench so that it would not dig into his legs. For the lateral pull-down, David sat on two 25kg weight plates, because the seat was too low for him to sit upright. With the limited range of motion in his knee joints, being seated too close to the floor caused him to lean backwards, when an upright position was required for the exercise. For the 45° leg press, a slightly deflated volleyball was placed between David's knees to ensure correct alignment of the knees during the exercise. Without the ball, the spasticity in David's adductors caused his knees to come together and would not enable him to perform the exercise using correct technique. For the seated leg curl, a weight belt, placed mid-shin, was used to strap David's legs onto the machine. David needed assistance to get into position for each exercise, and some help to execute the exercises.

During each session, David performed three sets for each of the three exercises. The targeted repetition range was 8–12 repetitions. Following the performance of these exercises, David was stretched with the assistance of the trainers. The major stretches were for quadriceps, hamstrings and adductors.

Outcomes

Because this case study was part of a research project and not a clinical consultation, the outcome measures were targeted towards addressing the research questions of the project rather than the expressed needs of the client. David agreed to participate in the research knowing that it involved engaging in a general weight training program, responding to psychosocially orientated questionnaires and undertaking strength tests, and being interviewed about his life and the exercise program. Although, during the interviews, he discussed his desire to be able to walk again, the research project was not designed to assist him to attempt this goal. The primary outcomes, then, were changes in strength and psychosocial functioning, as well as impressions of David and his thoughts on the program gained through the interviews.

Measures of strength on three exercises (Smith machine bench press, lateral pull-down, 45° leg press) were taken at weeks 3 and 10. The first measure of strength was taken at week 3, rather than during week 1, so that David had time to become comfortable with the exercises. Familiarisation sessions are recommended when changes in strength are being tracked over time, so as to increase the likelihood that any changes will be due to physiological adaptations (ACSM 2005), and not to learning effects. In the first 2 weeks of the program, David learned, and had an opportunity to practice, each exercise used in the strength test. The testing was designed to find David's three repetition maximum (3RM) on each exercise. Testing for David's 3RM on each exercise, rather than his 1RM, was conducted for safety reasons.

David increased his 3RM between weeks 3 and 10 for all three exercises. He increased his 3RM on the Smith machine bench press by 36% (from 70kg to 95kg), lateral pull-down by 56% (from 64kg to 100kg), and 45° leg press by 50% (from 180kg to 270kg).

Standard measures of several areas of psychosocial functioning (eg: mood, physical self-efficacy, social support) were administered at weeks 1, 5 and 9. David's scores at all three time points were highly favourable (eg: high physical self-efficacy) compared with other people with cerebral palsy (Gaskin & Morris 2008). These scores were at odds with stories of his struggles during his life (e.g., long periods of depressed mood), which he told during the interviews. At the time of the exercise program, David said that he was trying to think positively about life, which probably affected how he responded to the psychosocial measures. Accordingly, little was learned from David's scores on these measures about the possible effects of weight training programs on the psychosocial functioning of people with cerebral palsy.

From the interviews, it was clear that David's positive relationships with the trainers also seemed to enhance his motivation to persist with the exercise program during the 10 weeks. In his life, David experienced limited support from his father, medical practitioners, and teachers, and did not seem to have a strong network of friends. In contrast, David seemed to enjoy the respect, encouragement, and support he received from the trainers. Through participating in the research, David maintained the hope that he may, one day, walk again and attract a romantic partner.

Summary of key lessons

- Cerebral palsy presentations differ markedly between individuals.
- Exercise is of considerable benefit for improving and maintaining quality of life in people with cerebral palsy.
- Clinical exercise practitioners need to pay attention to individual needs, aspirations, and physical capabilities when planning exercise programs for people with cerebral palsy.

DISCUSSION Questions

- Is understanding a client's motivation to exercise important? If so, how might a therapist elicit and use such information?

- Consider a client with severe quadriplegic cerebral palsy who is dependent on others for performing ADL. What forms of exercise may be possible when working with such a client?

- Consider a client with mild hemiplegic cerebral palsy affecting the left side of her body. What strategies could be employed to assist her in performing exercises in the gym?

- Consider the role of *hope* in exercise therapy. Is it important to give clients hope that they will meet their goals? What about false hope?

REFERENCES

American College of Sports Medicine (ACSM) (2004) Exercise and Hypertension. Position Stand: Medicine & Science in Sports & Exercise

—— (2005) *ACSM's Health-Related Physical Fitness Assessment Manual*. Philadelphia: Lippincott Williams & Wilkins

American Heart Association (2007) *Resistance Exercise in Individuals With and Without Cardiovascular Disease. Benefits, Rationale, Safety and Prescription*. Online. Available: www.circulationaha.org (accessed 24 August 2010)

Blotzer MA (1995) Glimpses of lives: Stories of brief treatment. In: Blotzer MA, Ruth R (eds) *Sometimes You Just Want to Feel Like a Human Being: Case Studies of Empowering Psychotherapy with People with Disabilities*. Baltimore: Brookes, pp 151–62

Donovan K (1995) Sally: Recovery of our missing pieces. In: Blotzer MA, Ruth R (eds) *Sometimes You Just Want to Feel Like a Human Being: Case Studies of Empowering Psychotherapy with People with Disabilities*. Baltimore: Brookes, pp 183–90

Gaskin CJ, Morris T (2008) Physical activity, health-related quality of life, and psychosocial functioning of adults with cerebral palsy. *Journal of Physical Activity and Health*, 5:146–57

Gordon NF, Gulanick M, Costa C, et al (2004) Physical Activity and Exercise Recommendations for Stroke Survivors. An American Heart Association Scientific Statement From the Council on Clinical Cardiology, Subcommittee on Exercise, Cardiac Rehabilitation, and Prevention; the Council on Cardiovascular Nursing; the Council on Nutrition, Physical Activity, and Metabolism; and the Stroke Council. *Stroke* 2004;35;1230–40. DOI: 10.1161/01.STR.0000127303.19261.19

Krach LE (2001) Pharmacotherapy of spasticity: oral medications and intrathecal baclofen. *Journal of Child Neurology*, 16:31–6

Laskin JJ (2003) *Cerebral Palsy*. In: American College of Sports Medicine, *ACSM's Exercise Management for Persons With Chronic Diseases and Disabilities* (2nd ed). Champaign, IL: Human Kinetics, pp 288–94

Lindsay KW, Bone I (2004) *Neurology and Neurosurgery Illustrated* (4th ed). Edinburgh: Churchill Livingstone

National Stroke Foundation [Australia] (2010) Clinical Guidelines for Stroke Management 2010. Available: www.strokefoundation.com.au/clinical guidelines (accessed 31 August 2010)

Olkin R (1995) Matthew: therapy with a teenager with a disability. In: Blotzer MA, Ruth R (eds) *Sometimes You Just Want to Feel Like a Human Being: Case Studies of Empowering Psychotherapy with People with Disabilities*. Baltimore: Brookes, pp 37–51

Paneth N, Hong T, Korzeniewski S (2006) The descriptive epidemiology of cerebral palsy. *Clinics in Perinatology*, 33:251–67

Shuttleworth RP (2000) The search for sexual intimacy for men with cerebral palsy. *Sexuality and Disability*, 18:263–82

Stanley F, Blair E, Alberman E (2000) *Cerebral Palsies: Epidemiology and Causal Pathways*. London: Mac Keith Press

Taylor NF, Dodd KJ, Shields N, et al (2007) Therapeutic exercise in physiotherapy practice is beneficial: a summary of systematic reviews 2002–2005. *Australian Journal of Physiotherapy*, 53:7–16

The Australian and New Zealand Perinatal Societies (1995) The origins of cerebral palsy: a consensus statement. *Medical Journal of Australia*, 162:85–90

Williams MA, Haskell WL, Ades PA, et al (2007) Resistance Exercise In Individuals With And Without Cardiovascular Disease 2007 Update. A Scientific Statement From the American Heart Association Council on Clinical Cardiology and Council on Nutrition, Physical Activity, and Metabolism. *Circulation* 2007;116;572-584. DOI: 10.1161/CIRCULATIONAHA.107.185214

Chapter 16

Case studies in exercise as therapy for metabolic conditions

Steve Selig, Itamar Levinger, Helena Teede* and Amanda Deeks*

INTRODUCTION

In this chapter we present four case studies using exercise as therapy, or part of a broader therapeutic regimen, for metabolic conditions. As explained in Chapter 6, exercise is a powerful 'pill' for the management of metabolic conditions that alter glucose control. More, exercise is treatment with very few risks or side-effects in these clients because low to moderate intensity exercise is typically sufficient to afford some clinical change and gradual progression of exercise affords further improvements.

CASE STUDY 1: DIABETES MELLITUS AND A HISTORY OF MYOCARDIAL INFARCTION

Subjective

JL is a 52-year-old female who had developed obesity by 1996 — body mass index (BMI) is now 37.5 — and was diagnosed with type 2 diabetes mellitus (T2DM) in 2000. The diagnosis of T2DM was a chance event as she had attended the general practice for a prescription of Mogadon for insomnia, but the alert general practitioner (GP) took the opportunity to perform routine cardiovascular and metabolic observations and collected a random (non-fasted) blood sample

that returned an elevated blood glucose of 12.3mmol.l⁻¹. The diagnosis was confirmed when JL was persuaded by the GP to undertake an oral glucose tolerance test that showed a 2-hour post-prandial blood glucose of 9mmol.l⁻¹. JL has smoked since she was 15, with a smoking history of 45 pack-years and is both a regular and binge drinker who gets drunk at least once per week. She was employed as a shift worker in a food processing plant, and apart from occupational exercise of standing, walking, carrying and some lifting, she did little other exercise. Her diet was largely comprised of processed and take-away foods and she rarely (< 2 per week) cooks a fresh meal of meat and vegetables or eats fruit.

At the time of her T2DM diagnosis, JL was prescribed metformin by her GP who at the same time handed her pamphlets on exercise, nutrition, smoking cessation and alcohol dependence. At that stage the GP did not refer JL to allied health professionals such as a diabetes educator, dietitian or clinical exercise practitioner, as the GP believed that JL would not respond well to multiple interventions. Instead, the GP came to the view that the best initial course of action was to manage JL with metformin for the first couple of months, and then to refer to other allied health professionals once blood glucose control had improved. The GP felt that it was also possible that JL's early response to metformin may result in some desirable weight loss.

*These authors gratefully acknowledge the contribution of Dr Nigel Stepto for his expertise and assistance with case studies 3 and 4.

JL did not even read the pamphlets and lacked motivation to modify any of her risk factors for cardiovascular disease and diabetes. She also had a very poor understanding of the possible health impacts of diabetes and saw the condition as little more than a 'sugar problem'. JL soon became poorly compliant to metformin and stopped taking the medication altogether after the first three repeats. JL did not return to the GP again in 2000 and so was not referred to other health professionals to assist her to manage her diabetes.

In late 2004, JL woke up at 4 a.m. feeling very unwell with sweating, chest pain and nausea. Apart from taking pain killers and an antacid, she did nothing until later in the morning and then finally called her neighbour who looked after her for the next few days at home. JL did not attend hospital during or after this episode.

Twelve months after this health scare, JL lodged a workers' compensation claim for a stress-related illness. While on a return-to-work plan, JL volunteered for an 8-week exercise intervention study for people living with both diabetes and cardiovascular disease, and as such came under the care of a clinical exercise practitioner.

Objective

The clinical exercise practitioner conducted an initial exercise symptom-limited graded exercise test on a cycle ergometer for the assessment of aerobic power (VO_{2peak}). The clinical exercise practitioner recorded this pre-exercise ECG (see Figure 16.1). This was the first ECG since JL's chest pain episode in 2004.

The clinical exercise practitioner proceeded with the 8-week exercise intervention once safety

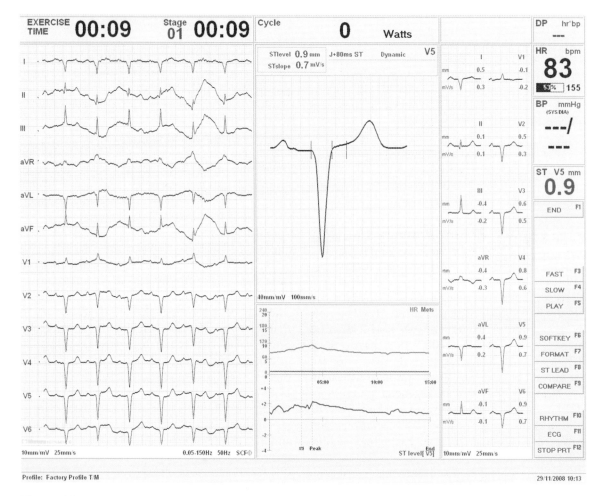

Figure 16.1 Pre-exercise ECG trace

had been established. A pre-intervention exercise study was conducted on a cycle ergometer, and an extract of the test is summarised in Table 16.1.

Assessment

In summary, the exercise test confirmed evidence of an old and extensive myocardial infarction, but current ischaemic heart disease was very unlikely, making it safe for her to participate in both the study and self-directed exercise. Breathlessness and hypoxia are barriers to her participation and these will need to be managed.

A second series of resistance exercise tests was conducted, using seven movement patterns involving all major joints. The client was asked to perform a 3RM test for each pattern; 3RM was considered safer than 1RM for this client. (3RM refers to the maximal load that can be lifted for three, but not more than three, repetitions; 1RM

is a similar term identifying loads that be lifted just once.) To eliminate an order effect, the same tests were repeated over the next few weeks using alternative sequences. An average of the results for three of the seven movement patterns is reported in Table 16.2.

Barriers to exercise intervention

JL has had a lifetime aversion to exercise and healthy lifestyle in general. This has contributed substantially to her current predicament of serious chronic cardiovascular and metabolic disease, and is likely to adversely affect her future quality of life (QoL) and longevity if she continues with her current lifestyle.

If JL had current angina, then this would have prevented her from participating in the exercise study, and been an absolute contraindication for participation in exercise and physical activity

---

Table 16.1 Results of pre-intervention cycle ergometry test

Stage	Watts	VO$_2$ (% peak)[1]	HR (% peak)	HbO$_2$sat%	RPE[2]	RPB[3]	ECG[4]	Comment
Rest (pre-exercise)	–	–	81 (47%)	99	–	–	SR; path Q in anterior and lateral leads	ECG evidence of old extensive myocardial infarction
Sub-maximal exercise	30	6.8 (49%)	115 (67%)	95	11	12	SR, no VEs, no ST↓	RPB ahead of RPE
Peak exercise	60	10.5 (75%)	144 (84%)	92	16	18	SR, some (<6) monomorphic VEs in last minute; no ST↓	Became very breathless at 60W with O$_2$sat% dropping to 91%; no ischaemia
1 min recovery	–	–	124 (72%)	95	–	–	SR, a few AEs, no ST↓	Slow recovery in heart rate
10 min recovery	–	–	88 (51%)	98	–	–	SR, no VEs, no ST↓	

[1] Peak exercise for this test occurred at a heart rate of 144, below the predicted maximal heart rate of 172 for a 52-year-old female not on medications. Based on HR$_{peak}$ = 172, VO$_{2peak}$ was predicted to be 14 ml.kg^{-1}.min^{-1}.

[2] RPE = ratings of perceived exertion, using Borg 6–20 point scale.

[3] RPB = ratings of perceived breathlessness, using a 6–20 point scale.

[4] ECG key: SR = sinus rhythm; AE = atrial ectopic; VE = ventricular ectopic; ST↓ = ST depression [possible ischaemia]; path Q = Q wave ≥ 25% of R amplitude [suggestive of previous full wall thickness infarct = Q infarct].

Table 16.2 Mean results of three 3RM tests

Stage[1]	HR(% peak)	RPE	RPB	Comment
Rest (pre-exercise)	85 (49%)	–	–	
Upper limb: bilateral elbow flexion and/or extension	155 (90%)	16	14	Upper limb exercises causes heart rate to rise higher, relative to similar intensities of exercise for lower limb and trunk. Client was relatively untroubled by breathlessness, compared to aerobic exercise test above
Lower limb: bilateral knee extension and/or flexion	142 (83%)	17	16	
Trunk: sit-ups with disc weight across chest	145 (84%)	17	17	

[1] Heart rate was permitted to return to within 10 b.min^{-1} of pre-exercise levels before commencing the next pattern.

programs. It was very important in this case that current angina was ruled out by the absence of signs and symptoms during her VO_{2peak} test and further risk analysis. There is a slight risk due to the fact that she was so limited by breathlessness that she was not able to reach her age-predicted HR_{peak}, but safety of participation is likely due to the exercise intervention being no greater than the peak exercise intensities reached during the pre-intervention exercise tests (both aerobic and resistance).

Enablers to exercise intervention

JL recently nursed her father, who had emphysema and a previous myocardial infarction, until his death from COPD. Her father died shortly before JL volunteered for the exercise study and was the 'final straw' in motivating JL to change her lifestyle. Although very painful for JL, witnessing the slow and uncomfortable demise of her father had become a motivating factor, at least for now. It also acted as a significant lever for the clinical exercise practitioner and other health professionals to support JL to make the necessary changes to her lifestyle to reduce her risks of increased chronic morbidity and early death.

Plan

Practitioner goals were for JL to get through the screening procedures in order to participate fully in the exercise study. This will enable JL to engage in exercise and physical activity on most days of the week. Client goals were to engage in regular exercise and lose weight (see intermediate goals, below).

Immediate exercise strategies

JL's glycaemic control was determined at rest (fasting blood glucose) and her involvement in the study was conditional on her resuming metformin; she agreed to comply with this. At this stage, there was no need to measure blood glucose during and following exercise, as her very low exercise capacity meant that it was very unlikely that she would be troubled by hypoglycaemia related to large volumes of exercise. Nevertheless, she was advised by the clinical exercise practitioner not to undertake more than 30 minutes of continuous moderate intensity exercise or 15 minutes of high intensity exercise, and was educated on the signs and symptoms of hypoglycaemia. JL was further advised to contact the clinical exercise practitioner in the event that any of these appear as a result of exercise or her participation in the study.

Regarding her breathlessness, JL was counselled that this is to be expected for smokers who have not exercised for extended periods, and gradually this will improve. It was recognised by both practitioner and client that multiple interventions (commencing participation in exercise, smoking cessation, medication compliance all at the same time) would quickly overwhelm JL, and so the immediate strategy was to focus on medication and exercise at this stage. If and when JL made medium-term gains with these, smoking and alcohol could be addressed.

Intermediate goals of exercise intervention

Practitioner goals included using exercise and metformin to improve glycaemic control at rest, and during and after exercise. Related to this, the clinical exercise practitioner supported JL to improve her knowledge and understanding of T2DM and its strong connections with cardiovascular morbidity and mortality. She currently thought of diabetes as no more than a 'sugar problem'. Further, the clinical exercise practitioner wanted JL to commit to preventing further deterioration of her metabolic and cardiovascular conditions, and even to improve her clinical status through healthy lifestyle and medication compliance.

Client goals were to improve fitness, lose weight, give up smoking and cut down on alcohol consumption. JL wanted to change jobs eventually to an office job, and to achieve this she enrolled in a Certificate 2 course in Information Technology. JL also wanted to lose 2kg per week for the first 4 months; the clinical exercise practitioner counselled JL that this goal was probably unachievable and certainly unsustainable, and even if this rapid weight loss could be achieved, undesirable muscle and body water would make up much of the weight loss.

Both practitioner and client wanted the client to experience the mood elevating benefits of daily exercise and physical activity participation. JL was becoming stronger in her attempts to cut down smoking with a view to quitting. To assist her with smoking cessation, she was advised to go for a 5–10 minute walk instead of a 'smoko' and arrangements were made to permit this at her workplace.

Intermediate exercise strategies

The emphasis in this stage was to plan, do, reinforce, and improve upon the immediate strategies outlined above, with a gradual shift from practitioner-driven to client-driven management of the program and lifestyle. The clinical exercise practitioner provided a weekly plan that if followed would achieve a weekly weight loss of 0.5kg for the next 6 months.

Long-term goals of exercise intervention

JL gradually became more engaged in her lifestyle program and long-term health. The practitioner and client goals began to coincide for the first time, with the overall aim to arrest the progression of metabolic and cardiovascular disease, and to prevent another acute cardiovascular event such as a myocardial infarction or stroke. The main functional aims of the program were to improve fitness and QoL. Smoking cessation and alcohol dependence were addressed, and the client was referred to programs with proven efficacy. In the meantime and as an interim measure, JL was counselled that mortality in smokers with a high level of VO_{2peak} was lower than in non-smokers with low VO_{2peak}, based on the work of Blair et al (1996). Long-term exercise strategies were continuations of the medium-term strategies, with gradual transfers to self-management and self-efficacy.

Outcome

JL lost only modest amounts of weight, but gained 25% in VO_{2peak} and managed to cut down on smoking to a fraction of her previous habit.

Discussion

Progression from obesity to diabetes to myocardial infarction, with a high risk of mortality, is accelerated in those who are non-compliant with prescribed medications or fail to change their unhealthy lifestyles. Ignoring signs and symptoms of an acute myocardial infarction results in a worse prognosis than those who call for emergency medical services. People living with diabetes mellitus often underplay the severity of their conditions and are unaware of the prognosis. For people with obesity-related diabetes, weight loss needs to be slow and sustainable. The biggest challenge for health professionals who work with people living with chronic medical conditions and complex care needs is that clients often lack both the motivation and knowledge needed to make the lifestyle changes to improve their long-term clinical status. Prescribing an evidence-based exercise program is the easy part; this by itself rarely results in long-term behaviour change. Interventions applied to clients with multiple cardiovascular and metabolic risk factors need to be applied in a logical sequence that the client can relate to; multiple interventions applied simultaneously tend to be overwhelming for clients and rarely result in long-term behaviour change.

Summary of key lessons

- Progression from obesity to diabetes to myocardial infarction, with a high risk of mortality, is accelerated in those who are non-compliant with prescribed medications or fail to change their unhealthy lifestyles.

- Ignoring signs and symptoms of an acute myocardial infarction results in a worse prognosis than those who call for emergency medical services.

- People living with diabetes mellitus often underplay the severity of their conditions and are unaware of the prognosis.

- For people with obesity-related diabetes, weight loss needs to be slow and sustainable.

- The biggest challenge for health professionals who work with people living with chronic medical conditions and complex care needs is that clients often lack both the motivation and knowledge needed to make the lifestyle changes to improve their long-term clinical status. Prescribing an evidence-based exercise program is the easy part; this by itself rarely results in long-term behaviour change.

- Interventions applied to clients with multiple cardiovascular and metabolic risk factors need to be applied in a logical sequence that the client can relate to; multiple interventions applied simultaneously rarely results in long-term behaviour change.

DISCUSSION Questions

1. What are the main risks with participation in exercise and physical activity for this client?
2. What are the main benefits with participation in exercise and physical activity for this client?
3. Outline the referral and service networks that will be needed to support this client.

CASE STUDY 2: RESISTANCE TRAINING FOR METABOLIC SYNDROME

Subjective

Rowena is a 53-year-old woman who is a teacher with metabolic syndrome (MetS). Currently Rowena is treated with lipitor (anti-cholesterol) and hormone replacement therapy. In addition, Rowena damaged her ligaments (knees) 15 years ago when she played sport. Her medical family history (mother) includes hypertension, dyslipideamia, diabetes and stroke. Rowena does not participate in exercise on a regular basis and her hobbies include computer games and watching TV. She is, however, keen to change her lifestyle as she does not want to became 'like my mum' (ie: to have diabetes and a stroke). In addition, Rowena has a poor diet which includes high caloric, high fat food and snacks such as potato-chips and chocolate. During the interview, Rowena seems to be keen and full of motivation to start an exercise program. Rowena prefers to start with resistance exercises and not aerobic exercises because in past attempts to perform activities such as cycling and power walking she felt some discomfort in the knees and in the lower back. Also, she prefers not to change her diet and exercise at once.

Objective

Prior to any exercise and functional assessments, Rowena was medically cleared by her general practitioner (GP) to participate in an exercise program. In addition, Rowena did not have any documented heart disease and her fitness test (aerobic power) included ECG monitoring. No ST changes, arrhythmias or any other contraindications for exercise were found. Rowena underwent anthropometric measurements, fasting blood test and functional capacities and QoL assessments. Rowena's metabolic risk factors include obesity (BMI = 39.9kg·m^{-2}), increased fasting glucose levels (6.9mmol·L^{-1}), hypertension (144/86mmHg) and high triglycerides levels (1.9mmol·L^{-1}). In addition, it took Rowena longer to complete activities of daily living (ADLs), compared to healthy women (37.03 sec versus 27.6 sec respectively) and she had low self-perceived QoL, both physical and mental aspects of the SF-36, compared to the mean scores of the general population (physical aspect = 29 versus 50.3 and mental aspect 43 versus 50.9). Data for the general population were taken from the Australian Bureau of Statistics, National Health Survey: SF-36 norms (ABS 1995). Finally, Rowena had a high score (103) in the Cardiac Depression Scale (CDS), which put her in the category of major depression (>100) (Wise et al 2006).

Assessment

Rowena has MetS and concomitant depression, and she is at a high risk for developing diabetes, heart disease and stroke. Although Rowena is genetically predisposed to have diabetes due to her family history, it is clear that her lack of physical activity (sedentary lifestyle) and poor diet also contribute to her clinical profile. The main objectives of the intervention are to improve Rowena's clinical profile and also to improve her self-perceived QoL through improvement in lifestyle, an increase physical activity level and modify energy intake.

Plan

Rowena has a sedentary lifestyle which increased her risk for T2DM and heart disease. As such the immediate goal was to increase her physical activity level. As Rowena preferred not to perform aerobic exercise (at least in the beginning of the program) she started with resistance training for 10 weeks. Rowena prefers to perform resistance training and not aerobic training. It is expected that resistance training will improve Rowena's glycaemic control, blood pressure (Castaneda et al 2002; Dunstan et al 2002) and muscle strength, muscle mass and QoL (Levinger et al 2007). The resistance training program was based on the recommendations of the American College of Sport Medicine (ACSM) for individuals with insulin resistance and T2DM (ACSM 2000). Rowena attended the gym 3 days a week. Training commenced with two sets of 15–20 repetitions (40–50% of on repetition maximum, 1RM). Then, the number of sets was increased to three while the number of repetitions was 12–15 (60–70% of 1RM). In the last 4 weeks of training, Rowena performed 3 sets of 8–12 repetitions (75–85% of 1RM). The intermediate goals and long-term goals will be to include aerobic exercise (to increase cardiopulmonary fitness and to 'burn' more energy) and alter her diet.

Outcome

Rowena attended to 90% of her training sessions (27/30). She was motivated and enjoyed the training sessions. Two main things motivated Rowena to come to the training sessions: (1) she felt good with her self; and (2) the social interaction with the trainer and other gym users.

Anthropometric

Training increased lean body mass (2.3kg) and reduced fat mass (1kg) and fat percentage (1.7%). No change in total body mass was observed. This finding emphasises the point that measurement of body mass and/or BMI following exercise training may be misleading as it does not distinguish between lean body mass and fat mass.

Clinical outcomes

The two main clinical benefits were a reduction in fasting glucose level by 10.1% (from 6.9 to 6.2mmol·L^{-1}) and a reduction in triglyceride levels by 31.6% (from 1.9 to 1.3mmol·L^{-1}). There was an increase in LDL from 2.7 to 3.0mmol·L^{-1}. However, both LDL values are within the normal range. No change was observed in blood pressure.

Functional outcomes

Both maximal muscle strength (sum of seven exercises) and the capacity to perform ADLs were improved (39% and -21.8% respectively). No change, and even small reduction (-4.6%), was found in VO$_{2peak}$.

Quality of life outcomes

Quality of life improved dramatically following training. Both self-perceived physical health and mental health of the SF-36 were improved (79.3% and 60.5% respectively). In addition, depression score was reduced from 103 to 75 (-27.2%). This score (75) is not considered as depression as it is lower than 90 (mild depression) (Wise et al 2006).

Summary of key lessons

- Measurement of body mass as an indicator for a successful intervention may be inadequate. Resistance training can change body composition (i.e. increase lean body mass and decrease fat mass) without altering absolute body mass. Improvement in body composition can lead to improvement in clinical outcome (i.e. lower glucose and triglycerides levels) even in the absence of changes in body mass.

- Resistance training as a single intervention has the capacity to improve clinical measures if the clinical measures are higher than the recommended levels. In Rowena's case, resistance training improved glucose levels and triglyceride levels as they were elevated, compared to the recommended values (fasting glucose <5.6 = mmol $\cdot$ L-1 and triglyceride <1.7 mmol $\cdot$ L-1) as published by the International Diabetes Federation (IDF) (Zimmet et al 2005).

- Resistance training is not a 'silver bullet' for all metabolic risk factors. In Rowena's case, resistance training had no effects on blood pressure, HDL or LDL. In order to target these metabolic risk factors, Rowena will probably need to include some aerobic exercises in her program (3–5 days a week) as well as modify her diet. These changes should be part of the intermediate and long-terms goals. In addition, resistance training had no effects on VO_2peak probably because this type of training is mostly anaerobic activity in nature and it aims to increase muscle strength rather than aerobic fitness. The inclusion of aerobic exercise should lead to an improvement in VO_2peak.

- An important lesson is that resistance training as a single intervention can improve the capacity to perform ADL, self-perceived QoL and reduce depression score independently to changes in aerobic fitness or body mass. Many ADL tasks do not depend on high levels of aerobic fitness, but are usually characterised by short bursts of effort (such as rising from a chair, climbing stairs and carrying groceries), and as such they depend more on muscular strength than aerobic fitness (Levinger et al 2007).

DISCUSSION Question

Rowena did not alter her blood pressure, HDL, or LDL levels with resistance training alone. She did, however, make some gains in strength and ADL, and she now perceives herself to be much healthier physically and mentally. Consider how you might encourage Rowena to extend her exercise program given she does not appear motivated to engage in aerobic training, and she has already achieved her goal of greatest personal importance (ie: feeling healthier).

CASE STUDY 3: POLYCYSTIC OVARY SYNDROME, INFERTILITY, AND GESTATIONAL DIABETES

Subjective

Kelly, a 32-year-old woman, is a stay-at-home mum with one child aged 4 years. Kelly's lifestyle is not ideal and she eats poorly and often binge eats, she has no regular exercise and has little incidental activity. She gained 10kg after the birth of her first child and has continued to gain weight since.

Kelly also reveals that she has been trying to conceive a second child for over 12 months. It took Kelly and her partner 6 months to conceive their first child and so she thought it may take some time to conceive again. However, Kelly is now becoming concerned and thinks she may need assisted fertility treatment. Kelly reports that she has always experienced irregular cycles, gains weight very easily, she says due to her 'poor metabolism', and regularly experiences acne on her face and upper back.

Trying to have another baby is putting a strain on her relationship, and she feels that her increased body weight makes her very unattractive to her partner: they have sex just to conceive. Kelly reports that she feels depressed and frustrated.

Objective

Kelly has just seen her general practitioner (GP) who provides a report of test results. Use of a standardised test for anxiety and depression (Hospital Anxiety and Depression Scale) reveals that she is suffering from mild to moderate depression. A transabdominal ultrasound shows multiple follicles on both ovaries. Fasting blood glucose = 4.4mmol/L (normal range <6) and 2-hour blood glucose is 6.9mmo/L (normal range <7.9). Kelly has a normal lipid profile, serum testosterone 2.9nmol/L (<2.4nmol/L usual in women), SHBG 27 (normal range 30–90) and she also has an elevated free androgen index (FAI) of 10% (normal range 1–5%). With these features Kelly has been diagnosed with polycystic ovary syndrome (PCOS), and exercise and lifestyle change is recommended.

On assessment, Kelly has a BMI of 31 and a waist circumference of 114cm. Kelly feels too self-conscious to exercise and will not wear bathers in public. For many reasons, including her anxiety and depression, Kelly is unmotivated. Guilt and limitations with child care as well as low self-esteem are all key barriers to exercise. Financial considerations are also barriers to formalised activity. Kelly has no past injuries and expressed no specific interest in types of activities.

Assessment

It is likely that Kelly has PCOS and her difficulty in conceiving is a consequence of this. She has significant barriers to lifestyle change and yet lifestyle change is critical to treatment of her PCOS, including cycle regularity and infertility, management of her weight, general wellbeing and prevention of long-term complications including diabetes.

Plan

Management of this complex case requires a multidisciplinary team. A treatment plan should first address sustainable lifestyle changes with the aim of increasing physical fitness and incorporating regular physical exercise and increasing incidental activity. She will need to aim to loose 5–10% of her body weight to improve fertility. This small weight loss is likely to promote ovulation and increase cycle regularity thus increasing her chances of conception. A physical activity plan may include increasing her daily activity such as increasing distance walked in a day, to joining community exercise groups. At home some inventive means of increasing physical activity could entail encouraging her to walk with her partner and/or close friends on a daily basis. In addition, innovative resistance training can be encouraged such that during her daily dose of television she could be active by undertaking some light resistance training using a fit ball and hand weights. Once her confidence is increased there may be the opportunity to join a community-based fitness centre (eg: YMCA) to undertake group exercises such as walking, aqua-aerobics or any other type of exercise class she has been inspired to try. It may seem obvious but it is important to remember that Kelly should enjoy or at least like any physical activity she does; this will be helped in a socially supportive environment.

Psychological support and counselling is critically important in Kelly's case with her psychological status being a major barrier to effective sustainable lifestyle change, and also impacting on her relationship with her husband. Relationship counselling may also be helpful. Even one visit to a psychologist where her partner is able to hear Kelly's fears and concerns about her body and self-confidence can be very beneficial. Kelly's partner needs to be engaged to support her lifestyle change rather than being unsupportive or undermining the process.

Kelly will also benefit from a visit to a dietitian once she has been reviewed by the psychologist. A meal plan and food diary may be helpful along with energy restriction. A modest goal of 3–5% of body weight is set initially as not only will it provide health benefits, it is achievable.

Progress

Kelly is seen by the psychologist, the dietitian and the clinical exercise practitioner over the next 12 weeks and progresses well. She is increasingly motivated as her barriers to lifestyle change are addressed and she is now aware that lifestyle is her key to fertility — a particularly motivating goal. Over 12 weeks, Kelly lost 4kg and after a further two cycles has confirmed she is now 6 weeks pregnant. She is very excited, but also worried about her health and that of her baby.

Plan update

It is vital that Kelly continues to maintain her lifestyle changes, including watching her diet and focusing on continuing her physical activity in her daily routine. Discussion and education around the problems and risks associated with obesity in pregnancy and the safety and levels of exercise in pregnancy is important.

Kelly's obstetrician has discussed the risks and Kelly has done further reading and is aware that in pregnancy potential risks of her excess weight include: miscarriage; fetal abnormalities; hypertension; and pre-eclampsia. Gestational diabetes and thrombosis are also raised. Women who are obese and pregnant are also more likely to have induced labour, caesarean sections, and perioperative complications. Fetal problems include fetal distress, birth injuries, macrosomia, perinatal morbidity and mortality. Kelly is understandably concerned, anxious and guilt ridden, but her commitment to lifestyle slips initially.

Reassurance that exercise can be maintained during pregnancy and that minimisation of weight gain is safe and has benefits is critically important at this stage. Provision of guidelines on weight gain in pregnancy can provide goals for Kelly to work towards and minimise a negative focus on potential outcomes.

Progress

Kelly did try to adhere to a lower calorie diet, however, she found she was often so tired she did not maintain ideal physical activity. Kelly has managed to control her weight gain in pregnancy, however, Kelly had a standard oral glucose tolerance test at 26 weeks in her pregnancy and has been told that she has gestational diabetes mellitus (GDM). GDM occurs in up to 10% of pregnancies and once again poses potential health risks to mother and baby. Risks include a 50–60% chance of the mother going on to develop type 2 diabetes, with premature birth, birth complications and obesity and diabetes rates higher in offspring of mothers with GDM (Crowther et al 2005; Ross 2006).

Plan update

Kelly will be referred to the high-risk pregnancy support service at her local hospital and/or community health centre. Also a tailored diet and physical activity plan needs to be developed for Kelly. Diet is covered by the multidisciplinary pregnancy team but no exercise advice is provided. The clinical exercise practitioner develops a physical activity plan, incorporating Kelly's limitations around her third trimester of pregnancy and her tiredness. This may include Kelly maintaining and/or re-invigorating her walking program or any community-based exercise she has enjoyed, especially with her partner (ie: her exercise regimen could have been maintained or restarted in her first trimester). During the second and third trimester when joints become more lax and tiredness becomes an issue, Kelly should be encouraged to maintain light aerobic exercise such as walking, aqua-aerobics and/or recumbent cycle ergometry. Kelly does not need to complete 40–60 minutes in a session but can break it into smaller 10–15 minute bouts. Most importantly, Kelly needs to be given strict guidelines about hydration and not exercising in high heat conditions.

Progress

Kelly manages through exercise and diet to control her GDM without insulin therapy and is pleased with her ability to manage her condition. Over her pregnancy she gains only 6kg and, after delivery, is 8kg down on her pre-pregnancy weight and is far fitter, with a much improved lifestyle. Kelly is well aware that she is at increased risk of type 2 diabetes and that this is preventable with a sustained healthy lifestyle, which Kelly needs to address as a lifelong priority.

Discussion

PCOS and obesity impact negatively on fertility and increase the risk of diabetes both during pregnancy and afterwards. Management of these conditions should begin with a multidisciplinary plan and, most importantly, sustainable lifestyle change. GDM poses significant complications and future risks for both mother and baby. Sustainable supportive education and maintenance dietary and exercise programs should be tailored to each individual woman. A positive mental state and positive emotional wellbeing will be vital to the success of any treatment plans.

Thorough evaluation, discussion, education and individualised treatment plans are critical to outcomes in PCOS-related infertility and GDM. Many therapeutic options are available to women including:

- lifestyle advice
- regular exercise
- small to moderate weight loss
- psychological advice and support
- metformin
- targeted infertility advice and treatments
- insulin therapy for GDM.

PCOS and obesity

Lifestyle change is first-line therapy and is critical in all overweight women with PCOS. Weight loss of 5–10% has major clinical benefits, including improving psychological outcomes (self-esteem, anxiety, mean depression scores and scores on general health questionnaire) (Galletly et al 1996), reproductive features (menstrual cycles, ovulation and fertility) (Clark et al 1998; Huber-Buchholz et al 1999) and metabolic outcomes (insulin resistance [IR]; metabolic syndrome [MetS]). It is critical to realise and to counsel clients that small achievable goals make a large impact, despite them remaining clinically overweight or obese (Clark et al 1998; Hamilton-Fairley et al 1993; Wahrenberg et al 1999). No specific dietary regimen has been proven superior in PCOS and although a low GI diet may offer theoretical advantages it is yet to be adequately researched in PCOS.

Structured moderate exercise (three times per week for 40 minutes) is more effective than diet alone, inducing greater improvements in androgens, insulin resistance and ovulation, and a trend to increased pregnancy rate with exercise versus diet alone in PCOS, despite a greater weight loss with diet alone. Translation of current evidence into practice suggests a combination of exercise with overall sustainable reduction in caloric intake through long-term behavioural change.

Obesity independently causes infertility and should be addressed with healthy lifestyle (lifestyle change is effective and critical, with small changes in weight having major benefits). PCOS is the most common cause of anovulatory infertility. Of women who attend infertility clinics for anovulation, 90–95% have PCOS. Of women with PCOS, 40% will take longer than 12 months to conceive, if they conceive at all, and 90% of women with infertility issues are overweight. Risks for both mother and baby in obese and obese PCOS women are increased. Be wary of age-related infertility and, if possible, plan a family before the age of 35 years. If BMI increases above 32 debate continues as to whether invitro fertilisation (IVF) should be used or is appropriate.

A sustainable physical activity program for women who are infertile may include aerobic and/ or resistance training depending on their personal preferences and barriers. The exercise programs while for the most part should be at a moderate intensity; if possible this should also include some high-intensity exercise to promote muscle adaptation.

A sustainable physical activity program for women with GDM will vary depending on each woman's capabilities, but should always include low to moderate intensity exercise. Early in pregnancy women can maintain exercise that would be prescribed to a normal but overweight woman, but avoiding high intensity exercise. As pregnancy progresses into the second and third trimesters the body's physiology and biomechanics change drastically and such exercise programs must be altered. Much more stringent guidelines (Artal & O'Toole 2003) should be followed, which means hydration needs to be maintained, exercise should be low impact and low intensity, and exercise in hot environments must be avoided. This may mean that short bouts of exercise more often during the day may be required to attain the recommended 30–60 minutes of exercise a day. Finally, if exercise is maintained during pregnancy the delivery is generally of shorter duration and the greater fitness levels will help in the final stages of the delivery (normal/vaginal).

The impact of the physical symptoms of PCOS, infertility, and GDM on mood are likely to be considerable. Infertility, long-term health concerns such as risk of T2DM and cardiovascular disease (CVD), challenges to feminine identity such as acne and hirsutism, negative body image, and low self-esteem take their toll on psychological wellbeing. Kelly experienced mild depression, negative body image and low self-esteem, which also impacted on her relationship with her partner. Even a few counselling sessions to educate, normalise and provide strategies to deal with body image and self-esteem issues can be very helpful to women with PCOS.

Limited studies of psychological wellbeing and infertility mostly focus on psychological influences of treatment such as IVF (Coyle & Smith 2005; Kee et al 2000; Yong et al 2000), and a small number of studies have found that infertile women have increased anxiety and depressive symptoms (Kee et al 2000; Fido 2004; Matsubayashi et al 2001), and the longer infertility continues the higher the levels of distress (Yong et al 2000; Domar et al 1993). The chronic impact of psychological distress on overall wellbeing means that the ability of these women to make sustainable lifestyle changes may be compromised. The value of physical activity in improving mood and overall ability to cope should not be underestimated. At a time when women at risk of GDM most need to increase their physical activity they often report that they are too tired to do so or are anxious about the effects on the baby. Reduction of this anxiety through education programs will be vital in the delivery of any physical activity program, while highlighting the benefits of physical activity on mood.

Summary of key lessons

- The journey to diagnosis for women with PCOS is often long and fraught with frustration and a sense of helplessness. One of the most difficult things for women is the lack of knowledge that both the community and many health professionals have of PCOS.

- PCOS is a complex condition that brings together matters of overweight and obesity, poor body image, infertility, and increased risk of other chronic conditions, particularly type 2 diabetes. Exercise is a potent intervention for addressing each of these issues, and low to moderate intensity exercise affords many benefits.

DISCUSSION Questions

1 What opportunities for low to moderate intensity exercises are available to a stay-at-home mum who has full-time responsibility for a pre-school aged child and little or no disposable income?

2 Given that Kelly is unlikely to afford the fees for many private consultations or monitored exercise sessions, what are your suggestions for her independent, self-monitored exercise?

CASE STUDY 4: USING EXERCISE AS THERAPY IN POLYCYSTIC OVARY SYNDROME

Subjective

Lucy is a 27-year-old woman who is currently completing her PhD in the area of property law. She has always been above average weight, however, in the last 2 years she has gained 20kg and is now 106kg (height 169cms). Lucy describes her diet as 'healthy' although she craves sweet foods, finds little time for exercise and admits that sitting at her computer for hours at a time is not ideal. Sometimes Lucy finds that she is short of breath, is aware her heart is racing and reports that a feeling of dread 'washes' over her. Lucy does not like going out in public places, she feels that people are looking at her because she is so overweight. Lucy is worried about her appearance and is concerned that her weight is getting out of control. Lucy also notes irregular periods (cycle length 42–100 days), hair growth on her upper lip and chin, which she waxes regularly, and moderate acne. No one has ever been able to explain to her why her periods are so irregular and she is concerned about underlying medical problems and future fertility.

Objective

To clarify Lucy's medical and psychological status Lucy is reviewed by her general practitioner (GP) and a transvaginal ultrasound reveals multiple follicles on both ovaries. Fasting blood glucose = 6.4mmol/L (normal range <6) and 2-hour blood glucose on an oral glucose tolerance test is 8.9mmo/L (normal range >9), while Lucy also has an elevated free androgen index (FAI) of 8% (normal range 1–5%).

Lifestyle and health assessment reveals that Lucy is obese and has a BMI of 37 with central/abdominal adiposity (waist circumference = 103cm). A comprehensive assessment finds that Lucy does not exercise at all and her incidental levels of activity are minimal with little or no housework, walking or work-related activity. Eighty percent of Lucy's energy needs come from fats and carbohydrates in her diet while 20% is from protein. Psychological review suggests agoraphobic tendencies and moderate anxiety. Lucy is referred for an exercise stress test, where she attained a VO_{2peak} of 19mL.kg^{-1}.min^{-1} with a normal ECG trace.

Assessment

Lucy fits the international Androgen Excess Society (AES) and the Rotterdam criteria (Group TREACw 2004; Azziz et al 2006) for polycystic ovary syndrome (PCOS), including the three criteria of: oligomenorrhea, clinical features confirmed by bloods of hyperandrogenism, and pelvic ultrasound confirmation (see Figure 16.2). Lucy also has impaired glucose tolerance (IGT) or prediabetes, which puts her at further high risk of type 2 diabetes melitis (T2DM) and cardiovascular disease (CVD). For many women PCOS is part of a continuum of metabolic disease (see Figure 16.3). Lucy has adverse lifestyle, obesity, PCOS and IGT already. Due to her PCOS, Lucy is also likely to experience problems with fertility and mood disorders such as depression and and/or anxiety, poor self-esteem and negative body image. The reproductive metabolic and psychological features of PCOS are all exacerbated by her obesity. Other investigations were undertaken, including follicle-stimulating hormone (FSH), luteinising hormone (LH), thyroid-stimulating hormone (TSH) and serum prolactin were within normal ranges (therefore ruling out other rarer causes of her symptoms, such as Cushing's syndrome and hypothyroidism, for example).

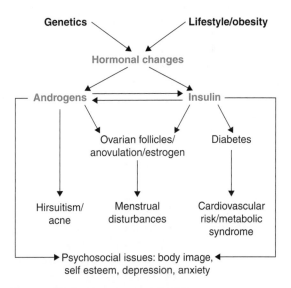

Figure 16.2 Features of PCOS

(Reproduced with permission from the RACGP CHECK program, Polycystic Ovary Syndrome, Unit 432, March 2008)

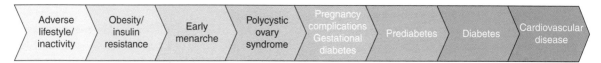

Figure 16.3 The continuum of lifestyle related metabolic disease across the female lifecycle

Plan

A treatment plan should first address education and understanding of PCOS and IGT. First-line treatment is sustainable lifestyle changes. This may include nutrition and diet tailored specifically for women with PCOS along with increasing frequency and intensity of physical activity. Assessment of psychological functioning should take place as impaired function is likely to impact on the success of any treatment or intervention plan. Medical therapy may also be important, particularly in cases where women have IGT or T2DM.

Discussion

Three-quarters of women with PCOS are likely to be overweight or obese. This weight increases the manifestations of all features of PCOS including psychological, reproduction and metabolic (see Figure 16.3), lifestyle change and risks of hyperinsulinemia, T2DM and CVD. There is a significantly increased risk of T2DM in women with PCOS (Wild et al 2000) and double the risk of CVD (Shaw et al 2008). Importantly, obesity affects psychological functioning and consequent ability to change behaviours. Mood and self-confidence are predictive of success at weight control. Depression, anxiety and social dysfunction are increased in women who are overweight and are known to improve with weight loss (Bradshaw et al 2004; Wadden et al 2006). Even a small to moderate weight loss (5–10kg/or 5–10% of initial weight) over 6 months has been shown to:

- improve reproductive features — menstrual cycles and fertility
- significantly ($\approx$ 60%) reduce the risk of T2DM in women with IGT
- improve metabolic features — reduce CVD risk factors (through decreased dyslipideamia and blood pressure, for example) and decrease long-term risk of CVD
- improve psychological wellbeing (anxiety, depression, poor self-esteem and negative body image) and overall QoL.

A referral to a dietitian is recommended for overweight women with PCOS, especially those with IGT (and is recognised in Australia under Medicare, as PCOS is a condition with obesity-related comorbidities). There is currently no one diet plan recommended for women with PCOS, rather a nutritionally adequate diet that contains: moderate protein (~15%); high complex carbohydrate (~55%) with increased fibre-rich breads, cereals, fruits and vegetables; and low fat (~30% of energy) (Moran et al 2008). Interestingly, both low and high protein dietary approaches have had similar outcomes in women with PCOS (Teede et al 2007). Sustainable changes through behavioural changes are critical and health coaching principles are important.

Physical activity is pivotal in the treatment plan of women with PCOS. Even without weight loss, increased physical activity will improve metabolic risk factors such as insulin resistance (IR) and IGT (National Health and Medical Research Council [NHMRC] 2003) improves menstrual cycles and fertility and improves psychological wellbeing (Stear 2003). The exercise intervention should include assessment and management of barriers to exercise including a sedentary job, agoraphobia, and low self-esteem in Lucy's case. Immediate goals include dealing with these psychological barriers, increasing Lucy's confidence to engage in exercise/physical activity, and introducing feasible exercise regularly to increase her fitness.

Short-term strategies (6–12 weeks): Lucy needs to increase physical activity under close supervision in a private one-on-one environment to increase her fitness levels that may incorporate both light resistance and endurance training twice a week with some home/office activities for the other days of the week.

Intermediate strategies (12 weeks to 12 months): Following intensive supervised training and confidence building Lucy needs to be encouraged to take the first steps into undertaking physical activity and/or exercise outdoors. This should include, in addition to the formal supervised exercise regimen, challenging her to start walking during breaks or after work by starting to walk up and down the street close to home or the office, and progressing to greater and greater distances away from home or office. Initially these activities may need to be supervised until Lucy's confidence is sufficient to undertake these activities on her own.

Long-term strategies (12 months onwards): For lifetime benefit, Lucy needs to be encouraged to take ownership of her physical activity plan and exercise training. This should include investigating the types of exercise activities she enjoys and then join small group exercise classes (eg: walking groups, aqua-aerobics, spinning classes, women-only fitness centres) which may include women in similar situations.

During all phases in increasing Lucy's physical activity, formal and informal exercise tasks should be included at regular intervals (monthly) to demonstrate to Lucy that all her exercise has benefited her life and health. Tests might include strength tests, 6-minute walk test (6MWT), sub-maximal estimations of VO_{2peak}, on cycle ergometer or step test.

Moderate physical activity should be incorporated daily (at least 30 mins/day) while education around increasing incidental physical activity is also important. This may include walking rather than driving short distances, viewing gardening and house cleaning as important increased activity, parking the car further away from shopping centres or work destinations, using stairs where possible, volunteering to get up and get something or meet someone.

Mood disorders such as anxiety and depression are higher in women with PCOS than in the general population (Ching et al 2007). It is not clear yet whether the physical aspects of PCOS cause depression and anxiety as is common with many physical illnesses, or if a diagnosis brings on increased mood disorders. Regardless of the origin of psychological dysfunction, it is important that psychological support and treatment is given to women with PCOS as required. As stated previously, impaired mood may compromise the ability to make lifestyle and behaviour changes or follow treatment regimens. Lucy reported in her first session that she experiences shortness of breath and feelings of dread along with avoidance of social situations. Lucy may be describing agoraphobia with panic attacks. Referral to a psychologist even for one or two sessions of education and assessment may help with motivation and self-efficacy in order to improve overall success of treatment plans, as well as investigate the possible use of other psychological therapies (eg: cognitive behavioural therapy) for concomitant psychological concerns.

Summary of key lessons

- Exercise prescription for women with PCOS, especially with additional psycho-social problems is challenging, however, most women have an activity they like doing or wish they could do. These activities and goals should be encouraged by developing an achievable individual exercise plan.

- Exercise training may involve starting with simple exercise tasks to develop fitness, mobility and confidence before a more complex training exercise regimen can be implemented to achieve true exercise goals.

- Physical activity promotes feelings of wellbeing and promotes good mental health, therefore it is likely that exercise will go some way to alleviate Lucy's metabolic, reproductive and psycho-social problems.

DISCUSSION Questions

1 How might you assist women with PCOS to understand their future health risks and the important role of lifestyle change?

2 How might you recommend that Lucy increase her incidental activity?

REFERENCES

American College of Sports Medicine [ACSM] (2000) Exercise and type 2 diabetes: position stand of the American College of Sports Medicine. *Medicine and Science in Sports and Exercise*, 32(7):1345–60

Artal R, O'Toole M (2003) Guidelines of the American College of Obstetricians and Gynecologists for exercise during pregnancy and the postpartum period. *British Journal of Sports Medicine*, 37:6–12

Australian Bureau of Statistics (ABS) (1995) *National Health Survey*. ABS, Canberra

Azziz R, Carmina E, Dewailly D, et al (2006) Criteria for defining polycystic ovary syndrome as a predominantly hyperandrogenic syndrome: an Androgen Excess Society Guideline. *J Clin Endocrinol Metab*, 91:4237–45

Blair SN, Kampert JB, Paffenbarger RS, et al (1996) Influences of cardiorespiratory fitness and other precursors on cardiovascular disease and all-cause mortality in men and women. *The Journal of the American Medical Association*, 276(3):205–10

Bradshaw A, Katzer L, Horwath CC, et al (2004) A randomised trial of three non-dieting programs for overweight women. *Asia Pac J Clin Nutr*, 13(Suppl): S43

Castaneda C, Layne JE, Munoz-Orians L, et al (2002) A randomized controlled trial of resistance exercise training to improve glycemic control in older adults with type 2 diabetes. *Diabetes Care*, 25:2335–41

Ching HL, Burke V, Stuckey BGA (2007) Quality of life and psychological morbidity in women with polycystic ovary syndrome: body mass index, age and the provision of patient information are significant modifiers. *Clinical Endocrinology*, 66(3):373–9

Clark AM, Thornley B, Tomlinson L, et al (1998) Weight loss in obese infertile women results in improvement in reproductive outcome for all forms of fertility treatment. *Human Reproduction*, 13(6):1502–5

Coyle M, Smith C (2005) A survey comparing TCM diagnosis, health status and medical diagnosis in women undergoing assisted reproduction. *Accupunt Med*, 23(2):62–9

Crowther CA, Hiller JE, Moss JR, et al (2005) Australian Carbohydrate Intolerance Study in Pregnant Women (ACHOIS) Trial Group. Effect of treatment of gestational diabetes mellitus on pregnancy outcomes *New England Journal of Medicine*, 352(24):2477–86

Domar AD, Broome A, Zuttermeister PC, et al (1993) The prevalence and predictability of depression in infertile women. *International Journal of Gynecology & Obstetrics*, 42(2):220–1

Dunstan DW, Daly RM, Owen N, et al (2002) High-intensity resistance training improves glycemic control in older patients with type 2 diabetes. *Diabetes Care*, 25(10):1729–37

Fido A (2004) Emotional distress in infertile women in Kuwait. *Int J Fert Womens Med*, 49(1):24–8

Galletly C, Clark A, Tomlinson L, et al (1996) A group program for obese, infertile women: weight loss and improved psychological health. *J Psychosom Obstet Gynecol*, 17(2):125–8

Group TREACw (2004) Revised 2003 consensus on diagnostic criteria and long-term health risks related to polycystic ovary syndrome. *Fertility and Sterility*, 81:19–25

Hamilton-Fairley D, Kiddy D, Anyaoku V, et al (1993) Response of sex hormone binding globulin and insulin-like growth factor binding protein-1 to an oral glucose tolerance test in obese women with polycystic ovary syndrome before and after calorie restriction. *Clin Endocrinol (Oxf)*, 39(3):363–7

Huber-Buchholz MM, Carey DG, Norman RJ (1999) Restoration of reproductive potential by lifestyle modification in obese polycystic ovary syndrome: role of insulin sensitivity and luteinising hormone. *J Clin Endocrinol Metab*, 84(4):1470–4

Kee BS, Jung BJ, Lee SH (2000) A study on psychological strain in IVF patients. *J Assist Reprod Genet*, 17(8):445–8

Levinger I, Goodman C, Hare DL, et al (2007) The effect of resistance training on functional capacity and quality of life in individuals with high and low numbers of metabolic risk factors. *Diabetes Care*, 30(9), 2205–10

Matsubayashi H, Hosaka T, Izumi S, et al (2001) Emotional distress of infertile women in Japan. *Human Reproduction*, 16(5):966–99

Moran LJ, Pasquali R, Teede HJ, et al (2008) Androgen Excess and Polycystic Ovary Syndrome International Position Statement. Lifestyle in PCOS. *Fertility and Sterility*, 92:1966–82

National Health and Medical Research Council (NHMRC) (2003) *Clinical Practice Guidelines for the Management of Overweight and Obesity in Adults*. Canberra: NHMRC

Ross G (2006) Gestational diabetes. *Australian Family Physician*, 35(6):392–6

Shaw LJ, Bairey Merz CN, et al (2008) Postmenopausal women with a history of irregular menses and elevated androgen measurements at high risk for worsening cardiovascular event-free survival: results from the National Institutes of Health — National Heart, Lung, and Blood Institute sponsored Women's Ischemia Syndrome Evaluation. *Journal of Clinical Endocrinology & Metabolism* 93:1276–84

Stear S (2003) Health and fitness series 1. The importance of physical activity for health. *J Family Health Care*, 13(1): 10–13

Teede H, Hutchison SK, Zoungas S (2007) The management of insulin resistance in Polycystic Ovary Syndrome. *Trends Endocrin Metab*, 18:273–9

Wadden TA, Butryn ML, Sarwer DB, et al (2006) Comparison of psychosocial status in treatment seeking women with class III vs class I-II obesity. *Obesity (Silver Spring)*, Suppl 2:90S–98S

Wahrenberg H, Ek I, Reynisdottir S, et al (1999) Divergent effects of weight reduction and oral anticonception treatment on adrenergic lipolysis regulation in obese women with the polycystic ovary syndrome. *J Clin Endocrinol Metab*, 84(6):2182–7

Wild S, Pierpoint T, McKeigue P, et al (2000) Cardiovascular disease in women with polycystic ovary syndrome at long-term follow-up: a retrospective cohort study. *Clin Endocrinol (Oxf)*, 52:595–600

Wise FM, Harris DW, Carter LM (2006) Validation of the Cardiac Depression Scale in a cardiac rehabilitation population. *Journal of Psychosomatic Research*, 60(2):177–83

Yong P, Martin C, Thong J (2000) A comparison of psychological functioning in women at different stages of in vitro fertilisation treatment using the mean affect adjective check list. *J Assist Reprod Genet*, 17(10): 553–6

Zimmet PZ, Alberti KG, Shaw JE (2005) Mainstreaming the metabolic syndrome: a definitive definition. This new definition should assist both researchers and clinicians. *Medical Journal of Australia*, 183(4):175–6

Chapter 17

Case studies in exercise as therapy for clients requiring special care

Melainie Cameron, Loretta Konjarski and Natalie Chahine

INTRODUCTION

In this chapter we have drawn together several case studies of clients who might be considered to have special care needs: children, elderly people and the chronically ill. We also explore the ethical complexities of giving special care. One tale tells of caring for one of those we love the most and explores how special care is manifest in a family; another tale explores therapy in a group setting and uncovers the difficulties of treating all participants the same way. In these tales we have digressed from the usual SOAP notes format (ie: subjective, objective, assessment, plan) in favour of a narrative style. These are real stories drawn from family life as well as from work, and they do not always fit neatly into the usual package of clinical records.

Carrolle's story is written posthumously, largely from memory, with limited access to formal clinical records. The author is her daughter. Some details may be 'rose coloured' because they were viewed by a child.

Marg's story is written with her full consent and collaboration with her healthcare practitioners. We are grateful to both Marg and her treating practitioners for their willingness to be involved in this venture.

The third story is that of a group of children who took part in a university program to promote physical activity amongst children with intellectual and physical handicaps. No individual children are identified. This program, although not

intended as 'therapy', has therapeutic effects on the participants, and this case study demonstrates that teachers and other serving professionals are able to deliver exercise with health benefits.

CASE STUDY 1: CARROLLE

Carrolle was 27 and pregnant with her third child when she was involved in a motor vehicle accident. She was stopped in a line of cars at traffic lights when a car struck her car in the rear and propelled it into the vehicle immediately in front. Although her car was unable to be driven, Carrolle was declared fit and well by ambulance paramedics, allowed to leave the scene of the accident, and was taken home by a friend. The day following the accident Carrolle woke with neck pain that subsided somewhat over the following few days. A few days later she developed bilateral hand pain that she attributed to the accident.

Over several weeks Carrolle's hand pain developed a consistent pattern. She woke with hand pain and stiffness in the small joints of both hands. After an hour or so, the pain and stiffness subsided to enable most normal hand functions throughout the day, but returned with extensive vigorous activity (eg: heavy gardening) or prolonged inactivity (eg: afternoon nap). Also, Carrolle felt much more tired than normal, and experienced some episodes of cramping and 'pins and needles' sensations in her fingers. Carrolle consulted several medical practitioners, who dismissed her pain as being largely unexplained and possibly fictitious. One practitioner told her she had Raynaud's phenomenon, because her hands turned white when cold, and pain, cyanosis, and hyperemia followed. Unfortunately, that practitioner could offer no further explanation of the cause of Raynaud's phenomenon. Carrolle became disgruntled with these incomplete and sometimes accusatory responses. She stopped seeking medical care.

Carrolle's blood pressure rose later in the pregnancy. Carrolle was admitted to hospital for 2 weeks before the baby was born to control this pre-eclampsia, and her healthy baby girl, was born without incident via normal vaginal delivery. Carrolle's hand pain and stiffness continued, but she ignored it because she was fully occupied by the demands of mothering a newborn. A few years later Carrolle had a fourth child. Her daily life was filled with the demands of raising children and keeping a home. She complained little, but her hand pain continued. The same symptoms of stiffness, pain, pins and needles, and cramping began in her feet. Again she sought a medical opinion, but felt dismissed by doctors who suggested she was simply tired, or worse, making up her symptoms.

Carrolle had a curvaceous figure. During pregnancies she gained weight easily, and exercised vigorously to reduce her weight afterwards. After the birth of her youngest child she resumed her hobbies of landscape gardening, bushwalking and tennis, but found that hand and foot pain limited her participation in these activities. Carrolle struggled to find comfortable footwear. I remember her bushwalking in 'masseur' sandals in a vain attempt to be active with us as children despite her constant foot pain.

Despite difficulty engaging in exercise, and no particular changes to her diet, Carrolle lost much weight over the next few years. Several of her friends commented that she was 'looking well', although she felt very unwell with joint pain and cramping in hands and feet, and persistent, unshakable fatigue, which was getting worse.

One winter Carrolle developed a persistent chest infection (bronchitis). For almost 15 years she had rejected mainstream medical care, and made lifestyle adaptations as her symptoms changed or worsened, so she had no ongoing relationship with a medical practitioner. She attended a local general practice to see the first available doctor, who immediately identified classic, advanced signs of progressive systemic sclerosis including thickening and hardening of the skin of her fingers, forearms, and face, and thinning of her hair with patchy hair loss. I remember a telephone call from her when she asked 'What's scleroderma? …because my doctor thinks I have it.' I was studying to be a healthcare practitioner, and had just started learning about some of the rarer arthritides and auto-immune diseases.

'What is scleroderma? … because my doctor thinks I have it …'

Scleroderma (progressive systemic sclerosis) is an autoimmune disorder of unknown cause, and because of the involvement of small joints in the hands and feet, it is usually classified as one of the arthritides. Scleroderma means 'hardening of the skin', but it is a disease with many presentations, including changes to skin and many internal organs. Presenting symptoms differ among patients, but all presentations of the disease derive from increased formation of collagen, in skin, internal organs, and blood vessel walls.

Carrolle re-entered the healthcare system, took an appointment with a rheumatologist, and underwent an assessment to determine the extent of her condition. Carrolle had widespread, progressive systemic sclerosis (scleroderma) with CREST features: calcific deposits in fingers and toes, Raynaud's phenomenon in hands and feet, esophageal dysmotility, sclerodactyly, and telangiectasia.

A definitive diagnosis for a condition that had become known in our family as 'Mum's disease' was a landmark in Carrolle's journey. Prior to diagnosis Carrolle had made changes to her activities out of necessity, when she felt she could no longer continue as before. With diagnosis came information, some understanding of what to expect in the natural history of this condition, and Carrolle made deliberate and considered choices about daily activities, work, exercise, food, clothing and footwear.

Carrolle learned that progressive systemic sclerosis is a chronic disease in which the functions of elastic connective tissues are compromised by the proliferation of fibrous connective tissues, and of fibrous components within tissues. She understood that this process could eventually affect vital organs. In particular, Carrolle learned that she was predisposed to chest infections because some sclerosis had commenced in her lungs. She learned that restrictive lung disease is a serious, and eventually fatal, sequela of scleroderma.

People with progressive systemic sclerosis may experience: joint pain, swelling, stiffness and deformity; osteoporosis caused by immobilised joints; shortening of the fingers caused by reabsorption of bone (osteolysis); muscle atrophy and weakness; thickening of the tendons; neural compression including symptoms of carpal tunnel syndrome; dry eyes, mouth, and skin as collagen formation damages sweat and saliva glands (Sjogren's syndrome); and digestive problems as the muscles in the oesophagus may become weak, causing difficulty with swallowing. The more Carrolle learned about this rare but serious chronic disease, the more she could understand her symptoms. 'Mum's disease', with sore hands and feet, pins and needles, weight loss, 'pointing around corners', coughing, and walking slowly finally made sense, but the news was serious. Carrolle determined to live as fully as possible, and to stay well for as long as she could.

Exercise plans

Carrolle decided that she was 'not going to let this bloody disease' take her job, so she began a deliberate program of exercises to maintain her work function. Carrolle worked as a senior office manager for the state government. She had fixed working hours in a pleasant office environment and a reasonable degree of autonomy over how she ordered her day. Carrolle continued to type, despite the evolution of voice-activated software and the opportunity to delegate typing tasks to more junior staff members. Carrolle decided that typing was gentle regular exercise that was likely to help her maintain hand function. She was correct. Carrolle could type up to 90 words per minute until a few weeks before she died. The training effects of this exercise, however, may have been task specific; Carrolle's handwriting declined as the scleroderma progressed, although her typing ability remained.

By the time of diagnosis Carrolle had already reduced her walking activities due to foot pain and difficulty finding comfortable footwear, but she learned that she needed to engage in some regular cardiovascular activity to preserve lung and heart function. Carrolle modified her travel to work,

regularly walking uphill from the train station to her office. She wore flat shoes to walk, and changed them when she arrived in the office. Also, she was able to arrange her working day so that she could rest for 30 minutes after walking. Carrolle became proficient at hiding her physical difficulties in the workplace — none of her colleagues realised that she experienced difficulties walking.

Disease progression

As the scleroderma progressed, Carrolle experienced difficulty in swallowing. She elected softer foods and always kept a glass of water at hand. Carrolle continued to lose weight. Loss of muscle function in her mouth and oesophagus contributed to difficulty with swallowing. Reduced gastrointestinal function produced nausea and abdominal cramps, which contributed to her reluctance to eat. In the last few months of her life, Carrolle lost most of her bowel function and developed faecal incontinence.

Despite Carrolle's persistence with walking as exercise, restrictive lung disease progressed. She developed a persistent cough and shortness of breath, initially on exertion and, subsequently, at rest. The winter before she died, Carrolle developed pneumonia. She presented to me with pain around the base of her chest cage on the right side and hoped that a little manual therapy and some breathing exercises might have her kicking along again. Unfortunately, her lung function declined continuously and rapidly from that time. Eight months later Carrolle died in pulmonary hypertension.

Discussion

I was a child when my mother first experienced symptoms of scleroderma. I was a teenager the first time she spoke with me about the possibility of her dying young. By the time she received a definitive diagnosis I was an adult, studying for a degree in healthcare. For my entire clinical career I have known my mother as a 'patient'. My interest in chronic illness, and in arthritic diseases in particular, springs from that mixed background of being both a child and a practitioner. It is messy territory, including both my love for my mother, and my desire to 'fix' her in the face of a progressive disease with no known cause or cure.

I couldn't fix my mother, and I can't fix other chronically ill clients either. It is the very nature of chronic diseases that they progress and worsen. Eventually, we lose.

But we also win. Exercise is a powerful tool for slowing the progress of chronic illnesses. People who engage in exercise can experience training related increases in muscle strength, power, endurance, hypertrophy, bone mass, cardiac efficiency, and respiratory function. These gains do not always outweigh the deficits caused by disease, but in almost all cases, they go some way to moderating disease effects.

Parents raise children by caring for their needs, and gradually setting them on courses of independence. When parents become ill or needy, adult children may be asked to return some of that care and attention. Although this shifting of roles as parents age happens to many children, healthcare practitioners are particularly vulnerable. Choosing to enter healthcare practice may have been borne from a desire to help, a satisfaction associated with assisting others. People with this character trait find it difficult to 'say no' at the best of times. When a parent becomes ill, it is not the best of times. I could not fix my mother, but neither could I tell her that I couldn't fix her. She kept asking for my assistance and advice, and I kept offering her what meagre help I could.

Clean, clear models of behaviour change show us that people move through stages, from preparation to action to maintenance, in their adoption of exercise. In chronic illness these maps are of limited usefulness: the map is not the territory. Carrolle adopted some forms of exercise (typing and walking) with sheer determination following diagnosis. She also rejected other forms of exercise as things she 'couldn't do anymore'.

Summary of key lessons

- Expected physiological effects of exercise occur in people with chronic disease much as they do in healthy people, but improvements may be slower, and in aggressive disease, exercise-related gains are eventually overcome by disease processes.

- Improvements gained from exercise may be highly specific, associated only with trained tasks. For example, Carrolle's typing ability persisted well beyond other dextrous hand functions.

- Clinical exercise practitioners working with chronically and terminally ill clients can expect to face the challenges of clients' declining physical function and eventual death.

DISCUSSION Question

Have you ever had a family member seek you out as a client? Recall this encounter. How did this encounter differ from your typical work?

CASE STUDY 2: MULTIPLE COMORBIDITIES (OR, WHEN EVERYTHING SEEMS TO BE GOING WRONG)

Subjective

Marg is an 80-year-old woman living alone in her family home. She is a war widow and has a very supportive family. Marg was referred to physiotherapy at a community health centre after complaining of bilateral knee pain. She had surgery approximately 10 years prior to this and is suffering general deconditioning. Marg was then referred to an exercise group run at the community health centre by a physiotherapist. Marg also suffers from a past history of pneumonia, anxiety and depression, angina, hypertension, chronic obstructive pulmonary disease, cerebrovascular accident, gastro-oesophageal reflux, osteoporosis and shortness of breath. She has also had a left total knee replacement in the past. Her main goals for attending the exercise group were to increase self-efficacy and confidence, improve balance, to start a home exercise program, and socialisation.

A year later Marg required a right total knee replacement. She was referred to a private physiotherapist for treatment following surgery. Marg re-presents to the community health centre a year later as she was concerned about the flexibility of her right knee almost 8 months post-knee surgery. She was encouraged by her exercise physiologist to make an appointment with the physiotherapist to discuss her concerns. In the meantime Marg continues to attend the weekly exercise group that is now being run by an exercise physiologist.

Marg is worried about falling, so she does not walk outside very often and has not been completing her home exercises. She has had no falls since the right total knee replacement. Marg receives home help with cleaning once a fortnight. She does not take regular medication for pain. Her main medication at the moment is aspirin 100mg, bricanyl inhaler, natrilix SR 1.5mg, nexium 40mg, ostelin vitamin D and calcium 500IU, and panamax 500mg as required.

Marg was also referred to a clinical exercise practitioner by her general practitioner (GP) for advice and management of recent blood test results indicating an increase in blood sugar levels and cholesterol.

Assessment

Marg has stiffness in the right knee following her total knee replacement but little obvious impairment to daily function. She is participating in an exercise class once a week for improving strength, balance and social interaction.

Plan

Marg is advised to participate in her exercise group once a week and complete her home exercise program provided by the physiotherapist. Her home exercises focus on improving knee flexion. The exercise class runs continuously for 1 hour each week. Marg is transported to and from the class by the local council service. Marg is able to liaise with the exercise leader during class to monitor her progress and ask any questions. Marg is encouraged to continue her home exercise program and get together with other participants in the group throughout the week for local walks.

Outcome

Marg participates in all her exercise classes each week. She looks forward to being picked up by community transport with a friend she has made in class. Marg has made marked improvement in being able to use an exercise bike, get in and out of a chair and improve her balance walking in the street. She feels more confident outside of her home and makes use of her walking stick if required. Marg has mentioned to her friend that she enjoys coming to the exercise class because she gets to catch up with everyone. She particularly enjoys catching up with a few of the participants after the class for morning tea at the local café.

Summary of key lessons

- Elderly clients can present with multiple comorbidities and this may present some challenges to participating in exercise. With this in mind, exercise needs to be gentle, progressed slowly, be interactive with other older adults and performed safely.

- Elderly people may not see exercise as an important part of their life; they may be more interested in the social interaction with other clients. Social interaction is an important role in maintaining good mental health in the elderly and is still an outcome of attending an exercise group, even if physical function is not improved.

- Elderly people need to feel comfortable coming to an exercise group by reducing barriers to attendance. Barriers may include access to transport, cost and time of the day, so it is important to take these factors into consideration when starting a group.

DISCUSSION Questions

1 Marg has approached you and asked for more variety in exercises outside the group. She doesn't want to do this alone. What can you suggest for Marg to do?

2 Is there any concern about Marg's current medication list and contraindications to exercise?

3 How can you progress Marg's exercises to ensure that her knee does not become stiff again and cause her lack of confidence in walking outside the home?

4 Marg re-presents to you after having a review with her orthopaedic specialist. On assessment you identified that Marg had 65° knee flexion and -5° knee extension. Her quadriceps control was reasonable and she was able to step up and down on a step, leading with the right leg. You have concern as to whether Marg can regain further knee flexion or whether there is a mechanical issue with the knee or soft tissue restriction that is restricting her movement. How do you approach this issue with her surgeon? Who do you consult? How do you progress further with this?

CASE STUDY 3: ADAPTED AQUATICS PROGRAM

Introduction

This case study draws on observations of the Adapted Aquatics program that is a Higher Education elective unit in the undergraduate course at the School of Sport and Exercise Science at Victoria University (VU). The course runs over a 12-week period in which VU students attend 12 1-hour lectures and participate in 12 2-hour 'Learning in the Workplace and Community' practical sessions with primary aged clients from the Croxton Special School in a unique 1:1 teaching/learning environment. During this time students from VU fulfil the competencies of the AUSTSWIM Teacher of People with a Disability certificate (see references at the end of this chapter), explore many other methods of teaching and communication for clients with a disability, and have 'hands-on' teaching experience in working with clients with an intellectual disability in an aquatic environment (as per Doremus 1992).

The clients from Croxton Special School are from the primary department of the school. While the medical records of each participating student are not made available due to privacy reasons, the school has determined the suitability of each child to participate in the aquatic program.

Clients who participate in the program must be able to toilet themselves and be deemed physically competent enough by the family doctor to participate. It is not necessary that the students be verbal, but being able to respond to simple commands is important as far as safety is concerned.

Most clients in this program have an intellectual disability — Autism, Asperger's syndrome, or Down's syndrome — and there are many students who have non-specific intellectual disabilities.

Clients who access this program have previously, in some cases, experienced disengagement from swimming programs delivered in the community. Often due to costs involved with staffing, clients are left sitting ('waiting for a turn', due to safety reasons) while the swimming teacher works with one or two students at a time. Many leisure centre staff may not have been trained in working with people with a disability and therefore may not provide programs suitable for the individual needs.

These primary aged clients are encouraged to learn to swim, and in most cases are able to perform some of the basic survival sequences such as falling into the pool forwards, rolling onto their backs and kicking to the edge of the pool. The aquatics program incorporates the basic principles of the Halliwick program (a program designed primarily for people with a physical disability; Tirosh et al

2008; Grosse 2010), including the progressive development of client autonomy.

Objective

The main objective of this program is to teach the clients basic swimming strokes wherever possible, teach and develop survival skills in the water, and to encourage a love of the aquatic environment. The other critically important outcome is the relationship that is formed between the client and the VU student teacher. It is this relationship that makes this program so special to the clients, the VU teachers, the staff from Croxton Special School, and the parents of the clients.

In terms of testing pre- and post-program, there is a strong recognition of the fact that many of these clients have spent a great deal of time in medical situations, and it is this fact that drives the need for this program to be a 'learn to swim and survive' program rather than a therapeutic program.

Given this understanding, the type of testing that is done to acknowledge the outcomes within the program is based on the Lifesaving Victoria's Swim and Survive sequence and the Halliwick principles (Tirosh et al 2008; Grosse 2010). No invasive physical testing of any kind is appropriate in this program as the rapport and relationships that are built between client and VU student are just as important as the physical outcomes.

Assessment

Clients with disabilities have the same water safety requirements as those children and adults without a disability. Although teachers and/or swimming teachers may not always be privy to the medical label and/or diagnosis given to a client, they are challenged to develop programs suitable to clients' specific needs.

The likely benefits for the clients accessing this program would be a combination of three main elements:

1 learning how to move in the water, progressing to swimming and water safety

2 the physical benefits of exercising in a safe, aquatic environment

3 the social benefits of participating in such a unique program.

Barriers to exercise intervention

There are several barriers that exist for clients with a disability, and especially young clients with a disability. In most cases if swimming lessons are sought by a Special school, the school must find a facility that can accommodate the school's needs. That is, does the centre have qualified swim teachers who have the experience to work with the client's or do they have the AUSTSWIM Teacher of People with a Disability certificate? Being able to confidently attend a centre where quality lessons are available is a challenge.

Immediate goals of exercise intervention

The immediate goal of the program is water familiarisation. Once the clients are familiar and comfortable with the water then the instructors can begin to use the Halliwick method of teaching people with a disability or, if the clients are more advanced, begin a 'learn to swim' and water safety program.

Immediate exercise strategies

Wherever possible the instructors are encouraged to keep the clients as active as possible through varying means. Walking, running and using pool aids to assist movement in the water are excellent means of exercising in the water, even if the client is not able to 'swim'.

Long-term goals of exercise intervention

The long-term goal of the program is to teach the clients to become familiar with the aquatic environment so they can access learn to swim programs in the community, or gain the necessary skills to be able to safely and confidently move and/or swim in the water.

Long-term exercise strategies

As the client becomes more confident and gains more skills in the water the idea would be to encourage this form of exercise as a safe, inexpensive and enjoyable means of exercising, both in youth and as the client ages.

Discussion

The Adapted Aquatics program has been an outstanding success from all aspects. The student/instructors from VU have gained invaluable experience through the interactions they have had with the student/clients from Croxton Special

School. The week-by-week teaching on a 1:1 ratio has allowed for a rapport to be established between the VU student and the Croxton client, an element of the program identified by both groups as *the* most important.

Although aquatic therapy has been one of the preferred therapies for children with neuromuscular conditions 'little research has been documented which establishes specific outcome effects' (Getz et al 2007:928). We do know that the aquatic environment allows for movements that may not be possible for some children with a disability on land, and that in some cases, where the water is warm, this will help if children have high muscle tone because the warm water will aid in relaxing muscles.

One of the most valued outcomes of the program at VU was the rapport established between student teacher and client. This is supported by a study conducted by Getz et al (2007) where it was reported that clients in aquatic therapy or an aquatic class showed an increase in social acceptance and 'the children were able to initiate multiple social interactions with their instructors and other children' (Getz et al 2007:936).

The Getz study also reported that 'the aquatic environment and treatment seem to lead to positive social interactions that carry over to daily life situations' (Getz et al 2007:936). This is precisely the feedback that the Adapted Aquatic program has had from Croxton Special School. The teachers from the school have indicated that the Croxton clients are very excited during the program, show an increased level of interaction when with their VU instructors and are often more engaged at school during the 12-week program.

Many times we have had excited staff members commenting on how animated some of the less verbal autistic students are in the aquatic environment. The Croxton clients' excitement could be due to many factors including the 'feel' of the water, experiencing buoyancy, the sounds in the pool area and extra stimulation from the one-to-one ratio and the noise associated with many children and instructors sharing a small space. The autistic students may also benefit from the repetitive nature of some of the activities and often like to repeat activities that they like to do. VU instructors are encouraged to use the 'Premack' principle, a teaching method used with people with intellectual disabilities where a non-preferred

activity is rewarded with a preferred activity. This often helps to motivate clients to try something new even when they really only want to do their preferred activity.

While there is evidence to suggest that 'physical activity is beneficial for youth with developmental disabilities' (Johnson 2009:166), and that 'aquatic therapy may have some benefit in improved respiratory function' (Johnson 2009:166), other aspects related to the benefits of aquatics for people with a disability have not been proven. There is a need for further research in this area, however, the difficulties may be that by doing further research the program may become medicalised and lose the important impact of trust, rapport and friendship.

It is clear that anecdotally, programs such as the Adapted Aquatics program at VU have benefits for the clients involved in the program and, add to that, provides a wonderful vehicle for pre-service teachers to hone teaching skills and learn to empathise and communicate with children/clients with disabilities. There is a clear need for further research to accurately pinpoint the benefits both physical and social so that programs like this are seen to be valuable rather than a 'time filler'.

Another benefit of this program is the ability to provide instruction on a one-to-one basis. When a student/client has the undivided attention of one instructor, the learning opportunities are increased just through that attention, and when this instruction is sustained over a 12-week period the opportunity for a deeper rapport grows. This rapport between client and instructor has been the most successful and critical element to the success of the Adapted Aquatics program at Victoria University. Students and clients form a real bond and in the last week of the program, when the clients are awarded certificates of achievement and presented with medals, the tears of joy and friendship flow freely.

Many of the VU students have described this unique experience as 'life changing' and perhaps the most 'valuable' unit they have undertaken in their degree. The reasons behind this are varied, but mostly have been attributed to the sense of doing something valuable, worthwhile and meaningful. Some VU students have been reported to believe that the experience in this unit has 'made them a better person'.

For all the talk about social interaction and bonding, the fact is that many of the clients have actually improved their aquatic skills. Clients have been assessed according to the Lifesaving Victoria Swim and Survive levels, a program that has levels of competence for both swimming ability and water safety skills. Using this assessment procedure we have been able to determine the level the clients are at, and have a clear plan for the challenges ahead.

The Adapted Aquatics program also makes use of the Halliwick program – a swimming program developed specifically for people with a physical disability. Some of the key concepts in the Halliwick program (there are 10; Tirosh et al 2008) are utilised by the VU instructors with the Croxton clients. An example of this would be the concept of disengagement. It is critical that while the students are supported in the water by the instructor, the clients are encouraged to 'disengage' from the instructor and from the use of buoyancy aids — to be independently mobile. This can be achieved by walking, paddling or swimming in an independent and safe fashion.

So while, in the technical sense, the Adapted Aquatics program is not considered a rehabilitation program, we know that it does indeed provide the clients, and in this case the instructors also, an opportunity to learn new skills, forge strong friendships/rapports, challenge and extend themselves and grow as a person. We know that 'evidence exists that physical activity is beneficial for youth with developmental disabilities' (Johnson 2009:166), which appear to be confirmed in the Adapted Aquatics program at VU.

Summary of key lessons

- Physical activity in groups affords both physiological and social health benefits, and although group recreation and play might not be intended as therapy, or delivered by clinical exercise practitioners, these interventions can be therapeutic.

- Group recreation and play-based therapies are of particular value in working with clients requiring special care, particularly children, frail and elderly adults, and people with disabilities because these clients commonly feel *excluded* (and sometime are actively excluded) from typical exercise and sporting environments.

DISCUSSION Questions

1 What are the perceived benefits of the Adapted Aquatics program at Victoria University for both pre-service teachers and clients?

2 Drawing on lessons from the Adapted Aquatics program, how might proponents of a 'regular' swimming program improve their learning outcomes for their clients?

3 Research the Halliwick swimming program for people with a disability. How can this program, designed primarily for people with a physical disability, be adapted for those with an intellectual disability? What are the benefits?

REFERENCES

Australian Council for the Teaching of Swimming and Water Safety (AUSTSWIM) Teacher of People with a Disability certificate. Online. Available: www.austswim.com.au/pages/p_teacher.htm#toad (accessed 31 August 2010)

Doremus WA (1992) Developmental aquatics: assessment and instructional programming. *Teaching Exceptional Children*, 24(4):6–10

Getz M, Hutzler Y, Vermeer A (2007) Effects of aquatic interventions in children with neuromotor impairments: a systematic review of the literature. *Clinical Rehabilitation*, 20:927–36

Grosse SJ (2010) Water freedom for all: The Halliwick Method. *International Journal of Aquatic Research and Education*, 4(2)

Johnson C (2009) The benefits of physical activity for youth with developmental disabilities: a systematic review. *American Journal of Health Promotion*, 23(3):157–67

Tirosh R, Katz-Leurer M, Getz M (2008) Halliwick based aquatic assessments: reliability and validity. *International Journal of Aquatic Research and Education*, 2(3)

Chapter 18

Case studies in exercise as therapy for athletes

Robert Robergs, Henry Pollard and Dennis Hemphill

INTRODUCTION

A high profile AFL athlete suffers an horrendous leg fracture during a televised football match. The graphic nature of the injury generates much media attention and an outpouring of public sympathy. Following surgery, which included the insertion of a titanium rod into his tibia, the long process of rehabilitation involves a roller coaster ride of heady optimism to anxious self-doubt about recovery and returning to the game. Team-mates do their best to support the injured player, but home visits decline as the team gets on with the business of finishing the season. The athlete becomes despondent after weeks of confinement with non-athletes in the local rehabilitation clinic, and from watching the team's games on television.

The body with football history

This athlete feels most 'at home' while on the football field. It is where the athlete is most comfortable, most in tune with his thoughts and actions, as well as those of his team-mates. It is on the field of play where the athlete feels the most knowledgeable, movement-articulate, and effective. While he has a number of outside interests, football is the athlete's principal source of identity, affirmed by his membership on the team and within the football community.

Injury as alienation

The player's injury is not simply about a broken limb; it is also about the damaged person. Thomas and Rintala (1989) argued that injury can produce alienation. For the injured athlete, there may be a rupture of mind–body unity ('mind is willing, but body is unable …'), an estrangement from team culture, a loss of identity, and/or a disconnection with a meaningful football future. Alienation may be so severe as to jeopardise the athlete's playing career.

Recovery

The 'body-as-machine' metaphor can be a useful one for, say, the surgeons, who attempt to reconstruct the broken limb of the footballer. Rehabilitation clinicians, according to Doolittle (1994), often mark recovery in terms of patients recovering basic functioning: limb strength, mobility, and independence. But patients often measure recovery in terms of how well and to what extent they can take up activities of concern, giving them identity and continuity with past, and a vision of a liveable future (Doolittle 1994). In this approach, therapy is as much about the recovery of the social body as it is repair of the injured limb.

Recovery may involve taking steps to re-establish the player's direct links with the team throughout the entire recovery process. For example, the player may be encouraged to undertake rehabilitation sessions at the team's training centres, support the recovery of other injured team-mates, train with the team, where appropriate, assist with coaching, sit with the team on game day, and to continue socialising with the team. Rather than seeing the injured athlete as 'bad luck' to have around, this approach normalises the injured athlete and affirms his identity on the team.

According to Nixon (1992) athletes are socialised to interpret and deal with pain and injury in ways that reflect a culture of risk in sport. As a result of this culture of risk, with slogans reinforcing heroic self-sacrifice (eg: 'playing with pain', 'there's no tomorrow', 'impossible is nothing'), athletes may under-report or deny the severity of their injuries or overestimate their recovery and readiness to return to play. Sport medicine personnel, who may themselves be immersed in this culture, may compromise the long-term health interests of the athlete in favour of short-term desires of the athlete or the team.

Moreover, the injured athlete may be so immersed in the footballer role and identify so strongly with the football way of life, and its culture of risk, that he cannot make a fully informed and voluntary choice about his playing future (Nixon 1992). This may serve as motivation for recovery, but it may also blind the athlete to more realistic timelines for recovery or to alternatives to football altogether. In a case like this, the athlete may benefit from advice about 'liveable futures' from medical staff and significant others outside the team or sport altogether (eg: player associations welfare officer, family members, friends).

The notions of 'identity,' 'culture of risk,' 'liveable futures' and 'alienation' can be used to illustrate how injury treatment is as much about the recovery or reconstruction of the social body as it is the physical one. It also reinforces the need for exercise and injury rehabilitation practitioners to be not only technically proficient, but also 'culturally competent'. That is, they need to be able to recognise and respond appropriately to the particular social reality that defines their clients.

CASE STUDY 1: UNEXPLAINED PRE-SYNCOPE DURING INTENSE EXERCISE

Subjective
Nicole is a 17-year-old female swim athlete from Albury, Western Australia. She currently weighs 59.0kg and is 159.4cm tall. Based on repeated email correspondence between the clinical exercise physiology team and Nicole's father regarding explanations of Nicole's symptoms, a more clear understanding was developed for Nicole's condition.

Nicole's symptoms consist of near loss of consciousness during extreme physical exertion. During swim racing, Nicole would complete the race but be incapable of leaving the pool. Parental explanations revealed a condition of near unconsciousness, with total loss of control of all limbs and voluntary movement. Symptoms were similar to a vaso-vagal response, but with no loss of consciousness or evidence of hypotension. This is the first reported presentation of such symptoms in a client to be tested in our facility.

Nicole's father explained that Nicole had completed numerous medical examinations with a cardiologist, pulmonologist and a neurologist. However, no clear medical diagnosis has been made of her condition, with no treatment outcome. Nicole has also completed a prior exercise test in Perth, revealing a maximal respiratory exchange ratio (RER) of approximately 1.0, and a maximal rate of oxygen consumption (VO_{2max}) measure of approximately 48mL/kg/min. The maximal RER value was lower than expected for the end of a maximal exercise test, indicating a condition that prevents Nicole reaching peak physiological and metabolic capacities. Such numbers also precluded an explanation of her condition to be metabolic acidosis, as Nicole is never able to exercise to the extent to develop metabolic acidosis which would coincide with RER values > 1.0.

We thought that due to the prior abnormal exercise test responses we should re-test Nicole again with added assessments of 12-lead electrocardiogram (ECG), haemoglobin saturation ($HbO_2sat\%$), and an additional lung function test to assess residual volume as an indirect marker of heart valve problems.

Objective
A series of different tests of physiological capacities and components of physical fitness were performed, and procedures and results are grouped by test category.

Pulmonary function
Nicole completed a spirometry and residual volume assessment using a computerised lung function analyser (Collins, Pulmonary Function Testing System, Braintree, MA), with residual volume measured by helium dilution. Results are presented in Table 18.1. All data were within normal limits for Nicole based on gender, age and height norms.

Table 18.1 Pulmonary function data

Measurement units	Test 1	Test 2	Averages
FVC (L)	3.82	3.92	3.87
FEV$_1$%	89.0	86.0	87.5
IC	3.15	3.09	3.12
ERC	0.84	0.96	0.9
TV	1.89	1.89	1.89
VC	3.98	4.05	4.02
FRC	1.77	1.87	1.82
RV	0.94	0.91	0.92
TLC	4.92	4.96	4.94
RV/TLC	19.05	18.31	18.68

Note: FVC = forced vital capacity; FEV1% = percentage of forced expiratory volume exhaled in one second; IC = inspiratory capacity; ERC = expiratory reserve volume; TV = tidal volume; VC = vital capacity; FRC = functional reserve capacity; RV = residual volume; TLC = total lung capacity.

Exercise testing

Based on the prior history and symptoms, it was decided that we would perform a standard clinical graded exercise test. To more clearly interpret the 12-lead electrocardiogram, we used a 20 Watt ramp cycle ergometer protocol. The bike test also made any occurrence of symptoms a safer situation for Nicole and test personnel.

We used a Quinton 12-lead ECG system, with heart rate signals integrated to our metabolic system, as described next. We performed breath-by-breath expired gas analysis indirect calorimetry to quantify ventilation and whole body metabolism, where heart rate was also acquired and aligned to each breath. We also recorded finger pulse oximetry from two oximetry systems; each one placed on the index finger of each hand. Oxyhaemoglobin saturation (HbO$_2$sat%) was recorded manually every 0.5 minute for each unit. Ratings of perceived exertion (6 to 20) were obtained every 2 minutes.

All metabolic and heart rate data was first screened for outliers, and then processed using a 15-breath average to remove excessive breath-by-breath variability. As data was inconsistent during the last 30s of the test due to near loss of consciousness, this data was removed. Results are presented in Table 18.2.

Figure 18.1 presents a stack plot of the respiratory analysis data of ventilation, oxygen consumption, RER, heart rate and the ventilatory equivalents for oxygen and carbon dioxide.

Summary of testing

The pulmonary function test went well, with normal values for all measures. The exercise test was performed with five test technicians responsible for the metabolic system, electrocardiography, blood pressure, pulse oximetry, and physical support for Nicole on the ergometer during the test. Nicole exercised for 9.25 minutes, with the test terminating due to near loss of consciousness and the need to physically lift and remove Nicole from the ergometer to a bench, where she recovered supine for almost 25 minutes. It is important to note that once in a supine posture after the test, Nicole remained

Table 18.2 Summary of exercise test results

Stage* Time (min)	Watts	RPE	BP mmHg	HR b/min	HbO$_2$sat%	VO$_2$ mL/kg/min
Seated rest			128/76	96	99	7.25
1	40			115	99	9.06
2	40		130/80	123	99	15.84
3	60	11		127	94	17.70
4	80	13	140/70	136	90	19.83
5	100	14		141	89	20.29
6	120	14	136/80	157	96	24.82
7	140	16		164	80	28.54
8	160			171	87	32.93
9	180			191	78	39.22
Pre- syncope at 9 minutes 19 seconds	186			196		40.30
Supine recovery						
IPE					99	
1					99	
2					99	
6			132/70		99	
9			122/68		99	

Note: Watts = power output during cycling; RPE = rating of perceived exertion; BP = systemic blood pressure; HR = heart rate; HbO$_2$sat% = arterial oxyhemoglobin saturation; VO$_2$ = rate of oxygen consumption; IPE = immediate post-exercise.

symptomatic, close to losing consciousness, for almost 5 minutes. Such symptoms gradually subsided over a period of 25 minutes. As such, the condition was not caused by post-exercise postural hypotension.

During the test we temporarily lost the ECG signal on two occasions due to a bad electrode. However, manual compression to the electrode and lead restored the signal. Such episodes can be seen in Figure 18.1d. Good heart rate signal remained through to the end of the exercise test and recovery.

Ventilation

Nicole had an apparently normal ventilatory response to exercise. However, as is consistent with a minimal development of metabolic acidosis, there was no large rate of increase in ventilation near the end of the test, nor did Nicole have a high peak rate of ventilation.

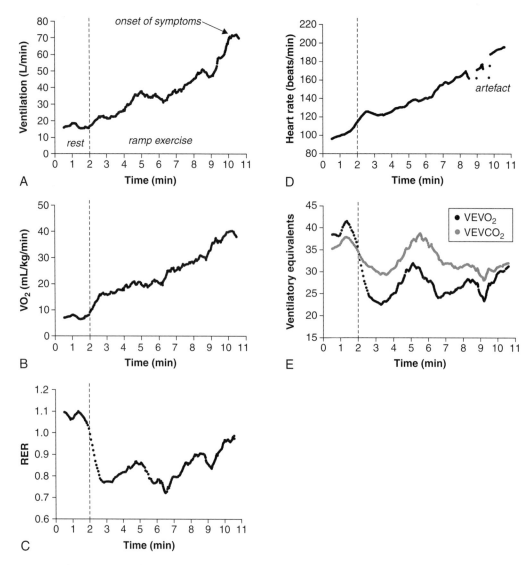

Figure 18.1 Stack plot of the metabolic and ventilatory responses to the incremental exercise protocol, showing (a) expired ventilation (stpd); (b) oxygen consumption, (c) respiratory exchange ratio (RER); (d) heart rate; and (e) ventilatory equivalents for oxygen and carbon dioxide

Oxygen consumption

The VO_{2max}, or VO_{2peak}, is the highest data point we measure after we process the data to remove the variability that is typical for breath-by-breath VO_2 analysis. In this instance, given the symptom limited nature of the exercise test, the label of VO_{2peak} is more correct. Nicole was prevented from attaining a true VO_{2max} due to her condition.

As shown in Figure 18.1b, Nicole's VO_{2peak} was measured at 40.3mL/kg/min. We can only estimate that a true VO_{2max} for Nicole would be

somewhere close to 50mL/kg/min. This would be a value typical for a well trained endurance swim athlete. As such despite Nicole's condition, she has been able to adapt normally to her swim training.

Ventilatory equivalents

Figure 18.1e shows the changes in the ventilatory equivalents. Note that during the last 2 minutes of the test, there was a trend for both measures to increase. The late increase in these variables, combined with the small increment and the low to moderate ventilation response to the exercise protocol all support a symptom limited, or premature end, to the exercise test. Clearly, Nicole's condition prevents her from exercising to her maximum capacity.

Respiratory exchange ratio (RER)

Figure 18.1c presents the RER data for the test. As with each of the ventilation, VO_2 and ventilatory equivalent data, the results indicate a premature end to the exercise test, with a peak RER of 0.99. Normally, we would measure values as high as 1.3 at the end of an incremental exercise test. Increases in RER above 1.0 indicate the onset of metabolic acidosis, and as such, it is clear that Nicole never developed a meaningful metabolic acidosis during the test, therefore ruling out acidosis as a trigger of her symptoms.

Heart rate

Figure 18.1c presents the data for heart rate. Nicole has an unusually high resting heart rate, as well as an atypically high heart rate response to exercise. The peak heart rate recorded was 196 beats/min, which is actually a few beats above her estimated maximal heart rate (estimated HRmax = 205.8 − (0.685 x age) = 194 beats/min). Note again that this is a high heart rate given that Nicole was not yet close to maximal exertion as defined by her measured physiological variables and estimated physiological capacities.

This heart rate response is deviant from Nicole's other physiological measurements. Most other measurements reveal lower than expected values, but heart rate is higher than expected. This abnormal result could reveal that heart rate is altered by her condition, suggestive of chronic dehydration, a contributor to her condition, or revealing a more complex central nervous system dysfunction causing her condition.

Blood pressure

Nicole had a small increase in systolic blood pressure during the exercise test, which is an abnormal response to incremental exercise. Diastolic blood pressure remained relatively stable, and we were unable to monitor blood pressure near the end of the test due to Nicole's symptoms. Recovery blood pressure was normal, with no evidence of profound hypotension (see Table 18.1).

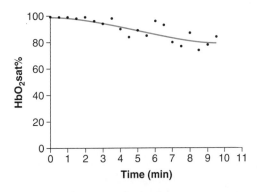

Figure 18.2 **The oxyhaemoglobin saturation ($HbO_2sat\%$) response to exercise**

Pulse oximetry

The haemoglobin oxygen saturation ($HbO_2sat\%$) data of Figure 18.2 are difficult to interpret. Finger pulse oximetry is not the most valid method of oximetry during exercise and, given Nicole's compromised function during exercise, we are unsure whether the observed decrease in $HbO_2sat\%$ is real or an artefact of an impaired peripheral circulation during exercise secondary to her condition. Despite these concerns, Nicole's $HbO_2sat\%$ immediately returned to normal values during recovery.

Electrocardiography

The 12-lead ECG was apparently normal throughout the test, with only an exaggerated heart rate response noted at rest and during exercise.

Assessment

We were able to do some literature research on Nicole's symptoms. As her symptoms were near classic for vaso-vagal syncope, we searched for research and medical commentary on exercise and syncope. Without too much effort, we were able to find research and medical case reports on athletes who experience syncope during intense exercise. While the physiological mechanism(s) of this response remain vague, there is some direction for future medical treatment that can be taken from this work, as will be explained next.

Basically, Nicole could have one of the following: vasodepressor syncope; postural tachycardia syndrome (POTS); or a third option of something different.

Vasodepressor syncope

We found a case study on a wrestler with similar symptoms to Nicole. However, the onset of syncope in this athlete was accompanied by a decreased heart rate, which Nicole has the opposite response to. This athlete was successfully treated with fludrocortisone, which increases sodium retention in the kidney, thereby expanding blood (plasma) volume. Interestingly, other published reports exist for exercise-induced syncope (Abe et al 1997; Bloomfield 2002; Grubb et al 1993; Hand 1997).

Postural tachycardia syndrome

We believe that this condition is most like Nicole's (Raj 2006). Individuals with POTS have a high heart rate, especially when moving from a supine to upright posture. For most activities and postures, the high heart rate prevents any hypotension, but for reasons that are not completely understood, there remains insufficient blood flow to the brain leading to symptoms of light headedness, exercise intolerance and, in extreme cases, pre-syncope. If this is Nicole's condition, she clearly has an extreme case.

What is also interesting is that approximately 80% of POTS patients are female and of menstruating age, with the role of oestrogen in fluid balance and hypovolaemia (dehydration) being an interesting contributor to symptom severity. Fludrocortisone administration has also been successful in decreasing symptoms of POTS.

Plan

We recommend that Nicole be seen once again by a cardiologist or neurologist who has been able to read this report and the articles that were identified to describe the condition. The cardiologist/neurologist will be able to decide on whether to follow a prescription of medications indicated by prior medical case study reports.

We hope that Nicole's parents pursue follow-up medical intervention as there is a reasonable expectation based on prior research and publications that correct medication therapy combined with a concerted effort to remain hydrated could completely remove Nicole's symptoms.

Discussion

This case study presents evidence of an atypical physiological condition of a young, apparently healthy athlete. A thorough assessment of underlying physiological capacities was essential to rule out dysfunction in oxygen transport that could possibly be caused by structural or functional abnormality in lung and/or cardiovascular function. The clear normality of Nicole's responses to spirometry testing and incremental exercise ruled out dysfunction in cardiopulmonary physiology.

As with all clinical exercise physiology assessments, tests and data interpretation need to be referenced as best as possible to prior research evidence. Investigation of prior published research and medical commentary on Nicole's symptoms was very helpful in interpreting Nicole's symptoms. It was important to realise that Nicole's condition had been reported in other athletes, and that there was medical evidence for combined pharmacological and nutritional intervention to remove symptoms. The possibility of continued exercise training and competition with minimal risk to health was a test result that both Nicole and her parents were hoping for.

Summary of key lessons

- Where possible, data from all prior medical and clinical exercise physiology assessments are essential for aiding in the detailed and accurate description of the symptoms and condition, as well as for result comparison.

- Clinical exercise practitioners need to know how to explore, understand and critically analyse prior published scientific and medical research. Such skills will invariably assist in data interpretation and a more evidence-based assessment and recommendation plan.

DISCUSSION Questions

1 What procedures and/or equipment could you standardise in your practice to ensure that you are going to always support receiving the most complete assessment of prior clinical history from your clients?

2 Do you have an emergency plan in place to deal with clients who experience pre-syncope during exercise testing?

3 How could you minimise clients' risk of falling and subsequent injury during exercise testing on a treadmill or cycle ergometer?

CASE STUDY 2: UNEXPLAINED POOR EXERCISE TOLERANCE IN A HIGH SCHOOL SWIMMER AND CROSS COUNTRY RUNNER

Subjective

Edwina is a 17-year-old female swim athlete from a local private school. She currently weighs 54.6kg and is 170cm tall. Edwina has a history of unexplained poor exercise tolerance, despite training and competing in competitive cross country running and swimming for several years. However, within the last year Edwina has had to reduce her cross country running training due to symptoms of fatigue in combination with other complications as will be explained below. Monitoring of post-exercise heart rate by her high school trainers revealed a very slow heart rate recovery, which in combination with declining swim performance suggested the need for physiological assessment follow-up. Consequently, Edwina was recommended for a complete graded exercise test in our facility by her coaching staff.

Consultation with Edwina's parents revealed that she has completed prior medical evaluations with a cardiologist and a pulmonologist. Cardiology assessment revealed a normal resting electrocardiogram (ECG), with no feedback given regarding auscultation and heart valve sounds. Edwina has not had a prior echocardiogram or exercise stress test with clinical assessments. Parental feedback of the diagnosis by the cardiologist was a confident conclusion of vocal cord dysfunction, resulting in a constriction of the upper airway, resulting in hypoventilation and a combined pulmonary and metabolic acidosis.

Pulmonary assessments have consisted of standard pulmonary function spirometric measures, as well as responses to pharmacological challenge and the assessment of exercise-induced broncho-constriction. Interpretation of a prior pulmonology report revealed a 14% improvement in $FEV_1\%$ following administration of albuterol post-exercise, and consequently, Edwina was prescribed bronchodilator therapy via an inhaler for administration as required.

Additional symptoms reported by Edwina and her father consisted of tingling sensations in her toes and fingers, especially after waking in the morning. The occurrence of these symptoms has been random with no apparent pattern. Edwina has also woken with red rash-like bumps on her feet and toes on numerous occasions, and has also observed a blue–purple colour tone to her fingers and toes. The tingling sensations and colour tone changes have also occurred in response to exercise stress.

Objective

Based on the prior history and symptoms, it was decided that we would perform a standard clinical graded exercise test on the treadmill using the Bruce protocol so that little movement artefact would occur on the 12-lead ECG. We used a Quinton diagnostic 12-lead ECG system, with heart rate signals integrated to our metabolic system, as described next. We performed breath-by-breath expired gas analysis indirect calorimetry to quantify ventilation and whole body metabolism, where heart rate was also acquired and aligned to each breath. We also recorded finger pulse oximetry from two oximetry systems; each one placed on the index finger of each hand. Oxyhaemoglobin saturation ($HbO_2sat\%$) was recorded manually every 0.5 minutes for each unit. Ratings of perceived exertion (6–20) were obtained at the end of each 3 minute stage. All measurements were continued through 4 minutes of an active recovery at 2.0 min/hr and 0% grade. Table 18.3 presents a summary of the test data.

Oxygen consumption

The VO_{2max} is the highest data point we measure after we process the data to remove the data variability that is typical for breath-by-breath VO_2 analysis. As shown in Figure 18.3a, Edwina's VO_{2max} was measured at 49mL/kg/min. Unfortunately, there are no suitable norms for VO_{2max} for young female endurance athletes. However, the normative data from the Cooper Clinic in Dallas reveals a rating of 'superior' for

a VO_{2max} >42mL/kg/min for women between 20 and 29 years of age for the general population. Nevertheless, our testing of athletes of equivalent training to Edwina's training status results in a rating of 'average' for this VO_{2max} value. Figure 18.3 presents a stack plot of the respiratory analysis data of oxygen consumption, ventilation, ventilatory equivalents and respiratory exchange ratio (RER; explained below).

Ventilation

Edwina had an apparently normal ventilatory response to exercise. Figure 18.3b shows a gradual increase in ventilation during the exercise protocol. Furthermore, Figure 18.3c depicts a ventilatory response leading to a typical profile for both ventilatory equivalents, where a threshold increase in ventilation divided by VO_2 (VE/VO_2) is typical for incremental exercise, and is called the ventilation threshold (VT). There is normally

Table 18.3 Summary of results for the exercise test

Stage[a] Stage:Time	Speed mi/hr	Grade %	est VO_2[b] mL/kg/min	RPE	BP mmHg	HR b/min	$HbO_2sat\%$	VO_2 mL/kg/min
Seated rest					112/78			
Stand rest					112/78	100	97	8.0(2.3)
1:1–3 min	2.5	12	24.1(6.9)	8	122/74	140	95	23(6.6)
2:3–6 min	3.4	14	33.2(9.5)	11	128/76	173	94	33(9.4)
3:6–9 min	4.2	15	41.3(11.8)	15	–	192	81	46(13.1)
4:9–9.5 min	5.2	15	42.8(12.2)	18	–	195	80	49(14.0)
Recovery[c] (min)								
1						166	96	
2						142	97	
3						139	96	
4						132	95	

[a] We started exercise at stage 2 of the Bruce protocol and could only increase % grade to 15% on our performance treadmill.
[b] From ACSM equations, mL/kg/min (METs).
[c] Active recovery at 2 min/hr, 0% grade.

a 1–2 minute delay in the threshold increase in ventilation divided by VCO_2 (VE/VCO_2). However, an endurance athlete should typically have this response occur above 80% of the VO_{2max} range. For Edwina, the VT occurred at 66% VO_{2max}, which can be classically interpreted as poor physical conditioning. An alternate interpretation is that an underlying cardiopulmonary condition is preventing Edwina from training and improving her physical conditioning.

The more important variable for assessing near maximal exercise effort is the ratio between carbon dioxide production (VCO_2) and VO_2. This is called the respiratory exchange ratio (RER). Values for RER in excess of 1.0 reveal metabolic acidosis and body metabolism associated with extreme exercise intensities. Figure 18.1d presents the RER data for Edwina's test. The RER response revealed a rapid increase in the transition to carbohydrate catabolism and the development of metabolic

acidosis early into the test (5.75 minutes and 60% VO_2max), supporting the VE/VO_2 and VE/VCO_2 data for the VT.

The combined VO_2, ventilation, VT and RER data reveal a compromised muscular endurance and/or cardiopulmonary capacity. Despite her years of training and current swim competition, Edwina has a maximal steady state (intensity above which metabolic acidosis and fatigue develops) that approximates a slow jog on level ground! The metabolic data reveal an abnormal response to exercise.

Heart rate, pulse oximetry and the 12-lead electrocardiogram

Figure 18.4a presents the data for heart rate, and Figure 18.4b presents the data for oxy-haemoglobin saturation. Edwina had a high resting (pre-exercise) heart rate (both seated and standing, ~100 beats/min), and had an abrupt

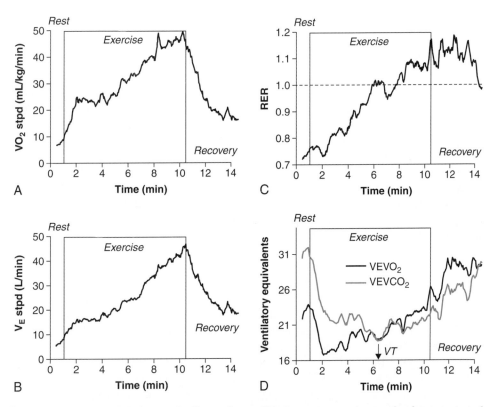

Figure 18.3 Stack plot of the metabolic and ventilatory responses to the incremental exercise protocol, showing: (a) oxygen consumption; (b) expired ventilation (stpd); (c) respiratory exchange ration (RER); and (d) ventilatory equivalents for oxygen and carbon dioxide

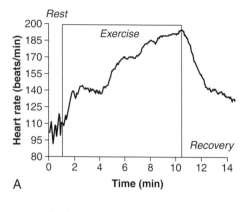

A

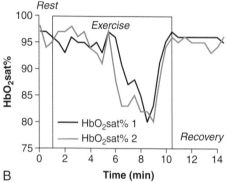

B

Figure 18.4 **The cardiopulmonary responses to the incremental exercise test for (a) heart rate and (b) oxy-haemoglobin saturation (HbO₂sat%)**

increase in heart rate during the exercise test. Heart rate had increased 40 beats/min to 140 beats/min during the first 3-minute stage of the protocol (second stage of the Bruce protocol), which is a slow walk up a moderate incline. This rapid response is highly irregular for a sedentary person, let alone a competitive endurance athlete.

An estimate of the maximal heart rate (HRmax) using 205.8 − (0.685 x age) reveals an estimated HRmax = 194 beats/min. Thus, the measured maximal heart rate of 195 beats/min was expected.

The HbO$_2$sat% data of Figure 18.4b are cause for concern. The HbO$_2$sat% decreased similarly in both measurement systems from expected values between 95% and 98%. The decreases occurred early, during the second stage of the protocol coinciding with a heart rate approximating 150 beats/min and at a metabolic intensity of 60 %VO$_{2max}$. Lowest readings occurred at the peak exercise intensity, and approximated 80%. As a decreasing HbO$_2$sat% reveals decreased

oxygen binding to haemoglobin, it also indicates an impairment in one of several physiological functions and anatomical locations of the heart and/or lungs that influences the partial pressure of oxygen in the arterial blood leaving the heart. These data, more than any other, indicate the urgent need for medical follow-up.

The 12-lead ECG also revealed indications of abnormality. Select traces have been scanned and are presented at the end of this report. We are concerned with the observation of tall peaked P-waves and irregular S-T segment and T-wave changes in specific (inferior) leads. However, as we are not a diagnostic medical facility, we are not allowed to clinically interpret the 12-lead ECG.

Assessment

Edwina has an unexpectedly poor metabolic capacity, an exaggerated heart rate response to exercise, and an early exercise onset reduction in her blood oxygen saturation (hypoxemia) accompanied by irregular ECG responses.

Plan

All data from this graded exercise test reveal poor physical conditioning and cardiopulmonary dysfunction. It is extremely important that Edwina undergo additional medical testing to further and more precisely evaluate heart and lung function, preferably in response to exercise stress.

Discussion

This case study is somewhat atypical in that exercise physiology testing occurred in response to inadequate prior medical testing and evaluation. In this context, inadequate refers to the inability for medical evaluation and testing to reveal the cause for unexplained premature exercise-induced fatigue.

The clinical exercise testing conducted in this evaluation also shows how beneficial clinical exercise testing is to clinical diagnoses. Superficially, the metabolic data from the exercise test appeared rather normal. However, quantification of a low metabolic threshold (ventilation threshold) revealed a relatively detrained condition. In combination with the pulse oximetry data, there is clearly a cardiopulmonary dysfunction, yet to be detected by medical evaluation, that is compromising the client's exercise capacities and tolerance.

Summary of key lessons

- It is possible for standard medical assessment of athletes to be incomplete and unable to diagnose causes of exercise dysfunction. Exercise testing or sport-specific testing may be required for a full assessment.
- A client's self-reporting is an important part of the clinical picture. Edwina reported that she was training frequently, but not achieving expected performance improvements. This report stood out against test results that suggested an untrained state.

DISCUSSION Questions

Consider how you might respond to a client whose self-reported training history appears inconsistent with exercise test results.

1 Who are you more inclined to believe: your client or the test data?

2 What are some of the more helpful and less helpful ways you could respond to your client in this situation?

CASE STUDY 3: A TALE OF TWO ATHLETES

Neck pain in a runner

Subjective

This case relates to a 45-year-old right-handed female accountant clerk who works 40 hours per week performing data entry and phone duties. She does not use a head set whilst performing data entry. She participates in recreational jogging running approximately 70km per week describing herself as a 'serious runner'. She complains of a 3-week history of right shoulder, elbow, and forearm pain. Additionally, she describes an increasing numbness in the right index finger the week prior to presentation.

The history revealed several sporadic short-term episodes of neck pain usually associated with a occipitofrontal headache without migrainous prodrome or other brainstem symptoms. The pain was typically similar in intensity but the duration of each episode has slowly increased over time. On review of the past history, there was a motor vehicle accident 17 years prior, resulting in a whiplash-associated disorder (WAD) classification 1 injury from a rear end collision with the head

facing forward. There is a past history of one to two acute episodes of pain without arm pain per year over the last few years. Pain resolved 2 weeks later after non-steroidal anti-inflammatory drugs (NSAIDs) and short-term spinal manipulation (chiropractic) treatment. Pain was aggravated by movement and work and relieved by rest and wearing a collar. She also had a case of left-sided 'shin splints' (medial tibial stress syndrome) approximately 2 years prior.

Objective

Pain was a constant 8/10 using the visual analogue scale (VAS) and the arm pain was 6/10. The pain had increased in intensity over the last 2 weeks. There was a doorbell sign (pressure over the intervertebral foramen [IVF] caused an increase in arm symptoms). The neck range of motion (ROM) was reduced in right lateral flexion greater than extension greater than rotation. Cervical distraction aggravated the pain and distraction relieved it. The Spurling and Soto-Hall manoeuvres were negative and the Valsalva was positive. Babinski and clonus testing was negative. Grip strength was reduced on the right by 30% compared with the left. Reflex testing revealed a reduced brachioradialis (+1), and decreased two point discrimination in the C_6 distribution. There were no lower limb symptoms.

Assessment

Due to the worsening nature of the symptoms and the referral of symptoms into the extremity, imaging was performed. Plain films revealed moderate degeneration at the C_{567} levels with reduced disc height and posterior osteophytic encroachment into the right C_{56} IVF. An MRI revealed a large posterolateral disc herniation with spurring into the right C_{56} IVF encroaching the C_6 nerve root.

Back pain in a bodybuilder
Subjective

A 39-year-old male right-handed store person presented with severe low back pain with antalgia to the right with pain and paraesthesia down the back of the left leg to the foot in the S_1 distribution. The paraesthesias were particularly noted in the fourth and fifth digits of the foot. The patient also participates in weight training 5 days per week as a bodybuilder.

The pain came on following heavy lifting all day at work. Pain came on slowly over a 2-hour timeframe after work. The patient had difficulty sleeping and the pain was worse the next morning. Pain was described as sharp on movement, particularly on weight-bearing of the left leg. The patient used a cane to ambulate. There were no bowel or bladder changes noted.

There is a past history of several acute episodes of pain without leg pain; approximately twice per year over the last few years. The pain typically resolved in 1–4 weeks without treatment being sought. The initial injury was sustained 9 years previously whilst performing a heavy awkward lift from the ground to above waist height. Past treatment has included NSAIDs, physiotherapy (short term), and wearing a brace at work. The pain is aggravated by sitting, bending and lifting and the cough and Valsalva manoeuvres. The pain is relieved by non weight-bearing, rest, heat, and lying down.

Objective

Examination revealed a 90kg, 180cm fit man who appeared to be in some distress, with guarded movement with right-sided antalgia.

He was unable to stand on his toes on the left and had positive Valsalva, slump and straight-leg raising (SLR) tests. The SLR was positive at 25°. The well-leg raise test was positive. The hip ROM revealed decreased left flexion and a positive left Scours test (hip flexion, adduction and internal rotation). There was a significantly reduced S_1 reflex. Sensory testing revealed a reduction in two-point discrimination on the lateral toes and lateral calf. There were negative Babinski and clonus findings and the motor testing of S_1 (gastrocnemius and soleus: standing on the toes) was 3/5. Lumbar ROM aggravated the leg pain especially in left lateral flexion, extension and flexion. Palpation was very sensitive at the lumbosacral region left greater than the right.

Assessment

Due to the worsening nature of the symptoms and the referral of symptoms into the extremity, imaging was performed, revealing degenerative change of a moderate to severe nature at L_5S_1 and of a moderate level at L_{45}. The magnetic resonance imaging (MRI) revealed a left L_5S_1 extruded L_5 disc that extended posteriorly and superiorly into the lumbosacral IVF on the left. There was a mild discal bulge at the left on the L_{45}.

Overall assessment

These two recreational athletes present with radiculopathy (nerve root compression) secondary to disc degeneration, the same condition but in differing regions of the spine.

Plan

The rehabilitation goals are similar for both clients, and are outlined below.

Phase 1: aims
- Reduction of pain and inflammation.
- Increase ROM.
- Prevent further damage.
- Concept of relative rest: remain active if movement does not cause increased pain.
- Use pain and disability questionnaires to quantify impairment, pain and disability: Oswestry disability questionnaire (lumbar), neck disability index (cervical) (Fairbank et al 2000; Vernon & Moir 1991).

Treatment

- Education of patient: the diagnosis, cause, sparing strategies, prognosis and aggravating and relieving factors for the condition.
- Postural advice. For the cervical case: sitting, lifting, computer use, sleeping, lifting and carrying objects off the shoulder and trapezius. For the lumbar case: moving from sit to stand, lying to sitting, lifting, sleeping, driving, pain-free postures.
- Lumbar and/or cervical brace may be provided in cases where lumbar and/or cervical instability is present or if there is severe pain. Supports such as these should only be used in the short term. It is important that the practitioner encourage early non-aggressive active therapy to prevent deconditioning (Dehner et al 2006).

Strength exercises

- Focus on ROM, not strength. Commence strength work in phase 2.

Mobility exercises

- ROM exercises for the neck (start with rotation then lateral flexion [side-bending] and flexion). Exercises to be performed in pain-free ROM initially.
- ROM exercises for the back (rotation) and flexion (knee to chest).
- Isometric contractions of the neck and lumbar ROM and especially the short flexors of the neck and the abdominals.
- Utilise McKenzie extension exercises if pain centralises. Discontinue if pain peripheralises (Hancock et al 2007).
- Pool walking (lumbar): walking in chest-high water. Caution should be taken not to continue walking until moderate fatigue or pain commences as the removal of the buoyancy when alighting the pool may aggravate the condition.

Clients are identified as ready to progress from phase 1 to phase 2 when they report decreases in pain and other symptoms, and demonstrate increased ROM and the capacity to perform exercises and activities of daily living (ADL) in a relatively pain-reduced state. For example, the clinical exercise practitioner could ask the client to demonstrate exercises and concurrently rate the pain on a scale of 0 (worst) to 10 (normal): Once a 7/10

can be achieved for a particular exercise, the client is progressed to the next level. Functional criteria, such as those captured in patient-specific functional scales, provide measures of ADL outcomes important to the client and should be used to document recovery (Binkley et al 1999; Stratford et al 2001).

Phase 2: aims

- Decrease pain and symptoms.
- Increase lumbar/cervical ROM.
- Improve functional capacity.
- Prevent deconditioning: perform some aerobic activity in addition to specific rehabilitation exercises.
- Identify yellow flags (ie: psychosocial markers for chronicity in spinal pain) using a questionnaire instrument (eg: Örebro Musculoskeletal Pain Questionnaire; Boersma & Linton 2004).

Strengthening exercises

- Continue phase 1 exercises.
- Supine cycling.
- Swiss ball abdominal roll in.
- Side bridge: commence side-lying, raise body as a plank from elbow to knees, elbow to feet, or hand to feet (Liebenson 2007).

Mobility exercises

- Continue phase 1 exercises.
- Seated lumbar flexion and extension.
- Stretching (*lumbar*: hamstrings, gluteal, gastro-soleus, tensor fascia lata; *cervical*: levator scapula, trapezius, scalenes, pectoralis major).
- Pool work (lumbar or cervical): walking and swimming as pain permits. If there is any aggravation, discontinue activity (Ariyoshi et al 1999).

Clients are identified as ready to progress from phase 2 to phase 3 when they report substantial decreases in pain and other symptoms, and demonstrate the capacity to perform basic-level stability exercises without pain. These clients will display largely normal locomotor patterns (ie: antalgic posture and gait abnormalities should have resolved).

Phase 3: aims

- Spinal stabilisation (ie: controlled spinal movement).
- Return to work and sport.

Strengthening exercises

Many variations and progressions exist for the basic exercise forms listed below. Commence with a simple form of the exercise that the client can perform without shuddering. Progress to a more difficult form of the exercise when the client reports that the exercise has become easy. Progressions may be made by adding load (weight), lengthening a limb lever, or increasing repetitions.

- Quadruped exercises: commence in four-point kneeling, raise upper/lower limbs to horizontal.
- 'Dead Bug' exercise: commence supine with thighs in 90 degree flexion, further flex or extend lower limbs.
- 'Superman' exercise: commence prone, extend spine without use of arms. Early progression places upper limbs in elevation (ie: as Superman flies) before extending spine.
- Side bridge (continue from phase 2).

Mobility exercises

- 'Cat-Camel' exercise: commence in four-point kneeling, flex spine fully, then extend spine fully.

Discussion

This spinal rehabilitation program is outcome oriented, based on a biopsychosocial model that promotes self-care and focuses on the client's functional goals (Liebenson 2007). In these features, it differs little from any evidence-based spinal rehabilitation program. These case studies demonstrate that musculoskeletal exercise rehabilitation in athletes commences similarly to that in non-athlete clients. (See DVD, case study 2, for further consideration of spinal exercise rehabilitation in an athlete.)

Athletes differ from other clients in that they have a high tolerance for (and enjoyment of) exercise, and may be expected to progress rapidly through the early phases of rehabilitation. Clinical exercise practitioners working with athletes need to become skilled in progressing mobility, strengthening, and spinal stabilisation exercises to continue to challenge athletes' exercise tolerances. More, athletes expect to return to sport. Clinical exercise practitioners working with athletes must be ready to progress rehabilitation exercises sufficiently to allow resumption of sporting activity.

A similar mindset may be found in the non-athlete worker. Work is important to people for many reasons (Heymans et al 2006). Income, activity, belonging, achievement as well as other issues are important to many clients and an early return to work may help motivate the client to resume normal ADL and promote healing in the process (Carleton et al 2009). Obviously a graded return to work is important in more severe cases.

A word of caution: not all athletes move rapidly through this type of rehabilitation program. Some of the strongest predictors of chronicity in musculoskeletal pain may be present with athletic injuries. For example, higher pain severity and longer pain duration at initial presentation, pain in multiple sites, and previous episodes of the same pain are all strong predictors of poor outcome (Mallen et al 2007) and possible in athletes; traumatic injuries may produce multiple sites and severe pain; overtraining injuries may lead to repeated episodes of pain and delays in care seeking. Some other predictors of chronicity are psychosocial (sometimes known as yellow flags) and appear to be at least as common in athletes as in other people: anxiety, depression, somatic perceptions, or distress associated with pain, as well as adverse coping strategies and low social support. In managing these yellow flags, which may lead to unhelpful beliefs about pain (Waddell et al 1993), Grotle et al (2006) recommends that if a patient is 'fearful' of exercise then 'graded exposures' to feared stimuli in a comfortable range may be helpful to disprove these beliefs. In such cases, returning workers often recommence work 3 days per week for reduced hours, with a day of rest in between. This is then progressed in hours and then days until a normal workload is achieved. In some cases this may take weeks or longer to achieve. Conversely, keeping one away from work may have deleterious effects on many psychosocial aspects of functioning that may hasten the progression of disability into chronicity (Nguyen & Randolph 2007).

Summary of key lessons

- Not all of the scientific evidence that is applicable in the management of athlete clients is drawn from studies on athletes. Many aspects of 'general' musculoskeletal exercise rehabilitation apply equally well to athlete clients, particularly in the early stages of injury and illness management.

- Athlete clients are distinguished from other clients by the expectation that they will return to sport as soon as possible; therefore, it is important to progress clinical exercises sufficiently to build sport performance tolerance.

DISCUSSION Questions

1 Sport is an activity of daily living (ADL) for athletes. Discuss how you might apply knowledge of an athlete's chosen sport in setting exercise progression goals.

2 Consider possible exercise goals for the two recreational athletes in this case study and how these goals might be individualised. For example, do you expect that both athletes will place the same importance on returning to running and/or weight training?

REFERENCES

Abe H, Iwami Y, Kohishi K, et al (1997) Exercise-induced neurally mediated syncope. *Japanese Heart Journal*, 38(4):535–9

Ariyoshi M, Sonoda K, Nagata K, et al (1999) Efficacy of aquatic exercises for patients with low-back pain. *Kurume Medical Journal*, 46:91–6

Binkley JM, Stratford PW, Lott SA, et al (1999) The lower extremity functional scale (LEFS): scale development, measurement properties, and clinical applications. *Physical Therapy*, 79:371–83

Bloomfield DM (2002) Strategy for management of vasovagal syncope. *Drugs Aging*, 19(3):179–202

Boersma K, Linton S (2004) Screening to identify patients at risk: Profiles of psychological risk factors for early intervention. *Clinical Journal of Pain*, 21:38–43

Carleton RN, Kachur SS, Abrams MP, et al (2009) Waddell's symptoms as indicators of psychological distress, perceived disability, and treatment outcome. *Journal of Occupational Rehabilitation*, 19(1):41–8

Dehner C, Hartwig E, Strobel P, et al (2006) Comparison of the relative benefits of 2 versus 10 days of soft collar cervical immobilization after acute whiplash injury. *Arch Phys Med Rehabil*. 87(11):1423–7

Doolittle N (1994) A clinical ethnography of stroke recovery. In: Benner P (ed.) *Interpretive Phenomenology: Embodiment, Caring, and Ethics in Health And Illness*. Thousand Oaks, CA: Sage Publications

Fairbank JCT, Pynsent PB (2000) The Oswestry Disability Index. *Spine*, 25(22):2940–53

González-Iglesias J, Fernández-de-las-Peñas C, Cleland JA, et al (2009) Thoracic spine manipulation for the management of patients with neck pain: a randomized clinical trial. *J Orthop Sports Phys Therapy*, 39(1):20–7

Grotle M, Vøllestad NK, Brox JI (2006) Clinical course and impact of fear-avoidance beliefs in low back pain: prospective cohort study of acute and chronic low back pain: II. *Spine*, 31(9):1038–46

Grubb BP, Temesy-Armos PN, Samoil D, et al (1993) Tilt table testing in evaluation and management of athletes with recurrent exercise-induced syncope. *Med Sci Sports Exerc*, 25(1):24–8

Hancock MJ, Maher CG, Latimer J, et al (2007) Systematic review of tests to identify the disc, SIJ or facet joint as the source of low back pain. *European Spine Journal*, 16(10):1539–50

Hand J (1997) Exercise-induced vasodepressor syncope in a collegiate wrestler: a case study. *J Athl Train*, 32(4):359–362

Heymans MW, de Vet HC, Knol DL, et al (2006) Workers' beliefs and expectations affect return to work over 12 months. *Journal of Occupational Rehabilitation*, 16(4):685–95

Liebenson C (ed.) (2007) *Rehabilitation of the Spine. A Practitioner's Manual*. Philadelphia, PA: Lippincott Williams & Wilkins

Mallen CD, Peat G, Thomas E, et al (2007) Prognostic factors for musculoskeletal pain in primary care: a systemic review. *British Journal of General Practice*, 57:655–61

Nguyen TH, Randolph DC (2007) Non-specific low back pain and return to work. *American Family Physician*, 76(10):1497–502

Nixon H (1992) A social network analysis of influences on athletes to play with pain and injury. *Journal of Sport and Social Issues*, 16(2):127–35

Raj SS (2006) The postural tachycardia syndrome (POTS): Pathophysiology, diagnosis and management. *Ind Pacing Electrophysiol J*, 6(2):84–99

Stratford P, Binkley JM, Stratford POW (2001) Development and initial validation of the upper extremity functional index. *Physiotherapy Canada*, Fall: 259–66, 281

Thomas C, Rintala J (1989) Injury as alienation in sport. *Journal of the Philosophy of Sport*, XVI, 44–58

Vernon H, Moir S (1991) The neck disability index: a study of reliability and validity. *J Manipulative & Physiological Therapeutics*, 14:409–15

Waddell G, Newton M, Henderson I, et al (1993) A Fear-Avoidance Beliefs Questionnaire (FABQ) and the role of fear-avoidance beliefs in chronic low back pain and disability. *Pain*, 52:157–68

Chapter 19

Case studies in exercise for occupational rehabilitation

Melainie Cameron, Ida Yiu, Garry Francis-Pester and Dennis Hemphill

INTRODUCTION

Occupational rehabilitation is often more complex and protracted than the clinical presentation alone would dictate. Clients with injuries or illness attributed to work are required to involve many people in their treatment and rehabilitation. Suddenly many people have an interest; stakeholders include not only the client and treating practitioners, but also employers, unions, insurers, colleagues, and regulatory authorities. In this chapter we present several case studies of injuries, illnesses, and incidents in workplaces. Some of these case studies are quite complex, with long and convoluted courses, so we have digressed from the structured SOAP (subjective, objective, assessment, plan) notes format. In other case studies, the injuries or illnesses themselves may seem to be quite straightforward conditions (eg: non-specific low back pain) for which exercise plays an important part in management, but management and progress to recovery may be complicated (and sometimes improved) by the involvement of many stakeholders.

Each case study deals with occupational rehabilitation from differing practitioner perspectives.

Private practice

In case study 1 Belinda seeks rehabilitation services from a private practitioner independent of her workplace or insurer. Fees for the practitioner's

Note: the case studies in this chapter are drawn from the authors' work with several organisations, including Jardine Lloyd Thompson, Parks Victoria, and Victoria University.

services are likely to be paid by a third party (workers' compensation insurer). In this case the clinical exercise practitioner acts independently of Belinda's employer, and is governed by relevant regional workers' compensation legislation only.

Managed care

Case studies 2A and 2B are complementary. In these case studies John and Peter are guided through occupational rehabilitation processes by a rehabilitation manager employed in their companies. Although she is qualified as a healthcare practitioner, the occupational rehabilitation manager does not provide clinical care as much as advocacy, support, and guidance to John and Peter. They receive clinical care in both the public health system (hospital emergency department, and hospital physiotherapy and occupational therapy outpatient clinics) and from 'panel doctors', practitioners associated with the relevant workers' compensation authority.

Occupational rehabilitation consultant

Case study 3 is written in the first person from the perspective of an occupational rehabilitation consultant working onsite for a large employer. In this case, the consultant acts both as a healthcare provider and a mediator between the injured employee and the employer.

Workplace culture

Case study 4 deals with a workplace culture that could (potentially) compromise return-to-work outcomes. The irony of this particular case study is that each of the employees is a clinical exercise practitioner in an organisation providing clinical exercise services, and the 'injured person' is a postgraduate student. Further, the organisation has an overt (written) commitment to health, wellbeing, and safety of all employees as well as clients. This case study, which includes neither a physical injury nor a plan for exercise rehabilitation intervention, is included in this chapter to raise awareness that harm in a workplace may be social, emotional, or relational, and that unhealthy workplace cultures can lead to disengagement from the working community.

CASE STUDY 1: PRIVATE PRACTICE

Subjective

Belinda, a 24-year-old woman working as a nurse in a large public hospital, presents to a clinical exercise practitioner complaining of acute low back pain that commenced yesterday after a fall in her workplace. Belinda, who stands only 158cm tall, was intending to assist with transfer of a patient in bed from one ward to another. In order to move the patient's bed from the ward, the door needed to be propped open. Belinda stood on a wheelchair in order to reach the door jam, but because she had not secured the brakes on the wheelchair, it moved from under her, and she fell to the floor, landing on her buttocks and back. This event was witnessed by another nurse, who assisted Belinda to stand after the fall. The event was reported to the nurse unit manager, and a written incident report completed and lodged. Belinda completed the work shift (40 minutes), and then drove home, where she took 2 × 500mg paracetamol, had a hot shower, put a heated wheat bag on her back, and retired to bed. Belinda reports that this morning she woke with bilateral back pain extending into both buttocks but no further down her legs. She did not attend work today, but telephoned her nurse unit manager to say that she had back pain, and then sought an appointment with a healthcare practitioner. Belinda reports that she took 2 × 500mg paracetamol 2 hours ago, and that her pain has subdued somewhat over that time. She reports no previous episodes of acute back pain and no previous history of work-related injury or illness.

Belinda smokes 10–15 cigarettes per day, and takes no regular exercise other than the physical activity involved in her work (ward nursing). She uses a triphasic oral contraceptive pill, but takes no other regular medication. Her medical history is otherwise unremarkable.

Objective

Belinda walks slowly, with her lumbar spine slightly flexed. She moves cautiously, but participates in the active examination. Her lumbar range of motion (ROM), assessed using a large arm goniometer, is limited to 50° flexion, 5° extension, and 15° side-bending right and left. Rotation is estimated at not more that 10° right and left. Physical examination reveals early bruising over both buttocks. Pain is reported at the end of all ROMs, particularly extension. Belinda reports tenderness to palpation through the muscles of the erector spinae and gluteal muscle groups bilaterally. Belinda rates her current pain using a 0–10 numerical rating scale at 6/10.

Assessment

Belinda has acute low back pain without evidence of radiculopathy. At this time Belinda's presentation does not fit any more stringent diagnostic classification than non-specific low back pain, although the progress (natural history) of her back pain may provide further clues. Belinda's back pain is temporally related to a known incident in her workplace, and an employee compensation claim is likely.

Plan

Belinda is advised to manage her back pain by staying as physically active as possible by continuing with activities of daily living (ADL; eg: eating, dressing, self-care), using over-the-counter simple analgesics (paracetamol) within the recommended dosage, and applying heat packs to the painful region as required. Belinda is also advised to keep a watching brief on symptoms, and to return for further investigations if symptoms worsen to include numbness or paresthesia in the saddle area, or pain, numbness, or paresthesia in the lower limbs. The negative sequelae of bed-rest and prolonged inactivity are discussed with Belinda and she is encouraged to commence a graduated return to work as soon as her walking tolerance allows.

Progress

Belinda is highly motivated to return to work. She commences a walking training program to increase her walking tolerance. After 2 weeks her back pain has subdued to 3/10, and her walking tolerance is 90 minutes. Belinda commences regular lumbar and abdominal strengthening exercises.

Belinda's nurse unit manager refuses to accommodate Belinda with reduced shift time or alternate duties that would allow a graduated return to work. The nurse unit manager argues that light duties are not possible in a busy nursing ward, and also that she does not want injured employees at work for fear of re-injury.

Belinda is frustrated by being unable to return to work. She feels that she is being punished for her error of standing on an un-braked wheelchair.

Belinda applies for, and secures, a part-time position (0.6) with a community nursing agency. This appointment requires that she work three 8-hour shifts each week, attending to patients in their own homes. She stands and walks for approximately 30 minutes at a time and carries a small case weighing 8kg. She drives between patients' homes. Belinda resigns her appointment at the public hospital.

Belinda continues with walking and strengthening exercises, increasing her walking tolerance to 2 hours continuous walking after 3 months of training. At this time she applies for an additional shift with the community nursing agency and her appointment is increased to 0.8. Several months later Belinda's appointment is increased to full-time.

Discussion

This case illustrates that sound clinical judgment and advice alone are not enough to generate successful clinical outcomes in occupational rehabilitation. Belinda is given sound clinical advice consistent with current evidence-based guidelines for management of acute non-specific low back pain, initially staying as active as possible, using simple analgesics and low-level heat wrap, watching for symptoms and signs of serious causes of back pain without avoiding movement due to fear (Australian Acute Musculoskeletal Pain Guidelines Group 2003). Belinda follows this advice and her back pain reduced quickly, allowing her to progress to specific aerobic and strengthening exercises, and rapidly regain some work capacity. Although Belinda has a functional capacity that would allow her to return to work, her immediate supervisor prevents her from doing so. Despite receiving evidence-based care for a work-related injury, Belinda does not return to her pre-injury employment.

Unfortunately, this occurrence is not uncommon; many employers maintain that graduated return to work cannot be accommodated in a given industry or in a particular workplace. The evidence for this claim is poor, but refusals of graduated return to work continue (see Chapter 9 regarding employers' attitudes to presenteeism). The potential loss to employers who refuse injured employees graduated return to work can be substantial. Belinda is a skilled young nurse. She has many working years ahead of her, and clinical skills transferable to many other areas of nursing. When she is refused graduated return to work, she elects to relocate herself from ward nursing to a new appointment in community nursing for the flexibility allowed in the new job. Lack of flexibility, and poor understanding of how work itself may be a form of training to increase work tolerance, has cost the nurse unit manager a valuable team member. Direct costs of this management decision are time and money that will need to be invested in replacing Belinda. Indirect costs are harder to measure, and may include reduction in nursing team morale among Belinda's colleagues should they realise that the nurse unit manager 'didn't want her back'.

Belinda's story ends on a high note because she took matters into her own hands, and sought a change in her working environment to allow a graduated return to work. Not all clients are as decisive or self-motivated as Belinda. While working part-time Belinda continued with an exercise program designed to increase her work capacity; clinical exercise practitioners can play an important role in assisting clients to use exercise to increase function regardless of access to graduated return to work.

Summary of key lessons

- Early assessment and intervention enhances the likelihood of positive outcomes in most clinical presentations, and particularly in cases of work-related injury.
- Early, graduated return to work may be used as a form of exercise training for work-injured clients. Early return to work has many advantages for employers and employees, but will only be successful if both parties contribute to the negotiations.
- Clients who are denied early, graduated return to work are able to increase work-related function through planned, targeted, graduated exercise.

DISCUSSION Question

Although Belinda was given sound advice for the management of non-specific back pain, many clients are not. How might you counter the false beliefs of a client who considers that back pain is best remedied by bed-rest and inactivity?

CASE STUDY 2A: MANAGED CARE — JOHN

John, a 46-year-old man, had been working as a mixer truck driver for a year in a construction company. John's duties included driving the mixer truck, loading and unloading cement, cleaning the hood and mixer, and occasionally (two or three times each year) using tools to peel off dried cement layers on the mixer. Sometimes, John needed to carry materials or tools with weight around 10–15kg. Prior to joining the construction company John had worked as a driver of a private car and a private van. John is the breadwinner of his family. He lives with his wife and two daughters (17 and 14 years old).

On 28 December, the second working day following Christmas, while John was cleaning the rear hoop and blade of the mixer truck with a water hose, the hose became trapped by the blade and John's right hand was caught under the blade. Immediately after the accident John was sent by ambulance to the accident and emergency department of a nearby hospital.

John was diagnosed with right index and middle finger crush injuries in which bones, tendons and nerves were damaged. John was admitted to the hospital and two reparative operations were

performed. Operations involved internal fixation of fractured bone, tendon and nerve repair. John was discharged with a hand splint on 5 January.

On the day after the accident John was contacted and visited by Betty, the rehabilitation manager for his company. During the first hospital visit, Betty had explained to John the nature of the injury, and a rehabilitation plan, return to work process, and possible outcomes. Also, Betty offered psychosocial support to John and his family.

On 18 January, Betty accompanied John to attend his allocated orthopaedic doctor, Dr Fu, for consultation. Dr Fu explained that John had a comminuted fracture of the right index finger and fractured head of the third metacarpal bone. Further, Dr Fu suggested that these are serious injuries and future stiffness and weakness is expected. Betty reassured John that he could expect to regain considerable hand function using ongoing exercises. She worked with John to agree to a series of ROM exercises to increase mobility in his right hand.

John underwent two further operations at hospital on 19 August and 15 November. The purpose of both operations was tendon release to allow greater ROM. In addition, John also attended the physiotherapy and occupational hand therapy clinics at the hospital. Betty encouraged John to continue with the exercises recommended by practitioners in these clinics.

The following January (13 months after the initial injury) Dr Fu requested a functional capacity evaluation (FCE) to determine John's physical capacity to return to his previous work. The FCE was carried out at an independent rehabilitation clinic. Results showed that John demonstrated work capacity to satisfy most of the physical demands of his previous job as a mixer truck driver, but John could not make a full-strength grip with his injured hand, so he may have difficulty in manoeuvring the wheel.

John had returned to modified duties at his original workplace on 13 February. The arrangement of the modified duties was based on the results of the FCE and Dr Fu's advice. From February to June, John carried out the following modified duties, gradually increasing duration and frequency of these activities: (a) stamping in-and-out tickets at the entrance of the mixer truck parking site; (b) driving private cars for colleagues; and (c) sitting beside his colleagues (mixer truck drivers) to act as assistant.

In mid-March, John undertook a truck driving course and test covering vehicle control, driving behaviour, road discipline, parking skill, driving attitude, hazard perception, and consideration for others. John gained satisfactory results in overall performance tests; his only problems were steering control and weakness during gear use. John commenced a specific exercise program to strengthen his right wrist, and hand.

In mid-June, John was scheduled to perform a test at a construction site. This test included items consistent with John's previous job requirements (eg: loading, unloading, cleaning, and driving the mixer truck). The test was assessed by his project manager and site safety officer. John returned to his previous job after passing this test at his construction site.

DISCUSSION Questions

If you were Betty:

1 What sort of questions would you ask John during the initial hospital visit (ie: initial interview)?

2 How would you introduce yourself, and explain your role, to John and his family?

3 How would you respond if John refused to do the driving test at the driving school?

4 How would you persuade John's employer of the merits of John returning to his previous job position as a mixer truck driver?

CASE STUDY 2B: MANAGED CARE — PETER

Peter, a 53-year-old man, was working as a manual labourer at an aged care facility (a seven storey building in Hong Kong). Work duties for Peter included daily maintenance tasks at the facility, and assisting his care attendant colleagues in bathing and care of the elderly people. Peter had been working in this job for 7 years.

On 5 June, while he was performing a building maintenance job, Peter fell from a stepladder around 60cm high. Immediately after the accident Peter was sent by ambulance to the accident and emergency department of a nearby hospital. Peter was diagnosed with a fractured skull, fractured right orbit, closed head injury, blunt eye trauma, bilateral fractures of distal radii and ulna styloid processes, and a left ulna fracture. Internal fixation of the multiple fractures of both upper limbs was performed during the hospitalisation. Peter was discharged to home after 2 weeks hospitalisation, and clinical exercise rehabilitation was arranged immediately after discharge.

Betty (rehabilitation manager for Peter's company) twice visited Peter in hospital. During her visits, Betty offered psychosocial support to Peter and his family and explained to Peter the nature of his injuries, rehabilitation plans, expectations of the return-to-work process, and possible outcomes.

Betty arranged for Peter to attend a panel orthopaedic doctor (Dr Fu) on 28 July. Dr Fu suggested that Peter would benefit from additional rehabilitation sessions. Consequently, Peter started an exercise rehabilitation program for mobility and general function in late July and a graduated work hardening program the following September. At a follow-up visit with Betty in September, Peter reported that he had hypertrophic scarring over both wrists, and he was referred to the public hospital for a pressure garment.

Peter returned to modified work duties in January, 7 months following his initial injury. Modified duties included morning deliveries of bread to different elderly centres, driving his private van, afternoon daily maintenance checks at the elderly home, and assisting in repairing damaged equipment. By mid-February Peter had gained sufficient confidence and work tolerance that he returned to his pre-injury duties. In early March Peter underwent a permanent impairment assessment that showed 6% permanent disability. He received a small lump sum compensation payment for this permanent impairment, and continued with his pre-injury employment.

DISCUSSION Questions

If you were Betty:

1 How would you explain Peter's medical condition to him during your first interview with him?

2 Would you prefer your contacts (particularly early contacts) with Peter to be by telephone, hospital visit, home visit, or a combination of these approaches? Why?

3 You might have more than a hundred clients (including some with long and complex cases). How would you allocate adequate time to Peter and prioritise his needs?

4 Consider how you could encourage Peter to return to modified duties, as recommended by Dr Fu, although he is still eligible for paid sick leave?

Combined discussion

These case studies highlight the potentially beneficial role of a rehabilitation manager as an advocate for an injured client. Occupational rehabilitation is a growing area of employment for clinical exercise practitioners. Practitioners working as client liaison require high-level interpersonal skills as well as sound clinical judgment. For example, Betty identified that Dr Fu's comments to John that stiffness and weakness were expected outcomes of a finger crush injury, although factual, could be unhelpful because they might lead John to accept reduced hand function rather than persisting with rehabilitation to as full a recovery as possible. Betty countered Dr Fu's suggestion, not with frank disagreement, but by using his opinion to emphasise to John the importance of adherence to an exercise program.

Over a protracted course of treatment including multiple surgeries, John persisted with exercise, and underwent considerable training and assessment. John continued with rehabilitation and made steady progress to an eventual return to full working duties. Why might John have persisted through prolonged occupational rehabilitation when many injured employees would have given up? In contrast to Belinda's experience (see case study 1), John's employer has supported John through (a) Betty's alliance with John, and (b) graduated return to work. Betty's support of John assisted in buoying him through the troughs and plateaus that are inevitable in rehabilitation, such that John did not become disgruntled with his employer or consider changing jobs.

Similarly Betty supported Peter, despite evidence of permanent impairment, to return to pre-injury duties. It is commendable that in Peter's case his company allowed Peter to progress with both a claim of permanent impairment and graduated return to work. Some employers consider these claims to be mutually exclusive, but Peter's story illustrates that that a client might be able, post-injury, to return to full employment, yet not be 100% recovered. Peter's story reminds us that not all work extends us to our full physical capacity.

Some managed care systems have been criticised for being overly directive and legislated, such that regulation can compromise clients' sense of control over their rehabilitation. These case studies give examples of a managed care system working well, seemingly due to the human face provided to workers' compensation by a skilled rehabilitation manager.

CASE STUDY 3: REHABILITATION CONSULTANT

This case study is divided into three distinct phases. Phase one is the post-incident acute and sub-acute phase. Phase two is the post-operative acute and sub-acute stage and phase three represents the functional restorative period. Over a two-and-a-half year period, clinical exercise in the context of a supportive work environment played a central role at every point of the rehabilitation process.

Phase 1
Subjective
A 37-year-old local government (parks and gardens) employee presented to me onsite with ongoing right leg and back pain following a lifting incident that occurred 11 days previously at the council depot. The specifics of the lifting incident involved lifting up a large lawn mower weighing 44kg from the ground level to the back of a utility truck. Although this event occurred at the worksite, the lawnmower was for private use (a longstanding privilege afforded to all employees).

On initial subjective assessment the client told me that his lumbar pain was intense and significantly restricted his movement but his right leg pain varied in terms of intensity and location. He reported that sometimes his right leg pain manifested as gluteal and hamstring tightness while at other times it developed as an unrelenting,

sleep disturbed right leg ache with accompanying pain when coughing and sneezing and a 'plastic' numbness feel to the dorsum of his right foot. He also described a high degree of irritability in terms of any slight aberrant movements, like a misplaced step, which would significantly exacerbate his back and leg pain. In summary, he described his movements as being careful and deliberate, especially with activities of daily living (ADL) such as sit to stand and walking. Past injury history included an episode in the absence of a known incident of less intense right 'sciatic pain a couple of years ago'. There was no other relevant medical history offered at the time.

Given the severity of the signs and symptoms, and in line with the employer's injury management procedures and workers' compensation regulations, the injured employee was sent to the local preferred medical provider where an expedited radiologist appointment was made and a magnetic resonance image (MRI) generated. Since I was the onsite treating practitioner the injured employee agreed that I was well placed to write continuing certificates of work capacity. An incident report and workers' compensation claim were lodged by the injured employee and subsequently accepted by the insurer. Certified restrictions consisted of no lifting, no repeated bending, with activities restricted to intervals of office work, which captured the main scope of his pre-injury duties.

Objective
On initial examination the injured employee demonstrated a careful somewhat antalgic gait pattern with some difficulty changing postures for the examination. Active range of movement was limited by lower back pain to only a few degrees of lumbar flexion and extension from a neutral standing position. Although bilateral active lumbar lateral flexion reproduced pain on the right, right lateral flexion was by far the more irritable direction. Lumbar facet joint palpation was essentially unremarkable, however, there was marked right lumbar para-spinal and gluteal muscle guarding. Lower limb neural tension was initially assessed via straight leg raise. Right straight leg raise was reduced to 30° compared with 70° on the left. Other routine neurological testing revealed that lower limb reflexes were normal although sensation

to sharp touch on the dorsum of the right foot was noticeably diminished compared to the left. Lower limb manual muscle testing demonstrated an estimated 25% decrease of right knee flexion/extension strength whilst all other lower limb movements, including plantar and dorsi-flexion strength, were bilaterally equal.

The first MRI report conclusion reads as follows:

> L5/S1 disc protrusion with posterior annular fissure contacting but not clearly compressing the descending S1 nerve root at the lateral recess bilaterally. Bilateral facet arthropathy, mild in nature. L4/5 central disc protrusion, non-neural compressive with mild bilateral facet arthropathy combining to result in a very mild central canal stenosis.

Assessment

Initially I viewed this report as somewhat puzzling in light of the clearly presenting discogenic clinical picture. With the exception of the L5/S1 disc protrusion associated with an annular fissure, the imaging highlighted in my view essentially incidental findings.

Plan

In the absence of clear annular nerve root impingement the decision was made to pursue conservative treatment in the form of an onsite and home program of therapeutic exercises under my guidance as the onsite consultant. My advice, in line with the preferred medical provider's view, was that a neurological opinion should be sought in order to explore more fully the source of the lumbar and leg pain. I arranged weekly onsite physiotherapy appointments for the first month and fortnightly for approximately 2 more months. In view of the irritability of the condition I made the decision to not employ passive joint mobilisation techniques but rather an active, gentle therapeutic movement approach that the injured employee could engage in and generally self-manage. Standing and prone trunk extension exercises were the focus initially, and once it was established that these exercises were in fact an easing factor, pain-free range of supine exercises involving lumbar rotation and paraspinal stretching were included. It was apparent at this stage that this fellow was motivated and therefore compliant with the exercise program. Clear guidelines relating exercise dosage to immediate and delayed pain response were discussed at length. His home program initially focused on walking and I asked him to gauge walking distance with regard to the onset of signs and symptoms and to be mindful of daily or activity patterns concerning pain behaviour. Other key advice offered in the acute/sub-acute stage was the importance of setting realistic goals in line with expected recovery and to expect challenging pain variability. In other words, expect some bad days. Exploring the nature of discogenic pain improvement with this injured employee appeared to make an impression. For example, the same pain for more activity must be seen in the context of improvement, not the often misconceived status quo.

Modest improvements in ADL were still accompanied with episodes of pain disturbed right leg pain. The only change I made to the exercise program was to introduce gentle right leg dural stretching that increased his back pain slightly but significantly improved straight leg raise to 80°. During this period a neurosurgeon twice injected steroid via an epidural approximately 2 months apart. This procedure facilitated only short-term improvement in both pain and ADL function. Given the lack of acceptable functional improvement the neurosurgeon offered a surgical nerve root decompression and this was agreed to by the injured employee once he was confident that he understood all the risks and benefits. Despite the certificate of capacity not changing there had been no work time lost with the exception of attending medical appointments.

Phase 2

An L4/5 microdiscectomy was performed via a microlaminectomy and the L5 nerve root was successfully decompressed. Interestingly there was a hook of bone from the L5 lamina that kept a large disc fragment compressed onto the L5 nerve root. This complicating factor was not evident on MRI and gives clarity regarding the persistent nature of the client's signs and symptoms. Inpatient physiotherapy consisted of post-operative education including mobilisation guidelines, initial transverse abdominus exercises and post-op precautions (no bending or twisting, no lifting > 1kg, limit sitting to < 20 minutes and no driving). Hands-on techniques were not indicated at this point and the client was referred back to me to address posture, improve gait quality and endurance, progress basic core stability exercises and to facilitate the return-to-work process.

Improvement in right leg pain was rapid allowing for a considerable improvement in walking endurance despite some lingering back discomfort. Hydrotherapy commenced with the emphasis on core stability following full wound healing. Convenient hydrotherapy was made possible by the use of one of the council pools and sufficient time was made available during work time to attend.

Phase 3

The neurosurgeon discharged the injured employee from his care approximately 1 year post the original lifting incident, advised him to return to full pre-injury duties and referred him back to me for further monitoring over the next 6 months. At the onsite clearance consultation he was extremely pleased with his progress and commented that he had 'never felt so good' and was now in full training for a 1km ocean swim. On examination he demonstrated full lumbar movement with only slight tightness restriction with flexion. Straight leg raise was now essentially bilaterally equal at 80° and his capacity for dynamic trunk stability had improved markedly. A gym program consisting of specific trunk strengthening, general resistance training and a significant aerobic component was arranged and reviewed by me and he is continuing to self-fund this initiative.

Discussion

This case study in my view offers some rich insights into the potentially critical role of clinical exercise within a biopsychosocial approach in an occupational rehabilitation setting. Firstly, effective communication between treating practitioners eventually led to the 'red flag' pathology being resolved. Although conservative management prior to the surgery could be seen as somewhat unsuccessful, the exercise component began to instil the ethic of self-responsibility and self-management, crucial attitudinal elements required for an effective long-term rehabilitation outcome. Further, the specific trunk strengthening and coordination gains and the ADL functional improvement that flowed from this must be viewed as a foundational benefit in a post-operative context.

Secondly, the importance of a supportive workplace culture cannot be overstated. The local management at this depot in effect gave full license to this approach in the form of trust to me as a practitioner and genuine concern for the long-term health and wellness of the injured employee. This is despite the fact that the actual injury event, although technically deemed a work accident, was essentially a task to appease a private errand. There was no pressure to return to the default adversarial approach to injury administration. The central injury management concern here is, why did this individual believe that lifting an awkward 44kg lawnmower from the ground to the utility truck was a viable task in terms of personal safety? Approximately 1 year prior to this event the employer invited me to run a series of work-team based manual handling training sessions. This was carried out with particular emphasis on relating safety consequences with safety behaviour decision making. In this case clearly training alone was not a sufficient barrier to stop this employee from making this critical moment error of judgment. A worksite assessment revealed there were a number of contributing factors to this lifting incident including a lack of personnel available due to the lateness of the day. Notwithstanding the shortcomings in the training, I consider this worksite-specific example, with the consent of the injured employee, to serve as a potent example to raise the efficacy of further injury prevention training and to reinforce the link between risk taking and personal health and wellness. The general learning from this event inspired vigorous workplace 'conversations'. Such workplace conversations, which generally included a positive reaction by the workforce in relation to the manner the line and injury management team responded to this incident, are extremely important because it can be argued that some of the long-term and unwritten cultural mores are formed within these conversations. The active, self-managed exercise approach to acute and persistent pain served as a form of occupational physical education; very different to the passive practitioner-dependent treatment they were familiar with in response to musculoskeletal injuries. This has now laid the foundations to use this onsite experience to roll out a task-specific exercise program as an injury prevention initiative.

The onsite nature of my injury management involvement with this organisation is of significant importance for a number of reasons. Firstly the practitioner/patient interaction dynamic has been altered in the direction of functional work outcomes. This is not an unreasonable direction, for while the injured employee's welfare remains central to all treatment considerations, my access to line management and understanding of how the work culture operates allows me to 'set the scene' through relentless communication to optimise and balance return to work and rehabilitative outcomes. This also meant that at no stage did the organisation lose control of the injured employee's progress. It is well established that injured workers that remain in contact with their employer have significantly improved rehabilitation outcomes. The cost benefit analysis in the short term relating to this single case study in terms of minimising external treatment costs and the positive insurance premium effect exceeded expectations.

The relevance of the psychosocial domain in setting and adjusting the prescription and dosage parameters of this onsite clinical exercise approach was further heightened when the injured employee informed me of his encroaching depression. With the help of professional counselling and onsite workplace support the injured employee used the goal setting and quantitative potential of exercise, especially the aerobic component of the program, as an adjunct antidote to depression. Persistent lumbar pain is fundamentally a lonely experience; there is no blood and no bandages, in fact few obvious signs that can relay the potential seriousness of the pathology to those around you and the consequent strength of character required to be positive is therefore also not readily evident. This timely mix of lumbar strengthening, dynamic trunk control and aerobic training together with ongoing emotional support had the combined effect of decreasing the further risk of injury and enhancing mental health at crucial points in the rehabilitation process. This employee now has an intrinsically motivated view towards health and wellness, especially with respect to the worth of a persistent and progressive approach to exercise and how this can enhance wellbeing in many facets of life.

In summary, this organisation, through determined and at times disruptive innovation, licensed the onsite exercise rehabilitation approach and as a result not only delivered a stunning rehabilitation outcome but also provided a consultative safety management improvement opportunity that has paid significant cultural dividends.

As a concluding remark, I view clinical exercise as a potent medicine. Like most potent medicines the risk of negative side-effects is high if the exercise prescriptions (ie: selection, dosage, timing) are not dispensed effectively. On the contrary, a targeted clinical exercise approach backed by sound clinical judgment can unlock the well-established psychological and biological effects of specific and general exercise and therefore has a great deal to offer in the rehabilitation of injured employees in an occupational setting.

DISCUSSION Questions

1 In this case study clinical exercise was used in preference to passive mobilisation. List the advantages of clinical exercise over passive treatment approaches in certain circumstances.

2 What do you think are the 'workplace settings' that led to such a successful outcome for this injured employee?

3 The success of clinical exercise is dependent on compliance. In this workplace example what are the key points that enhanced exercise compliance?

4 Why is the workplace potentially such a 'fertile' environment to roll out a therapeutic exercise intervention? What are the side benefits for the host organisation?

CASE STUDY 4: UNCOMFORTABLE WORKPLACE

Several members of an exercise rehabilitation unit at a university work together in an on-campus clinic. The clinic is staffed by senior academic practitioners, postgraduate clinical exercise science students on practicum, as well as a clinic manager, lab officers and technicians. This clinic provides professional services to staff and students, but mainly to clients who are referred to it by medical practitioners. Clients tend to be recovering from workplace or sport injuries, or managing chronic conditions such as obesity, diabetes or heart disease.

The clinic operates as a business and provides an authentic, 'real-life' teaching and learning setting for the student practitioners. It is a challenging environment, and the group works collaboratively to identify and solve problems presented by each client. The camaraderie of the group stems from the experience of working 'hands-on' with real clients and cases. A team approach is very much evident in the way the group works, especially with consultations, therapeutic sessions, and case reviews.

Camaraderie also stems from the opportunity to socialise at and outside work. The group meets daily for morning and afternoon coffee breaks, and occasionally for dinner or drinks at restaurants on the weekends. Their get-togethers involve a certain amount of 'shop talk' plus jocular banter among members of the group. Members frequently resort to good humoured 'bagging' of each other for slip-ups at work and for just about any other perceived shortcoming. During one coffee break a male staff member with a trendy floral shirt is chided as a 'poofter' and asked whether it was picked out by his boyfriend. Laughter ensues.

Conversation is at times laced with sexual innuendo. One senior male academic compliments a female postgraduate student on her sexy dress; then he bemoans the fact that he is still married. Another male clinician cries out that the dress should be the new standard uniform for female clinical staff. 'Put it back in your pants' yells another colleague. More laughter ensues.

One relatively new female postgraduate student in the group approaches a trusted senior female colleague after several such get-togethers, expressing her growing unease with some of the offensive and discriminatory remarks and behaviour of colleagues. The student feels the need to stand up for herself and approach the situation head on, but she is fearful of the consequences. After all, she is new to the clinic and wants to fit in. She opts to avoid the morning and afternoon coffee breaks when she can, but this too attracts unwanted attention and put-downs when she returns to the clinic.

Issues

This is a complex situation, but an all-too-familiar one in many workplaces. Joking and teasing behaviour can create a sense of belonging and allegiance to the group, however, the sexist and homophobic nature of some of the behaviour can reinforce male privilege and heterosexual norms, making work-life hostile or uncomfortable for others. There may have been no conscious attempt by members of the work-group to cause harm, but the environment may be intimidating and demeaning to others just the same.

There are other issues of power. The new female postgraduate student perceives that, as a new student clinician, she is very much dependent on supervisors for mentoring and on clinical staff to access consultation space, equipment and clients. This puts her in a vulnerable position, one where she is less likely to voice complaints for fear of losing access to needed support and other resources.

The offensive workplace behaviour may be considered sexual harassment under Victorian (see Victoria Equal Opportunity Act 1995) and Australian (see Human Rights and Equal Opportunity Commission Act 1986) equal opportunity and anti-discrimination legislation. Moreover, in this case, the employer and managers may be vicariously liable for the unlawful behaviour in the workplace.

Dealing with the issues

Organisational equal opportunity, harassment and anti-discrimination policies may make provisions for cases like these to be dealt with at the local departmental level before they progress to a more formal complaint at the institutional level. The situation is complicated by the fact that the 'issues raised' come from an anonymous source (via a senior staff member) to a head of school, and no-one specifically has been identified as the source of the alleged sexual harassment.

As a first step, care should be taken to support and protect the welfare of the student suggesting that the workplace behaviour is, at times, offensive. In this case, the student should be made aware that the concerns she has raised are being taken seriously and that efforts will be made to understand and, where appropriate, address the problem. She should be provided with a copy of the organisation's relevant policies and procedures in this regard and advised of her options to make a complaint or pursue other suitable options. The student should also be encouraged to continue liaising with her staff confidante, but also be made aware of the existence of confidential and impartial support services for students and employees.

One intervention strategy is for the head of school or manager to send a global email alerting staff to their rights and responsibilities to contribute to the maintenance of a safe and inclusive workplace. This action may serve notice, but it may also miss the mark. That is, a global message may go over the head of the work group in question, and it might be resented by staff members who are already doing the right thing by their colleagues and students.

Local level managers may instigate smaller work group discussions to raise the issue of workplace conduct, discrimination and harassment. However, this can backfire if staff members in a work group perceive that they are being singled out as potential perpetrators. Efforts may need to be made to ensure that it is known that small group discussions on the matter are being conducted across the department.

The postgraduate student concerned should be kept informed of the actions and interventions undertaken and asked to take notice and report any improvements in the workplace culture. If the harassing behaviour persists, and departmental level attempts to resolve the issue have been exhausted, the postgraduate student should again be advised of her right to pursue the matter through the organisation's discrimination and harassment policies and complaints procedures or an external commission or tribunal.

Prevention

A 'whole-of-organisation' approach may be what is needed to promote a safe and inclusive workplace. It should be made clear that the elimination and prevention of workplace harassment and discrimination is not just the responsibility of equity officers and managers, but of everyone in the organisation. In addition to clear legislation and policy statements, professional development is required at the school or department level to ensure that managers and staff members have the knowledge and skills to prevent and deal effectively with incidents of sexual harassment or discrimination.

Professional development activities may include seminars, workshops and on-line resources to ensure that managers, staff members and students are clear on what kinds of behaviours constitute sexual harassment and discrimination. All members of the organisation should be made aware of their rights and responsibilities under relevant harassment and anti-discrimination legislation and employment policies.

Professional development activities may also focus on how power imbalances, grounded as they often are in gender, rank or other characteristics, can create difficulties in workplace relationships, leaving some in the organisation more vulnerable than others. The organisation should also ensure that all students and staff members have clear and safe means to identify problems and voice concerns about workplace culture and behaviour.

A measure of workplace health and wellbeing may be the extent to which issues related to safety, equity and respect are mainstreamed; that is, integrated into the day-to-day operations at local levels of an organisation. It may mean that workplace health and wellbeing is a standing agenda item in department or group meetings, or it is added as a criterion for program reviews. In either case, it becomes a local matter of how people work together rather than as simply a legislative or policy compliance issue. In the long run, self-regulation may be preferable to top-down management interventions when it comes to changing workplace culture.

Summary of key lessons

- There may be discriminatory and demeaning behaviours in workplace cultures that go unrecognised as such by employees and managers.

- Employees and managers need to know their legal rights and responsibilities under relevant organisational equal opportunity, harassment and anti-discrimination policies.

- Intervention strategies at the local level can often be considered before allegations of staff misconduct proceed to a more formal complaints stage.

- A safe and inclusive workplace is the responsibility of both managers and employees.

- Educating staff for self-regulation may be preferable to 'top-down' compliance approaches to creating and sustaining safe and inclusive workplaces.

DISCUSSION Questions

1 Can you identify behaviours or other features of your workplace culture that some members may perceive as demeaning or discriminating?

2 Can you think about how gender, sexual orientation, occupational rank or other variables may constrain some members in a workplace from speaking out when they have an issue with workplace culture and behaviour?

3 What do you think are the pros and cons of 'self-regulation' versus 'top-down' management of equal opportunity and anti-discrimination issues in the workplace?

REFERENCES

Australian Acute Musculoskeletal Pain Guidelines Group (2003) *Evidence-based Management of Acute Musculoskeletal Pain*. Bowen Hills, Australia: Australian Academic Press

Government of Australia (2006) Human Rights and Equal Opportunity Commission Act 1986. Australian Government, Attorney-General's Office. Canberra

State Government of Victoria (2009) Victoria Equal Opportunity Act 1995. Victorian Equal Opportunity and Human Rights Commission. Melbourne, Victoria

Chapter 20

Case studies in learning from our mistakes

Dennis Hemphill, Melainie Cameron and Steve Selig

INTRODUCTION

In the wisdom of Aesop (620–564 BC), it is better to learn through the mistakes of others than through your own. As clinicians and teachers we have found that we learn a great deal from the times we have made errors, and in this chapter we present case studies of our mistakes as lessons. These lessons are not the only, or perhaps even the most important, lessons of clinical practice, but they are ours.

We have learned deeply because we own the errors, and integrate what we have learned into our work. It was Billy Joel who sang 'I'm not the only one who's made mistakes, but they're the only things I can truly call my own'. In this chapter we encourage all clinicians, particularly young practitioners, to see the value and importance of their mistakes. Do not 'bury them', as we often jest in medical circles, but admit them, study them, learn from them, and own them.

In this chapter, as in Chapter 10, we write personal tales and tell stories using individual voices. Also, we digress somewhat from the more structured format of Chapters 11 to 19. We have not edited out these differences in voice and style because we wish to own our stories, mistakes and all. In case studies 1 and 2 we recount clinical consultations where our mistakes were of a practical, clinical nature; an incorrect diagnosis, and a less than completely thorough clinical history. In case study 3 Dennis recalls his early days of work and reflects on his approach to skin-fold testing. To open this chapter and begin our discussion of mistakes, we consider a vignette from the field of

massage, a bodywork tale that could just as easily apply to clinical exercise practice.

VIGNETTE: THE HOLIDAY MASSAGE

As part of a weekend getaway, a young man books a therapeutic massage for his girlfriend at the hotel at which they were staying. During the massage, which is observed by a trainee therapist, the male therapist comments about a 'knot' in the woman's hamstrings and proceeds to massage the muscle starting from its origin under the buttocks. Upon completion of the massage, the boyfriend inquires as to how she enjoyed it. However, the girlfriend expresses her considerable discomfort at having her body parts exposed and especially about having her buttocks massaged. The more she thought about it, the more upset she became, eventually filing a sexual assault charge against the massage therapist and the hotel.

The gendered and sexual body

There are several ways to unpack this case. First, it may be useful to look at the body not simply as an object or machine, but as a social body. That is, the body is not neutral; rather, it comes inscribed with social meanings. For example, the gendered body sets up expectations (sometimes stereotypical) about the roles of men and women, plus their capabilities and accessibility.

Now, let's add touching into the equation. Touching another person without permission can be considered assault. Touching body parts is contentious; some are coded as sexual and more out of bounds than others. Permission to touch certain body parts is dependent on the nature of the relationship between people. Thus, the gendered and sexualised body can add tension to the therapeutic relationship. This, combined with the 'hands-on' nature of massage, can make ambiguous the difference between therapeutic and sexual touching.

There are three legal and ethical principles that can be used to judge and help guide professional conduct in this case, and others like it: informed consent, privacy, and confidentiality.

Informed consent

Ensuring informed consent means that clients are provided with sufficient information to make a knowledgeable and self-determined choice to participate. Prior to an evaluation or procedure (eg: therapeutic massage), participants should be made aware of the following: the purpose of an assessment or procedure; the methods to be employed, especially of a 'hands-on' or 'intrusive' nature (eg: massage, skin-fold test); the risks, if any, and how they will be managed; the right to withdraw consent and terminate the evaluation or procedure; and the method of keeping personal information and results confidential. Clients should be required to indicate that they understand the methods, risks and safeguards as part of the consent process.

Privacy

Care should be taken to provide a non-threatening setting for assessments or procedures. This is especially important in cases where clients may be required to partially undress or disclose private information. Practitioners should ensure suitable change areas, dressing gowns, and draping techniques, if disrobing is required; and the session should not be uninterrupted by others during assessments or consultations. Student trainees or other personnel should be allowed to observe or participate in the assessment or procedure only with the prior consent of the client; and personal particulars and health information requested should be limited to only that which is required for the assessment or procedure.

Confidentiality

Ensuring confidentiality means that care is taken to protect the identity of the client from unwarranted public access and potential misuse of assessment or consultation information. Confidentiality can be promoted by ensuring that personal particulars, health histories and assessment information are coded and stored in such a way as to protect the identity of the client; information is accessible only to those directly involved in ongoing evaluations or procedures; and names and personal details are not included on a mailing list for internal use or external distribution or sale without the permission of the client.

So, what can we say about the massage case above? The charge of sexual assault may have been avoided if the therapist had taken the time to inform the client beforehand about the rationale for a deep buttock massage; to ask whether the client was comfortable about being massaged in this way; to offer a substitute masseur, if she was not comfortable; and to ask the client's permission to have a trainee present during the massage.

Respecting 'personhood,' in this case, means providing the information and the opportunity to be self-determining prior to and during the practitioner–client relationship. It is creating a setting where the client is enabled to make an informed choice about a procedure that can affect her health and wellbeing.

CASE STUDY 1: MISDIAGNOSIS

Roslyn was a 49-year-old female with advanced progressive systemic sclerosis (PSS, formerly known as scleroderma) demonstrating full-blown CREST syndrome (calcinosis, Raynaud's phenomenon, esophogeal strictures, sclerodactyly, and telangietasia). Roslyn was a long-term client who appreciated my interest in rheumatological disease and valued my clinical judgment.

On this occasion Roslyn presented to me at short notice, complaining of an acute onset of generalised fatigue and a diffuse, erythematous, non-itching, macular rash. Her symptoms had commenced within the previous 24 hours, and had rapidly progressed. Roslyn was carried into the examination room by her husband because she was too fatigued to walk.

Roslyn consulted me rather than her general practitioner (GP) because it was a public holiday, and my practice was open and conveniently located near her home. I asked many questions, gathering a detailed clinical history, learning that in the preceding month Roslyn had developed an anal abscess for which her GP prescribed a course of Bactrim (sulfamethoxazole and trimethoprim). She had completed the course of antibiotics 3 full days prior to presentation, and reported no side-effects from the medication. She could not identify any particular cause for her fatigue or rash.

The most important aspect of Roslyn's past medical history was advanced PSS and related skin complaints (abscesses, cysts, calcinosis circumscripta, etc). Also, she had contracted a varicella zoster (chicken pox) virus infection at 40 years of age and scarred noticeably on her face and neck. The scarring was probably more marked due to the skin thinning and weakening effects of PSS.

I conducted a thorough physical examination of Roslyn, and found little to assist my diagnostic deliberations. Signs of PSS were obvious, but signs explaining the rash and fatigue were noticeable in their absence. The mucous membranes were free of Koplik's spots, and heart and lung sounds were normal. There were no vesicles forming within the rash. Spots did not appear to 'congregate' in the warmer regions of the body (groin, flexures, behind ears) as is typical in varicella zoster and measles infections, nor were they concentrated in contact areas as expected with a topical allergy.

In the absence of other signs, I concluded that Roslyn had probably acquired an acute viral infection, most likely rubella. I advised her to take 2–3 weeks rest, and to maintain fluid intake during this time. Given that the rash was not particularly itchy, and that Roslyn had very fragile and sensitive skin, I did not recommend any topical agents. Roslyn took my advice, and within two-and-a-half weeks had fully recovered and returned to all her usual activities, including full-time office work. As a courtesy, I notified her GP of my examination findings and advice.

PSS affects elastic tissues of the body, gradually replacing them with inelastic, fibrous tissue. The most apparent changes occur in the skin, which initially appears thickened, and later becomes taut and thinned and extremely fragile. Thinned, fragile, inelastic skin does not form an adequate barrier against infection, and is particularly vulnerable to trauma and irritation. Two weeks after returning to work, Roslyn experienced recurrence of the anal abscess, and consulted her GP, who prescribed a repeat course of Bactrim. Within hours of commencing the course of antibiotics, she developed a diffuse, erythematous, non-itching, macular rash, and began to feel fatigued.

I had overlooked a delayed hypersensitivity drug reaction in Roslyn. Her second allergic response to Bactrim (an antibiotic sulphonamide) was obvious and marked. She discontinued the medication immediately, but the profound inflammatory response in her skin produced burning, blistering and debridement of the skin of most of her body. She was hospitalised and placed on intravenous hydrocortisone for 2 days. Because PSS also affects the muscular and elastic tissue of blood vessel walls, leading to thinned, friable vessels, intravenous drug administration is not ideal. Roslyn was transferred to oral prednisolone as soon as possible.

Discussion

I was mortified! How could I have been so stupid? I had missed a common allergic response to sulphur-based drugs, and this omission cost Roslyn a serious second drug reaction which (if unchecked) could have killed her.

Allergies to antibiotic sulphonamides are common, with an overall incidence (occurrence of new cases) of approximately 3% (Choquet-Kastylevsky et al 2002). Some people, including those with slowed metabolisms, such as chronically ill and immunocompromised people (eg: Roslyn) are at higher risk of sulphur allergies. Skin reactions are the most common adverse reactions to sulphonamides, ranging from various benign rashes to life-threatening toxidermias such as epidermal necrolysis in which the epidermis (outermost layer of skin) dies and peels away. Other major adverse drug reactions include acute inflammatory responses in liver and lungs, and blood dyscrasias. More, there is a possibility that if the sulphonamide is continued (or re-administered) despite a mild rash, subsequent reactions may be more severe.

In time Roslyn recovered, and forgave me for my oversight. That Roslyn's GP also overlooked this event was of cold comfort — I was a young practitioner, new to the region, and I dearly wanted to impress the local medical establishment with my skill. In time, my ego recovered. I had missed this diagnosis, yes, but my advice to Roslyn for her general care (ie: rest, maintain fluids, apply no topical agents, seek medical help if worsening) had been reasonable in the circumstances.

Summary of key lessons

- This mistake refined my diagnostic skills. Never again will I exclude the possibility of drug reaction just because the client is no longer taking the medication.

- I have subsequently learned that reporting of drug allergies is a fraught area of clinical practice. Clinical records of drug allergies appear to influence practitioners' future recommendations for drug prescription only 30% of the time, and allergy reactions may be under- or over-reported by clients, calling into question the validity of allergy records (Lutomski et al 2008).

CASE STUDY 2: SCREENING BEFORE HIGH-INTENSITY EXERCISE

I had received a referral from a cardiologist to supervise a sign- and symptom-limited graded exercise test for the assessment of aerobic power (VO_{2peak}) for the purpose of providing a safe and effective exercise program and lifestyle plan for a patient. The client (Ian) was a 61-year-old professional football coach who had suffered an extensive anteroseptal myocardial infarction 2 years before. Fortunately, soon after the onset of chest pain he had called for an ambulance, and his early admittance to hospital limited the extent of myocardial damage as he underwent emergency angioplasty and a stent for another severely stenosed coronary artery. Ian was also fortunate that a subsequent cardiac arrest occurred whilst still in hospital, and he was successfully resuscitated. At the time he was not fitted with an implantable cardioverter defibrillator (ICD), but if this occurred today, he would fit the criteria for having such a device implanted.

Ian was left with moderate heart failure (60% cardiac function) and was given general lifestyle advice in hospital but did not return for phase 2 cardiac rehabilitation because he was 'involved in sport and could easily adopt a healthier lifestyle'. According to the information that he was required to provide to me in writing before the exercise test, his self-reported lifestyle since his heart attack was exemplary. He reported that he had developed enduring good habits regarding exercise, food and alcohol consumption and that he was currently participating in at least 14 hours of exercise and physical activity per week, some at high intensities.

I supervised a sign- and symptom-limited graded exercise test at 7 p.m. as part of a postgraduate student laboratory class with approximately 15 postgraduate students present, most of whom had current qualifications in cardiopulmonary resuscitation (CPR). The medical referral from the cardiologist stated that I did not need to arrange for a medical practitioner to be present at the test. The test proceeded normally and there were no adverse signs, symptoms or events during any of the exercise including exercise at VO_{2peak}. The first 10 minutes of recovery was also uneventful. At about this time, Ian told me that he was starting to feel unwell, and complained of feeling dizzy. We laid him on a gym mat on the floor, with feet elevated.

My initial management was to provide medical oxygen via a mask, to stay with him and to closely observe signs and symptoms (facial colour, ECG, heart rate, $HbO_2sat\%$, blood pressure, breathing depth and frequency) and to continue to reassure him. At this time, I assigned tasks to several students; these included recording all events against the time of day for the purposes of reporting, preparing to call for an ambulance using wall mounted instructions near the telephone, and to bring the automated defibrillator closer to the casualty. Over the next few minutes, Ian continued to deteriorate and became very light headed, nauseous, agitated and sweaty.

I needed to make a decision as to whether to call for an ambulance and decided not to at this stage, but to continue to use observation. My decision was based on my assessment of him suffering from a vaso-vagal episode rather than an acute cardiac event that would have required emergency medicine. He did not have any chest pain typical of angina and I confirmed with Ian that the feelings that he was experiencing were quite different from the symptoms that he experienced during his acute myocardial infarction. There were no changes to the ST segment or T wave on his ECG, and no other signs other than a persistent bradycardia and hypotension. Vaso-vagal episodes are common in exercise physiology laboratories that conduct maximal exercise intensity testing, and can normally be adequately managed by exercise physiologists who are trained in the recognition and management of the related signs and symptoms.

Ian slowly started to recover and so we gradually moved him to sitting upright, then standing, and then walking, all the time observing his vital signs including HbO$_2$sat% and blood pressure. After 75 minutes of continuous monitoring, I drove Ian home where his wife continued to observe him. I rang his home at 8 a.m. the next morning and his wife answered, and I was shocked when she told me that Ian had been taken to hospital by ambulance at 10.30 p.m. (1¼ hours after arriving home) after she was concerned about his condition. He had fainted at home after feeling worse again. He spent the night under observation in hospital where tests revealed that he had not suffered another myocardial infarction or any other acute coronary event. I rang Ian at 9 a.m. and he was feeling better and was being discharged from hospital. I rang him again in the evening and he had recovered.

Discussion

Ian had self-reported on his risk factor consent form to me that he was currently doing 14 hours of exercise and physical activity per week, with some of this at high intensities. However, Ian failed to tell me that this pattern had changed in the past few months due to heavy work commitments and that his exercise volume and intensities were now actually much lower. I conducted the exercise test to maximal relative intensity on the basis of his self-reported regular exercise participation and an exemplary lifestyle since his myocardial infarction and cardiac arrest.

The exercise test proceeded to 1–2 stages above what I have used as the termination criterion had I been aware of this recent cessation of regular exercise. Unaccustomed high-intensity exercise is a risk factor for vaso-vagal episodes, as well as a trigger for acute cardiac events in those with current coronary artery disease.

Summary of key lessons

- Clinical exercise practitioners rely on the provision of accurate information from their clients, particularly in relation to medical and lifestyle histories. This was not provided adequately in this case. As a result, I now cross-check written and verbal information provided by clients, and where possible also check the veracity of these against other information provided in the form of medical referrals and medical histories.

- Although I correctly interpreted the adverse signs and symptoms of this client as being consistent with a severe vaso-vagal episode, if this occurred again with someone with this medical history, then I would call an ambulance soon after the onset of signs and symptoms.

- The class was at night with few responsible people on the campus. It is safer to conduct such exercise tests during normal office hours where it is easier to manage emergencies.

CASE STUDY 3: EYES WIDE SHUT

As a recent exercise science graduate in my first 'real' job, I was keen to get started. There in front of me was the first cohort of 30 general staff members of a metropolitan hospital waiting for evaluations as part of their employee fitness and health program. Stations were set up in a section of the cafeteria to pre-test blood pressure, aerobic capacity and body fat. My job was to conduct a seven-point skin-fold calliper test to help determine each client's overall body fat.

I asked the first person in the line to record results for the group. One by one, I asked staff members to lift their T-shirts, remove their track pants, or roll up their shorts so that I could apply the spring-loaded metal callipers to the domed fat pinched between my fingers. For the men it was chest, back, bicep, abdomen, hip, front thigh and calf; for women it was bicep, tricep, abdomen, hip, front thigh, rear thigh and calf. As each measurement was taken I called out the result to my trusty recorder. It wasn't long before those in the queue were curious as to what was happening, and several crowded around to watch the proceedings.

In one case, a timid young woman was reluctant to expose any flesh for my measurements. Much time was spent explaining the benefits of having the skin-fold test done. After all, the test would provide the baseline data for her to see the fat loss at the end of the 12-week fitness program! After much cajoling, I managed to get the young woman to pull up her baggy track suit top just enough to expose a patch of skin on her abdomen. Just before I could get my index finger and thumb in there to pinch the fat, down comes the track suit top and a cry from the woman that she couldn't do it. Perplexed as to what all the fuss was about, I excused the woman from the testing.

Not long after this episode I was sitting in a medical clinic waiting room, looking around, and contemplating the ailment for which each patient was seeking treatment. One by one, each patient was called into the inner sanctum of the doctor's examination room, emerging some time later, stopping only to make a follow-up appointment or bidding the receptionist good-bye before departing the clinic. What happened behind those closed doors between doctor and patient was private and confidential, as it should be. I laughed to myself at the thought of a doctor openly discussing and addressing a patient's personal health issue right there in the middle of the waiting room. Then it struck me: something dubious like that would be not unlike what I had done in the case of the body fat assessments.

I had learned to do skin-fold calliper testing the year before in a Fitness Evaluation and Exercise Prescription module at university. We learned that fat loss could be a more useful indicator of fitness than weight loss, because exercise can lead to muscle gain. Learning to do the skin-fold calliper test was not the best indicator of body fat percentage, but it was considered a relatively good field test, especially when dealing with large numbers of people in a short period of time.

During our lab sessions, students were keen to learn and refine their measurement skills by testing each other. Being eager to learn the technique and also being relatively comfortable with our bodies, the male and female students thought nothing of stripping down to the bare minimum so that we could readily locate, pinch and measure fat at several sites on each other's bodies. Undertaking a rigorous fitness program and then retesting ourselves to see the fat loss only seemed to reinforce the usefulness of the skin-fold calliper measurement tool.

I brought into my new role as an exercise professional a scientific eye for the body, including its muscles, fat pattern, posture and gait, and I assumed that my clients would be interested in receiving useful feedback that could improve their fitness. However, in my zeal to help clients, I presumed to know what was best for them. The scientific outlook blinded me in this case to the impact of measuring body fat, especially of those who may not be so comfortable with their bodies.

The French existentialist philosopher, Jean-Paul Sartre (1956), considered 'the look' of others to be destructive of one's subjectivity. In psychological terms, 'the look' is one of surveillance, evaluation and judgment leading the looked-at person to feel increasingly self-conscious. Accordingly, the scrutiny of body fat, along with pinching and measuring it, was doubly intrusive, and could exacerbate the client's self-consciousness and embarrassment.

While exercise practitioners may have the client's best interests at heart when they undertake fitness assessments and exercise prescriptions, they must also be aware of client rights, integrity and welfare. In the case above, this includes informed consent, as well as respect for client privacy and confidentiality, similar to that provided by medical practitioners. Clients in this case should have been informed beforehand of the procedures, risks and safeguards (including a private room for partial disrobing and assessment), and their right to refuse or withdraw consent.

This case also illustrates the need for exercise practitioners to recognise the assumptions that underpin professional practice. For Tinning (1997) pervasive is the 'performance paradigm'; that is, the scientific framework where the body is seen as an object or machine to be measured, remodelled or fine-tuned. It may also require recognition of the social forces (eg: fashion, film and advertising industries) that can create unrealistic standards of physical attractiveness. Taken together, the body can become the prime site for excessive self-scrutiny and anxiety.

Summary of key lessons

This case illustrated how I became the unwitting accomplice in demeaning a client. The understanding of ethical principles (eg: informed consent, privacy, confidentiality), plus a critical awareness of the 'performance principle' and the body beautiful, could have gone some way to preventing it. So, with the benefit of hindsight, this case may alert practitioners to some dubious practices and help them conduct fitness testing or exercise prescription in a more humane manner.

DISCUSSION Question

To close this chapter, we offer a single discussion question, equally applicable to each case study. To err is human. Recall your last (remembered, acknowledged) mistake in your clinical work. What have you learned from this mistake?

REFERENCES

Choquet-Kastylevsky G, Vial T, Descotes J (2002) Allergic adverse reactions to sulfonamides. *Current Allergy and Asthma Reports*, 2:16–25

Lutomski DM, Lafollette JA, Biaglow MA, et al (2008) Antibiotic allergies in the medical record: effect on drug selection and assessment of validity. *Pharmacotherapy*, 28(11):1348–53

Sartre J-P (1956) *Being and Nothingness*. New York: Washington Square Press

Tinning R (1997) Performance and participation discourses in human movement: toward a socially critical physical education. In: Fernandez-Balboa J-M (ed.) *Critical Postmodernism in Human Movement, Physical Education and Sport*. Albany, New York: State University of New York Press

Appendix 1

Summaries of clinical classification and diagnostic criteria

Conditions are listed in alphabetical order. No priority or importance is implied in this listing.

DEPRESSION

Diagnostic criteria for depression

A Five (or more) of the following symptoms have been present during the same 2-week period and represent a change from previous functioning; at least one of the symptoms is either (1) depressed mood, or (2) loss of interest or pleasure. Do not include symptoms that are clearly due to a general medical condition, or mood-incongruent delusions or hallucinations.

(1) Depressed mood most of the day, nearly every day, as indicated by either subjective report (eg: feels sad or empty) or observation made by others (eg: appears tearful).
Note: In children and adolescents, can be irritable mood.

(2) Markedly diminished interest or pleasure in all, or almost all, activities most of the day, nearly every day (as indicated by either subjective account or observation made by others).

(3) Significant weight loss when not dieting or weight gain (eg: a change of more than 5% of body weight in a month), or decrease or increase in appetite nearly every day.
Note: In children, consider failure to make expected weight gains.

(4) Insomnia or hypersomnia nearly every day.

(5) Psychomotor agitation or retardation nearly every day (observable by others, not merely subjective feelings of restlessness or being slowed down).

(6) Fatigue or loss of energy nearly every day.

(7) Feelings of worthlessness or excessive or inappropriate guilt (which may be delusional) nearly every day (not merely self-reproach or guilt about being sick).

(8) Diminished ability to think or concentrate, or indecisiveness, nearly every day (either by subjective account or as observed by others).

(9) Recurrent thoughts of death (not just fear of dying), recurrent suicidal ideation without a specific plan, or a suicide attempt or a specific plan for committing suicide.

B The symptoms do not meet criteria for a mixed episode.

C The symptoms cause clinically significant distress or impairment in social, occupational, or other important areas of functioning.

D The symptoms are not due to the direct physiological effects of a substance (eg: a drug of abuse, a medication) or a general medical condition (eg: hypothyroidism).

E The symptoms are not better accounted for by bereavement (ie: after the loss of a loved one); the symptoms persist for longer than 2 months or are characterised by marked functional impairment, morbid preoccupation with worthlessness, suicidal ideation, psychotic symptoms, or psychomotor retardation.

REFERENCE

American Psychiatric Association (2000) Diagnostic and statistical manual of mental disorders (4th ed, text revised). Washington, DC: American Psychiatric Association

OSTEOARTHRITIS

Classification criteria for osteoarthritis of the hip

Combined clinical (history, physical examination, laboratory) and radiographic criteria, in the traditional format, comprises hip pain and at least 2 of the following 3 features:

1 ESR<20 mm/hour
2 radiographic femoral or acetabular osteophytes
3 radiographic joint space narrowing (superior, axial, and/or medial).

This classification method yields a sensitivity of 89% and a specificity of 91%.

REFERENCE

Altman R, Alarcon G, Appelrouth D, et al (1991) The American College of Rheumatology criteria for the classification and reporting of osteoarthritis of the hip. *Arthritis & Rheumatism*, 34:505–14

Classification criteria for idiopathic osteoarthritis (OA) of the knee

Clinical and laboratory knee pain	Clinical and radiographic knee pain	Clinical knee pain
+ at least 5 of 9: • Age > 50 years • Stiffness < 30 minutes • Crepitus • Bony Tenderness • Bony enlargement • No palpable warmth • ESR <40 mm/hour • RF <1:40 • SF OA	+ at least 1 of 3: • Age > 50 years • Stiffness < 30 minutes • Crepitus • + Osteophytes	+ at least 3 of 6: • Age > 50 years • Stiffness < 30 minutes • Crepitus • Bony Tenderness • Bony enlargement • No palpable warmth
92% sensitive	91% sensitive	95% sensitive
75% specific	86% specific	69% specific

Alternative for the clinical category would be 4 of 6, which is 84% sensitive and 89% specific.

REFERENCE

Altman R, Asch E, Bloch D, et al (1986) The American College of Rheumatology criteria for the classification and reporting of osteoarthritis of the knee. *Arthritis & Rheumatism*, 29:1039–49

Classification criteria for osteoarthritis of the hand

Hand pain, aching, or stiffness and 3 or 4 of the following features:

1 hard tissue enlargement of 2 or more of 10 selected joints
2 hard tissue enlargement of 2 or more DIP joints
3 fewer than 3 swollen MCP joints
4 deformity of at least 1 of 10 selected joints.

The 10 selected joints are the second and third distal interphalangeal (DIP), the second and third proximal interphalangeal, and the first carpometacarpal joints of both hands. This classification method yields a sensitivity of 94% and a specificity of 87%.

Abbreviations: ESR = erythrocyte sedimentation rate (Westergren); MCP = metacarpophalangeal; RF = rheumatoid factor; SF OA = synovial fluid signs of OA (clear, viscous, or white blood cell count <2000/mm^3).

REFERENCE

Altman R, Alarcon G, Appelrouth D, et al (1990) The American College of Rheumatology criteria for the classification and reporting of osteoarthritis of the hand. *Arthritis & Rheumatism*, 33:1601–10

OSTEOPOROSIS

Classification criteria for osteopenia and osteoporosis

Categories and clinical criteria for men and postmenopausal women aged 50 years and older using DXA measurements at the femoral neck appear below.

Classification	Criterion
Normal bone	T-score ≥ −1 SD
Osteopenia	T-score between −1 and −2.5
Osteoporosis	T-score ≤ −2.5 SD

Reference

Kanis JA, McCloskey EV, Johansson H, et al (2008) A reference standard for the description of osteoporosis. *Bone*, 42:467–75

PAIN

Pain is an unpleasant sensory and emotional experience associated with actual or potential tissue damage, or described in terms of such damage. The inability to communicate verbally does not negate the possibility that an individual is experiencing pain and is in need of appropriate pain-relieving treatment. Pain is always subjective. Each individual learns the application of the word through experiences related to injury in early life. Biologists recognise that those stimuli which cause pain are liable to damage tissue. Accordingly, pain is that experience we associate with actual or potential tissue damage. It is unquestionably a sensation in a part or parts of the body, but it is also always unpleasant and therefore also an emotional experience. Experiences which resemble pain but are not unpleasant (eg: pricking) should not be called pain. Unpleasant abnormal experiences (dysesthesias) may also be pain but are not necessarily so because, subjectively, they may not have the usual sensory qualities of pain.

Many people report pain in the absence of tissue damage or any likely pathophysiological cause; usually this happens for psychological reasons. There is usually no way to distinguish their experience from that due to tissue damage if we take the subjective report. If they regard their experience as pain and if they report it in the same ways as pain caused by tissue damage, it should be accepted as pain. This definition avoids tying pain to the stimulus. Activity induced in the nociceptor and nociceptive pathways by a noxious stimulus is not pain, which is always a psychological state, even though we may well appreciate that pain most often has a proximate physical cause.

Acute versus chronic pain

Classifications of pain based on time are arbitrary but widely used. In Australian guidelines for the management of acute musculoskeletal pain, acute pain is defined as pain that is present for fewer than three months, whereas chronic pain is present for longer than three months.

REFERENCES

Australian Acute Musculoskeletal Pain Guidelines Group (2003) *Evidence-based Management of Acute Musculoskeletal Pain*. Bowen Hills: Australian Academic Press
Merskey H, Bogduk N (eds) (1994) Part III: Pain Terms, A Current List with Definitions and Notes on Usage. In: *Classification of Chronic Pain* (2nd ed). IASP Task Force on Taxonomy. Seattle, USA: IASP Press, pp 209–14

PERIPHERAL ARTERIAL DISEASE

Classification criteria for peripheral arterial disease

Grade	Category	Clinical description	Objective criteria
0	0	Asymptomatic – no hemodynamically significant occlusive disease	Normal treadmill or reactive hyperemia test
	1	Mild claudication	Completes treadmill exercise[†] AP after exercise >50mmHg but at least 20mmHg lower than the resting value
I	2	Moderate claudication	Between categories 1 and 3
	3	Severe claudication	Cannot complete standard treadmill exercise[†] and AP after exercise <50mmHg
II[*]	4	Ischemic rest pain	Resting AP <40mmHg, flat or barely pulsatile ankle or metatarsal PVR; TP <30mmHg
III[*]	5	Minor tissue loss - Non healing ulcer, focal gangrene with diffuse pedal ischemia	Resting AP <60mmHg, ankle or metatarsal PVR flat or barely pulsatile; TP <40mmHg
	6	Major tissue loss – extending above TM level, functional foot no longer salvageable	Same as category 5

Key: AP: ankle pressure; PVR: pulse volume recording; TP: toe pressure; TM: transmetatarsal;

[*]Grades II and III, categories 4, 5 and 6 are embraced by the term chronic critical ischemia;

[†]Five minutes at 2mph (3.2km/h) on a 12% incline.

REFERENCE

Rutherford RB, D Baker JD, Ennst C, et al (1997) Recommended standards for reports dealing with lower extremity ischemia: Revised version. *Journal of Vascular Surgery*, 26:517–38

RHEUMATOID ARTHRITIS

Classification criteria for rheumatoid arthritis

Criterion	Definition
1. Morning stiffness	Morning stiffness in and around the joints, lasting at least 1 hour before maximal improvement
2. Arthritis of 3 or more joint areas	At least 3 joint areas simultaneously have had soft tissue swelling or fluid (not bony overgrowth alone) observed by a physician. The 14 possible areas are right or left PIP, MCP, wrist, elbow, knee, ankle, and MTP joints
3. Arthritis of hand joints	At least 1 area swollen (as defined above) in a wrist, MCP, or PIP joint
4. Symmetric arthritis	Simultaneous involvement of the same joint areas (as defined in 2) on both sides of the body (bilateral involvement of PIPs, MCPs, or MTPs is acceptable without absolute symmetry)
5. Rheumatoid nodules	Subcutaneous nodules, over bony prominences, or extensor surfaces, or in juxta-articular regions, observed by a physician
6. Serum rheumatoid factor	Demonstration of abnormal amounts of serum rheumatoid factor by any method for which the result has been positive in <5% of normal control subjects
7. Radiographic changes	Radiographic changes typical of rheumatoid arthritis on posteroanterior hand and wrist radiographs, which must include erosions or unequivocal bony decalcification localised in or most marked adjacent to the involved joints (osteoarthritis changes alone do not qualify)

For classification purposes, a person shall be said to have rheumatoid arthritis if he/she has satisfied at least 4 or these 7 criteria. Criteria 1 through 4 must have been present for at least 6 weeks. Patients with 2 clinical diagnoses are not excluded. Designation as classic, definite, or probable rheumatoid arthritis is *not* to be made.

REFERENCE

Arnett FC, Edworthy SM, Bloch DA, et al (1988) The American Rheumatism Association 1987 revised criteria for the classification of rheumatoid arthritis. *Arthritis & Rheumatism*, 31:315–24

Appendix 2

References for evidence-based clinical and exercise guidelines

Acute musculoskeletal pain

Australian Acute Musculoskeletal Pain Guidelines Group (2003) *Evidence-based Management of Acute Musculoskeletal Pain*. Bowen Hills: Australian Academic Press

Age and frailty

Chodzko-Zajko WJ, Proctor DN, Fiatarone-Singh M, et al (2009) American College of Sports Medicine position stand: exercise and physical activity for older adults. *Medicine and Science in Sports and Exercise*, 41:1510–30

Chronic heart failure (CHF)

Francis GS, Greenberg BH, Hsu DT, et al (2010) 2010 Clinical Competence Statement on Management of Patients With Advanced Heart Failure and Cardiac Transplant: a report of the ACCF/AHA/ACP Task Force on Clinical Competence and Training. *Journal of the American College of Cardiologists*, 56:424–53

Selig SE, Levinger I, Williams AD, et al (2010) Exercise & Sports Science Australia Position Statement on exercise training and chronic heart failure. *Journal of Science and Medicine in Sport*, 13:288–94

Coronary artery disease (CAD)

American College of Sports Medicine (ACSM) (1994) ACSM position stand. Exercise for patients with coronary artery disease. *Medicine and Science in Sports and Exercise*, 26:i–v

Fraker TD, Fihn SD, Gibbons RJ, et al (2007) Chronic Angina Focused Update of the ACC/AHA 2002 Guidelines for the Management of Patients with Chronic Stable Angina: a report of the American College of Cardiology/American Heart Association Task Force on practice guidelines writing group to develop the focused update of the 2002 Guidelines for the Management of Patients with Chronic Stable Angina. *Circulation*, 116:2762–72

Hypertension

Pescatello LS, Franklin BA, Fagard R, et al (2004) American College of Sports Medicine position stand: Exercise and hypertension. *Medicine and Science in Sports and Exercise*, 36:533–53

Sharman JE, Stowasser M (2009) Australian Association for Exercise and Sports Science position statement on exercise and hypertension. *Journal of Science and Medicine in Sport*, 12:252–7

Osteoarthritis

National Institute for Health and Clinical Excellence (2008) Nice Clinical Guideline 59. Osteoarthritis: the care and management of osteoarthritis in adults. London: National Institute for Health and Clinical Excellence

The Royal Australian College of General Practitioners (2009) Guideline for the non-surgical management of hip and knee osteoarthritis. Melbourne: Royal Australian College of General Practitioners

Osteoporosis

The Royal Australian College of General Practitioners (2010) Guideline for the prevention and treatment of osteoporosis in postmenopausal women and older men. Melbourne: Royal Australian College of General Practitioners

Rheumatoid arthritis

The Royal Australian College of General Practitioners (2009) Clinical guideline for the diagnosis and management of early rheumatoid arthritis. Melbourne: Royal Australian College of General Practitioners

Type II diabetes mellitus

Albright A, Franz M, Hornsby G, et al (2000) American College of Sports Medicine position stand: Exercise and Type 2 Diabetes. *Medicine and Science in Sports and Exercise*, 32:1345–60

Valvular disease

Bonow RO, Carabello BA, Chatterjee K, et al (2008) Focused update incorporated into the ACC/AHA 2006 guidelines for the management of patients with valvular heart disease: a report of the American College of Cardiology/American Heart Association Task Force on Practice Guidelines (Writing Committee to Revise the 1998 Guidelines for the Management of Patients With Valvular Heart Disease): endorsed by the Society of Cardiovascular Anesthesiologists, Society for Cardiovascular Angiography and Interventions, and Society of Thoracic Surgeons. *Circulation*, 118:e523–661

Appendix 3

Contraindications to exercise testing

CONTRAINDICATIONS AND PRECAUTIONS GROUPED BY INTERNATIONAL CLASSIFICATION OF DISEASE (ICD019) CODES

The risk of sudden death and morbidity from exercise stress testing, which is generally low, is greatly increased by failing to consider contraindications for testing.[1] The American College of Cardiology/American Heart Association (ACC/AHA),[2] American College of Sports Medicine (ACSM),[3] and the American Association of Cardiovascular and Pulmonary Rehabilitation (AACVPR)[4] generally agreed on concerns. The three sources cited a total of 29 concerns for exercise testing. The overwhelming proportion (70%) of concerns was circulatory. About half of the guidelines were considered absolute contraindications (ACI), whereas the other half were viewed as relative contraindications (RCI). These organisations also provide guidelines for terminating an exercise test.

A00-B99 Certain Infections and Parasitic Diseases

D50-D89 Diseases of Blood and Blood Forming Organs, and Certain Disorders

Issue	Level of concern	Sources	Qualification/rationale/comment
Acute infection	ACI	ACC/AHA[2,a] ACSM[3]	
Chronic infectious disease	RCI	ACSM[3]	(ie: mononucleosis, hepatitis, AIDS)
Infection	ACI	AACVPR[4,a,b]	The infection may affect exercise performance; exercise may aggravate the condition. Note: exercise with fever stresses the cardiopulmonary system, the immune system, and may be further complicated by dehydration.[5]

General note: sources indicate that risk and benefits should be weighed for an RCI.

[a]Relative acute myocarditis or pericarditis;

[b]Also active endocarditis.

Abbreviations: ACC/AHA, American College of Cardiology/American Heart Association; ACSM, American College of Sports Medicine; AACVPR, American Association of Cardiovascular and Pulmonary Rehabilitation; AI, absolute indications for terminating; RI, relative indication

E00-E90 Endocrine, Nutritional and Metabolic Diseases

Issue	Level of concern	Sources	Rationale/comment
Electrolyte abnormalities	RCI	ACC/AHA[2] ACSM[3] AACVPR[4]	(E.g., hypokalemia, hypomagnesemia) Note: hypokalemia may clinically present as hypotension, arrhythmias, ECG changes, and cardiac arrest (with 2.5 mEq/L serum potassium). Hypermagnesemia may be seen in chronic renal failure and clinically presents as bradycardia, weak pulse, hypotension, heart blocks, and cardiac arrest. Hypomagnesemia may clinically present as arrhythmias, hypotension, or sometimes hypertension.[6]
Metabolic disease (uncontrolled)	RCI	ACSM[3]	The patient's condition may affect exercise performance; exercise may aggravate the condition, eg: diabetes, thyrotoxicosis, myxedema.[7] Note: hypoglycemia (<50 mg/dL) may clinically present as tachycardia, convulsions, and coma. Severe hyperglycemia (>300 mg/dL) is a life-threatening metabolic condition that can lead to diabetic ketoacidosis or hypoglycemic hyperosmolar non-ketotic coma. In thyrotoxicosis, metabolism is elevated, sympathetic activity increased, and there is an increased risk of atrial fibrillations, congestive heart failure, and MIs.[7]

F00-F99 Mental and Behavioral Disorders

Issue	Level of concern	Sources	Rationale/comment
Mental impairment	RCI	ACC/AHA[2] AACVPR[4,a]	If leading to an inability to adequately exercise.

[a]Inability to cooperate.

00-I99 Diseases of the Circulatory System

Issue	Level of concern	Sources	Rationale/comment
Acute Myocardial Infarction (within 2 days)	ACI	AACVPR[4]	Note: in an early post-MI, there may be activity restrictions. Uncomplicated cases are progressed in physical activity, starting with *gentle exercises* in conjunction with adequate rest periods, within the first 24 hours.[8]
Active endocarditis	ACI	AACVPR[4]	Note: endocarditis is an infection of the endocardium, heart valves, or a cardiac prosthesis; treatment includes bed rest.[8]

Issue	Level of concern	Sources	Rationale/comment
Angina (unstable)	ACI	ACC/AHA[2,a] ACSM[3] AACVPR[4,b]	Note: if the patient presents with unstable angina, additional stress may induce an infarction.[9]
Aortic stenosis	ACI	ACC/AHA[2] ACSM[3] AACVPR[4,c]	If severe and symptomatic.
Cardiac arrhythmias	ACI	ACC/AHA[2] ACSM[3] AACVPR[4]	If uncontrolled, causing symptoms or hemodynamic compromise.[4] Note: exercise may increase an arrhythmia or may induce one by increasing myocardial oxygen demand or increasing sympathetic tone.[8,9]
Dissecting aneurysm	ACI	ACSM[3] ACC/AHA[2,e]	Known or suspected. Note: an aneurysm is an abnormal dilation of a vessel with a diameter 50% of normal. Weakness in the wall results in a permanent sac-like structure. A thoracic aortic aneurysm can rupture under the force of elevated blood pressure.[8,9]
Heart failure	ACI	ACC/AHA[2] ACSM[3] AACVPR[4,c]	If uncontrolled and symptomatic.
Myocarditis or pericarditis (acute)	ACI	ACC/AHA[2] ACSM[3] AACVPR[4,f]	Note: pericarditis is an inflammation of the double-layered membrane — the pericardium — that surrounds the heart. In constrictive pericarditis, the fibrotic tissue compresses the heart, reduces CO, and leads to cardiac failure. One of the treatments is bed rest when fever is present (for acute idiopathic, post-MI and post-thoracotomy pericarditis).[8,9] Myocarditis is a focal or diffuse inflammation of cardiac muscle; treatment includes modified bed rest to reduce the workload of the heart.[8,9]
Pulmonary embolus or infarction (acute)	ACI	ACC/AHA[2] ACSM[3] AACVPR[4]	
Resting ECG shows recent significant change	ACI	ACSM[3]	If findings suggest an acute cardiac event such as an MI within 2 days. Note: ST displacement (on ECG) is the period between complete depolarisation and beginning repolarisation of ventricular musculature. It may be elevated or depressed in angina (transient muscle ischemia) or in muscle injury. Elevation may suggest the early stages of an MI (ie: acute myocardial muscle damage).[8,9]

Issue	Level of concern	Sources	Rationale/comment
Arterial hypertension	RCI	ACC/AHA[2] ACSM[3] AACVPR[4]	If severe (ie: at rest systolic >200 mm Hg and/or diastolic >110 mm Hg).[4]
Atrial fibrillation	RCI	AACVPR[4]	With an uncontrolled ventricular rate. Note: atrial fibrillation is a chronic arrhythmia resulting in rapid irregular atrial myocardial contractions whereby blood remains in the atria. Blood flow is reduced; congestive heart failure and cardiac ischemia can develop.[8, 9]
Atrioventricular block	RCI	ACC/AHA[2] ACSM[3] AACVPR[4]	If high-degree.
Bradyarrhythmias	RCI	ACC/AHA[2] ACSM[3] AACVPR[4]	
Coronary stenosis	RCI	ACC/AHA[2] ACSM[3] AACVPR[4]	Left main artery or its equivalent.[2–4]
Hypertrophic cardiomyopathy	RCI	ACC/AHA[2] ACSM[3] AACVPR[4]	Note: cardiomyopathy is a condition that involves myocardial muscle fiber impairment that presents similarly to CHF and can result in sudden death. Avoid risk by eliminating strenuous exercises (eg: running, competitive sports).[8]
Other outflow tract obstructions	RCI	ACC/AHA[2] ACSM[3]	
Stenotic valvular heart disease (moderate)	RCI	ACC/AHA[2] ACSM[3] AACVPR[4]	Note: in severe aortic valvular heart disease, there is a low stress tolerance that is easily reached.[9]
Tachyarrhythmias	RCI	ACC/AHA[2] ACSM[3] AACVPR[4]	
Ventricular aneurysm	RCI	ACSM[2]	

[a] If not stabilised previously by medical therapy
[b] If high risk
[c] If decompensated, symptomatic
[d] Systolic BP >200 mm Hg and diastolic BP >110 mm Hg
[e] Acute
[f] Relative acute

N00-N99 Diseases of the Genitourinary System

Issue	Level of concern	Sources	Rationale/comment
Renal failure	ACI	AACVPR[4]	This condition may affect exercise performance; exercise may aggravate condition.[4] Note: with renal failure, the concern is exacerbating the existing medical conditions with exercise. Check for physiological stability (eg: potassium not >5 mEq/L).[10]

R00-R99 Symptoms, Signs (also possibly M00-M99 Diseases of the Musculoskeletal System and Connective Tissue or G00-G99 Diseases of the Nervous System)

Issue	Level of concern	Sources	Rationale/comment
Physical impairment	RCI ACI	ACC/AHA[2] AACVPR[4,a]	If resulting in an inability to adequately exercise.

[a]If safe and adequate performance is precluded

Procedural concerns

Issue	Level of concern	Sources	Rationale/comment
Disorders exacerbated by exercise	RCI ACI	ACSM[3] AACVPR[4,a]	If neuromuscular, musculoskeletal, rheumatoid.[3]
Informed consent not obtained	ACI	AACVPR[4]	

[a]If acute non-cardiac disorder that can be exacerbated by exercise (infection, thyrotoxicosis, renal failure)
Abbreviations: ACC/AHA, American College of Cardiology/American Heart Association; ACSM, American College of Sports Medicine; AACVPR, American Association of Cardiovascular and Pulmonary Rehabilitation

INDICATIONS FOR TERMINATING EXERCISE TESTING GROUPED BY INTERNATIONAL CLASSIFICATION OF DISEASE (ICD019) CODES

I00-I99 Diseases of the Circulatory System

R00-R99 Symptoms, Signs, and Abnormal Clinical & Laboratory Findings of the Circulatory System

Issue	Level of concern	Sources	Rationale/comment
Systolic BP drop from baseline ≥10 mm Hg 'despite increase workload, when accompanied by other evidence of ischemia'	AI	ACC/AHA[2,a] ACSM[3] AACVPR[4,a]	
Angina (moderate to severe)			Grade 3-4.[4]

Issue	Level of concern	Sources	Rationale/comment
Signs of poor perfusion			(Cyanosis, pallor).
Ventricular tachycardia (if sustained)			
'ST elevation ≥1.0 mm in leads without diagnostic Q-waves— other than V_1 or a V_R'			
Systolic BP drop from baseline ≥10 mm Hg 'despite increase workload, in absence of other evidence of ischemia'	RI	ACC/AHA[2,a] ACSM[3]	
'ST or QRS changes such as excessive ST depression (>2 mm horizontal or down sloping ST-segment depression) or marked axis shift'		AACVPR[4]	
'Arrhythmias—other than sustained ventricular tachycardia'			Arrhythmias such as multi-focal PVCs, triplets of PVCs, supraventricular tachycardia, heart block, bradyarrhythmias.[3]
Chest pain increasing			
Claudication			
Development of a 'bundle-branch block or intraventricular conduction delay, which can not be distinguished from ventricular tachycardia'	RI RI AI	ACC/AHA[2] ACSM[3] AACVPR[4,b]	
Hypertensive response	RI	ACC/AHA[2] ACSM[3]	Where systolic BP >250 mm Hg and/or diastolic BP >115 mm Hg when definitive evidence is lacking.[2]

[a] 10 mm Hg
[b] Only bundle-branch block mentioned

R00-T98 symptoms, signs, and abnormal clinical & laboratory findings (not elsewhere classified)

Issue	Level of concern	Sources	Rationale/comment
Nervous systems symptoms increase	AI	ACC/AHA[2] ACSM[3] AACVPR[4]	(eg: ataxia, dizziness, near syncope) AACVPR CNS symptoms.[4]

Issue	Level of concern	Sources	Rationale/comment
Fatigue	RI	ACC/AHA[2] ACSM[3] AACVPR[4]	
Shortness of breath Wheezing Leg cramps			

Procedural concerns

Issue	Level of concern	Sources	Rationale/comment
Technical difficulties monitoring (eg: ECG, systolic BP)	AI	ACC/AHA[2] ACSM[3] AACVPR[4]	
Client wishes to stop	AI	ACC/AHA[2] ACSM[3] AACVPR[4]	

Reproduced, with minor modifications, with permission from Bataviam (2006). *Contraindications in Physical Rehabilitation*. St Louis: Elsevier, Part II, Ch3, Exercise Testing

REFERENCES

1 Richard D, Birrer R (1988) Exercise stress testing [review]. *J Fam Pract*, 26(4):425–35
2 Gibbons RA, Balady GJ, Beasely JW, et al (1997) ACC/AHA guidelines for exercise testing. *J Am Coll Cardiol*, 30: 260–315
3 American College of Sports Medicine (ACSM) (2000) *ACSM's Guidelines for Exercise Testing and Prescription* (6th ed). Philadelphia: Lippincott Williams & Wilkins
4 American Association of Cardiovascular and Pulmonary Rehabilitation (AACVPR)(2004) *American Association of Cardiovascular and Pulmonary Rehabilitation Guidelines for Cardiac Rehabilitation and Secondary Prevention Programs* (4th ed). Champaign (IL): Human Kinetics
5 Appendix B: Guidelines for Activity and Exercise. In: Goodman CC, Boissonnault WG, Fuller KS (eds) (2003) *Pathology: Implications for the Physical Therapist*. Philadelphia: WB Saunders
6 Goodman CC, Snyder TEK (2003) Problems affecting multiple systems. In: Goodman CC, Boissonnault WG, Fuller KS (eds) *Pathology: Implications for the Physical Therapist*. Philadelphia: WB Saunders, pp 85–119
7 Goodman CC, Snyder TEK (2003) The endocrine and metabolic systems. In: Goodman CC, Boissonnault WG, Fuller KS (eds) *Pathology: Implications for the Physical Therapist*. Philadelphia: WB Saunders, pp 317–66
8 Professional Guide to Diseases (6th ed) (1998). Springhouse (PA): Springhouse Corp
9 Pagana KD, Pagana TJ (2002) *Mosby's Manual of Diagnostic and Laboratory Tests* (2nd ed). St Louis: Mosby
10 Boissonnault WG, Goodman CC (2003) The renal and urologic systems. In: Goodman CC, Boissonnault WG, Fuller KS (eds) *Pathology: Implications for the Physical Therapist*. Philadelphia: WB Saunders, pp 704–28

Index